Patrick Holford BSc, DipION, FBANT, NTCRP is a leading pioneer in new approaches to health and nutrition, and is widely regarded as Britain's leading spokesman on nutrition and mental health issues. He is also the author of over 30 health books, translated into over 20 languages and selling over a million copies worldwide.

Patrick Holford started his academic career in the field of psychology. In 1984 he founded the Institute for Optimum Nutrition (ION), an independent educational charity, with his mentor, twice Nobel Prize winner Dr Linus Pauling, as patron. ION has been researching and helping to define what it means to be optimally nourished for the past 25 years and is one of the most respected educational establishments for training nutritional therapists. At ION Patrick was involved in groundbreaking research showing that multivitamins can increase children's IQ scores – the subject of a *Horizon* documentary in the 1980s. He was one of the first promoters of the importance of zinc, antioxidants, essential fats, low-GL diets and homocysteine-lowering B vitamins.

He is Chief Executive of the Food for the Brain Foundation and director of the Brain Bio Centre, the Foundation's treatment centre. He is an honorary fellow of the British Association for Applied Nutrition and Nutritional Therapy, as well as a member of the Nutrition Therapy Council.

patrick
HOLFORD

with Liz Efiong

SAY
NO TO
CANCER

THE DRUG-FREE
GUIDE TO PREVENTING AND
HELPING FIGHT CANCER

piatkus

PIATKUS

First published in Great Britain in 1999 by Piatkus
Reprinted 2001, 2002, 2003, 2004, 2005, 2006, 2007 (twice), 2009

This updated and expanded version first published 2010
Copyright © Patrick Holford 1999, 2010

A CIP catalogue record for this book
is available from the British Library.

ISBN 978-0-7499-5411-6

Typeset in Berkeley by Phoenix Photosetting, Chatham, Kent
Printed and bound in Great Britain by CPI Mackays, Chatham, ME5 8TD.

Papers used by Piatkus are natural, renewable and recyclable
products sourced from well-managed forests and certified
in accordance with the rules of the Forest Stewardship Council.

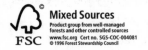

Mixed Sources
Product group from well-managed
forests and other controlled sources
www.fsc.org Cert no. SGS-COC-004081
© 1996 Forest Stewardship Council
FSC

Piatkus
An imprint of
Little, Brown Book Group
100 Victoria Embankment
London EC4Y 0DY

An Hachette UK Company
www.hachette.co.uk

www.piatkus.co.uk

Contents

Acknowledgements

Cancer is a complex subject and I am indebted to all the researchers whose work is contributing towards finding a way forward, including Dr Richard Passwater, Dr Balz Frei and colleagues at the Linus Pauling Institute and the World Cancer Research Fund, who have helped to put diet at the top of the anti-cancer agenda. I am also grateful for the research of Professors Jeff Holly, Jane Plant, Dan Burke and Gerry Potter. Most of all I am especially indebted to Liz Efiong, who has helped research and update this edition. My thanks also go to the team at Piatkus, and especially Jillian Stewart and Jan Cutler for their help editing this edition.

Guide to Abbreviations and Measures

1 gram (g) = 1,000 milligrams (mg) = 100,0000 micrograms (mcg or μg).

Most vitamins are measured in milligrams or micrograms. Vitamins A, D and E are also measured in International Units (iu), a measurement designed to standardise the different forms of these vitamins, which have different potencies.

1mcg of retinol (mcgRE) = 3.3iu of vitamin A (RE = retinol equivalents)

1mcgRE of beta-carotene = 6mcg of beta-carotene

100iu of vitamin D = 2.5mcg

100iu of vitamin E = 67mg

1 pound (lb) = 16 ounces (oz) 2.2lb = 1 kilogram (kg)

In this book calories means kilocalories (kcal)

CAUTION

If you have been diagnosed with cancer, you should not undertake an extensive nutritional strategy on your own. Cancer is a complex and life-threatening disease that requires professional medical care. Some alternative remedies may actually worsen cancer if they are not used appropriately. Therefore, if you want to use any of the alternative remedies discussed in this book, use only as part of a cancer-treatment programme that is guided and monitored by a qualified nutritional therapist, doctor or equivalent health professional who is experienced in cancer care and alternative medicine and who can work with your doctor to devise the most appropriate strategy for you. Simply because a substance is 'natural' doesn't mean it is never harmful. Very high doses of nutrients can have adverse effects; this is why you need a nutritional therapist to advise you and to run tests to find out what you need.

If you are taking medication, we recommend you check with your doctor if there are any contraindications between the medication and the supplements you wish to take. Check with your doctor before changing or stopping any conventional medical treatments or medications, and keep all of your doctors and/or alternative practitioners informed of all treatments that you are receiving.

The recommendations given in this book are solely intended as education and information, and should not be taken as medical advice. Neither the authors nor the publisher accept liability for readers who choose to self-prescribe.

All supplements should be kept out of reach of infants and children.

References and Further Sources of Information

Hundreds of references from respected scientific literature have been used in writing this book. Details of specific studies referred to are listed on pages 350–80. More details on most of these studies can be found on the Internet for those wishing to dig deeper. PubMed is a service of the US National Library of Medicine that includes over 18 million citations dating back to 1948. This is where you can access most of the studies mentioned (see http://www.ncbi.nlm.nih.gov/pubmed/). On page 397 you will also find a Recommended Reading list, which suggests the best books to read if you wish to find out more about the topics covered.

Introduction

No diagnosis strikes more fear into the hearts of patients than that of cancer. It is often perceived as incurable and of unknown cause – and in many ways viewed in the same way as the plague must have been in the 17th century: we live in fear of it and avoid talking about it. Meanwhile, as we hide our heads in the sand, cancer has grown to be the second most common cause of premature death in the Western world and is predicted to become the number-one cause of death within 20 years. It is already the primary killer of people under the age of 50. When this book was first published in 1999, it was predicted that within 15 years one in four people would be diagnosed with cancer at some point in their lives. And now, ten years later, it is already one in three! And it is predicted to be one in two by the year 2020! Although there have been great strides made in cancer treatment, what is badly needed is a way to prevent it ever occurring, or reoccurring.

Cancer is largely a 20th-century invention

It may surprise you to know that cancer is, for the most part, a 20th-century invention. The top five cancers – lung, breast, stomach, colorectal and prostate – were more or less unheard of before the early 20th century. The growth in the incidence of cancer parallels the industrialisation and chemicalisation of our world: the more developed a country, the more cancer there is. Indeed, the higher the per-capita income, the higher the incidence of cancer.[1]

This is because most cancers are primarily the result of changes we have made to our total chemical environment: what we eat, drink and breathe. Changing patterns of cancer in the economically developed world show that cancer rates are strongly influenced by environmental factors. According to one of Britain's top medical scientists, Sir Richard Doll, 90 per cent of all cancers are caused by this. The most conservative cancer experts say that at least 75 per cent of cancers are associated with environment and lifestyle.

However, probably 85 per cent of cancers are preventable. Research published in the *New England Journal of Medicine* describing a study involving 45,000 pairs of twins found that cancer is much more likely to be caused by diet and lifestyle choices – those things we can change – than by genes. Identical twins, who are genetically the same, had no more than a 15 per cent chance of developing the same cancer. This suggests that the cause of most cancers is about 85 per cent environmental – and that means it is down to factors such as diet, lifestyle and exposure to toxic chemicals. This study found that choices about diet, smoking and exercise accounted for 58 to 82 per cent of cancers studied.[2]

In the space of two generations, humankind has invented ten million new chemicals and unwittingly released thousands of them into the environment. Many are known to be carcinogens (that is, they are capable of causing cancer). And we take these into our bodies through our food, the air we breathe and the water we drink. Many are easily avoidable – although some are not.

What we eat is especially relevant. We have, it seems, been digging our own graves with our knives and forks. Today's diet of refined foods laced with chemicals and devoid of nutrients is now thought to be the greatest single contributor to cancer risk. Conversely, by eating the right diet you can cut your risk of cancer by up to 40 per cent, says the World Cancer Research Fund, and the European Commission estimates that a quarter of a million lives could be saved each year across the 27 member states through dietary changes alone. According to the Cancer Research Campaign, at least three out of four of all cancers are potentially preventable, but will only be avoided if the messages get through to people while they are young.

Cancer isn't only about diet, however. We unknowingly expose ourselves to many cancer-causing chemicals in our homes and workplaces. So, minimising this exposure can also greatly reduce our risk of cancer.

Boosting your immune system

Avoiding or reducing known cancer-initiating chemicals is just one piece of the equation. Another is preventing your exposure to cancer promoters. These include chemicals and foods, and even your body's own hormones, which, if out of balance, can encourage cancer cells to grow. The other critical piece of the jigsaw is strengthening your own defences. Carcinogens are nothing new. They exist in nature, even in everyday health-promoting foods, but they don't necessarily present a problem, because the body is designed to detoxify carcinogens. It's when your body's defences are weak, and you are exposed to too many carcinogens, that the trouble starts.

So, boosting your immune system and improving your liver's ability to detoxify carcinogens are clearly vital, as you'll see in Chapters 6 and 7. I believe your risk of developing cancer really can be massively reduced or entirely eliminated by putting all these pieces together: avoiding known carcinogens; eating the right diet; balancing your hormones; improving your liver's detoxification potential; and boosting your immune system. Such a prevention strategy forms the basis for preventing the recurrence of cancer and reversing the process of cancer cell growth. The evidence presented in this book strongly suggests that you genuinely can 'say no to cancer'.

Are we winning the cancer war?

Despite the fact that we already know how to drastically reduce cancer risk, the sad truth is that we are not taking the necessary action – with a few notable exceptions. The incidence of lung cancer, for example, is now decreasing in many countries as fewer and fewer people smoke. Cervical cancer and cancer of the stomach are also in decline. Despite this, the overall rate of cancer, which now strikes one in three and kills one in four, is still very much on the increase.

What is particularly worrying is the rise in hormone-related cancers. These are cancers of hormonally sensitive tissue, which, in men are cancer of the prostate and testes, and, in women are cancer of the breast, cervix, ovaries and womb (endometrium).

Take breast cancer, for example. Currently, one in nine women in the USA develops breast cancer – one in eight in the UK. Breast cancer incidence rates in the UK have increased by more than 50 per cent over the last 25 years. Prostate cancer rates have tripled over the last 30 years. In truth, these cancers are occurring more frequently and earlier in people's lives than they were a decade ago. It is highly likely that dietary changes and our exposure to environmental toxins play a significant role in this.

In 1992, a statement signed by 69 highly respected medical and scientific experts in the USA stated, 'Over the last decade, some five million Americans died of cancer and there is growing evidence that a substantial proportion of these deaths was avoidable.'[3] The reason for the statement was to protest against the failure of the policies of government and cancer institutions. In March 2010 a briefing by the *Journal of the American Medical Association* reported that there has been less than a 1 per cent decrease in the rate of new cancer diagnoses between 1999 and 2006, almost half of which is accounted for by reduced lung cancer diagnoses presumably from anti-smoking campaigns.[4] Nearly one in two men and more than one in three women in America will be diagnosed with cancer this year, they say. In America in 2009 there were 1.5 million cases of cancer and more than 560,000 deaths. This can hardly be called a success given that the American government have spent $100 billion on cancer research in the past forty years.

Are we even fighting it?

Has anything changed? Remarkably little research money is being spent on prevention, with most being directed towards variations on conventional treatment using surgery, chemotherapy or radiotherapy. Indeed, improvement in cancer treatment has reduced cancer mortality. Today, a breast cancer patient is likely to survive longer than 20 years ago. However, what these statistics don't always take into account is that people are often just being diagnosed earlier, and hence appear to survive longer.

However, conventional treatment, which is all rather medieval in concept (essentially to cut it out, burn it out or drug it out), is not truly addressing the underlying factors that lead cells to become cancer cells in the first place. This should be the first line of attack.

While prevention is obviously better than cure, the fact is that cancer prevention is not profitable. Interestingly, some of the main cancer charities receive funding from the pharmaceutical industry, which hardly encourages them to concentrate resources on tackling the true causes of cancer – namely our modern diet, lifestyle and over-exposure to cancer-causing chemicals. Before you donate money, ask how much of it is truly being spent on non-drug prevention research.

On a positive note, there is, however, a list of known factors associated with increasing cancer risk that we can all do our best to avoid. In this book these factors, and the necessary actions, will become clear.

Putting prevention into practice

Learning how we can prevent cancer is important for everyone. The easiest way to stay free of cancer is to do all the right things in the first place; people with an early diagnosis, or who have had cancer in the past, can often prevent its development or recurrence. Primary cancers are very rarely life threatening; it is the secondaries, the cancers that follow, that claim all too many victims.

I cannot stress enough that cancer must be looked at holistically, which means in terms of *all* the possible contributing factors, both internally and externally, not just in terms of the organ or area of the body it is affecting. Your body is a highly complex adaptive organism, but unfortunately most people treat their cars better than they do their bodies! Most cars get an annual service (or at least an oil change every now and then) but mention a 'detox' to most people and they run for the hills.

So, once diagnosed, it is absolutely essential to follow the right kind of diet, address hormonal imbalances, avoid carcinogens and boost your immune system. The purpose of this book is to explain what that means in practice. But first, it's worth knowing what causes cancer and how you can intervene to keep your body healthy.

How to use this book

Cancer is a complicated issue, so this book is structured to make it easy for you to understand what you need to do to reduce the risk.

Part 1 explains what cancer is, which factors cause normal cells to become cancer cells and then encourage their growth, and why you can expect almost complete protection by following the advice in this book.

Part 2 reveals the connections between different foods and the development or avoidance of cancer. Reading this section will help you understand the basis for the practical recommendations later in the book.

Part 3 identifies the lifestyle and environmental risk factors of cancer – with recommendations of ways you can cut your risk.

Part 4 shows you the evidence on how nutrients and other natural remedies can help you avoid cancer, and outlines some that may have a specific role to play if you already have cancer.

Part 5 offers clear, practical guidelines for staying free from cancer. If you read nothing else, read this. It includes your action list for developing a cancer-free diet and lifestyle.

Part 6 tells you what to do if you have cancer – how to use natural approaches alongside conventional treatments to maximise your recovery from chemotherapy, radiation and surgery, and how to reduce the risk of recurrence. It also contains specific advice for the two most common cancers: breast and prostate.

Part 7 gives you specific advice on risk factors, prevention and nutritional support for each kind of cancer.

Medical advice

Many of the strategies recommended here have been proven to be effective, but the recommendations in this book do not replace those of your doctor or cancer specialist. If you wish to change your medication or your treatment strategy, please consult your doctor. In Chapter 35 I discuss how to integrate conventional cancer treatment with the recommendations in this book.

Wishing you the best of health,

Patrick Holford

PART 1

WHAT CAUSES CANCER?

CHAPTER 1

What is Cancer?

It may surprise you to know that we all have cancer cells in our bodies. Cancer occurs when cells start to behave differently from normal – growing, multiplying and spreading. It is like a revolution within the body, when a group of cells stops working in harmony with the whole organism and start running riot. We all produce cancer cells, so the odd revolutionary cell is a common occurrence. The immune system of a healthy person simply isolates and destroys such offenders before they develop to form a cancer mass, or tumour. However, in cancer the immune system is overcome and the cancer spreads. Understanding how and why this happens is the key to preventing cancer.

An embryo turns into a baby, and eventually into a fully grown human, because our cells are programmed to multiply – 2, 4, 8, 16, and so on – until you have the 30 trillion or so cells that make up an adult. The early cells all look similar and then, as they develop, they start to look different from one another and take on specific roles in the body. Although most cells continue to be replaced throughout our lives, they generally stop growing or multiplying, and they basically settle down (like good citizens) to get on with their specific duties, respecting their neighbours.

Cells that change

If, however, a cell is damaged in some way, it can start to behave more primitively, growing and multiplying, not respecting its neighbours, nor carrying out its specific function. This is a cancer cell. Most cancer cells will be detected by the immune system and weeded out. Some, however, appear more resistant, or can flourish because the immune system is weak.

They may then go on to develop clusters of 'undifferentiated' cells. If the cells are not actually multiplying and do not pose an immediate risk, the growth is called a benign tumour. If, however, the cells are multiplying, it is called a malignant tumour.

In due course the multiplying cancer cells become a cancer mass. Like any other cells, they need food to keep working, and so the mass develops its own blood supply to provide this. This is called angiogenesis. Depending on where and how big the cancer mass is, symptoms may become apparent. During an autopsy after a death from a different cause, many people are found to have a cancer mass without ever having been aware of it.

These 'primary' cancers have different names, depending on the kind of tissue they occur in and their location. Most human cancers are carcinomas (carc = cancer; oma = tumour), which are malignant tumours that arise from epithelial cells (cells that form part of the covering or lining of a body surface). Melanomas (melano = black), for example, are cancerous growths of melanocytes, which are skin cells that produce the pigment melanin. Sarcoma is a general term for any cancer arising from muscle cells or connective tissues; for example, osteogenic sarcomas (osteo = bone; genic = origin), which are the most frequent type of childhood cancer, destroy bone tissue (connective tissue) and eventually spread to other areas of the body. Leukaemia is a cancer of blood-forming organs characterised by rapid growth and distorted development of leukocytes (white blood cells) and their precursors. Lymphoma is a malignant disease of lymphatic tissue; for example, lymph nodes. An example is Hodgkin's disease.

Primary and secondary cancers

'Primary' cancer is rarely likely to be fatal. However, at some point, a more mobile 'metastatic' cancer cell may develop. These metastatic

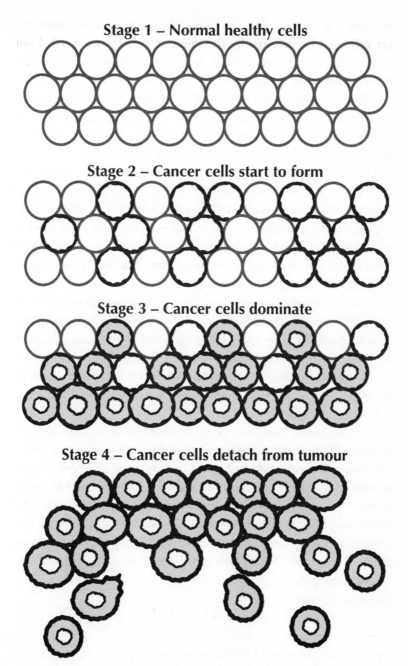

Stage 1 – Normal healthy cells

Stage 2 – Cancer cells start to form

Stage 3 – Cancer cells dominate

Stage 4 – Cancer cells detach from tumour

Normal cells versus cancer cells

cells can leave the original cancer mass and spread around the body, through the bloodstream or the lymphatic vessels. They can then lodge in different parts of the body and start multiplying there, resulting in what are known as 'secondary tumours'.

These secondaries are more insidious, and much harder to treat, and they tend to spread and grow more quickly. Consequently, the average chance of surviving, once secondaries appear, is much lower.

What's the aim of conventional treatment?

The main focus of conventional cancer treatment is the early detection and then annihilation of the tumours. The earlier a cancer is detected, the better the chances of eliminating the primary tumour before it metastasises (or spreads) and produces secondaries.

Early detection, however, is not without its problems. Mammograms, used to detect breast tumours, are capable of detecting micro calcifications (small calcium deposits) in the breasts, which could never be felt before. These micro calcifications may not be cancer as we know it; but whether or not they warrant treatment is a matter of debate.

Mammograms also expose a woman to radiation, thereby increasing cancer risk. Some scientists therefore believe that routine mammography under the age of 50 for symptom-free women is unwarranted. In fact, a recent study has suggested that as many as one in three breast cancers detected by mammogram may be harmless. Researchers from the Nordic Cochrane Centre in Denmark looked at a range of statistics from between 1971 and 1999 from five countries that had implemented screening programmes, including the UK. The results showed that some women had had treatment for cancers that were unlikely to kill them or spread.[1]

Once the cancer has been removed with surgery the most usual follow-on treatment for breast cancer is with the drug tamoxifen, yet many people who don't take it do just as well as those who do. Overall, it decreases mortality by less than 10 per cent (see page 320).

The options

There are three ways to annihilate a tumour: with surgery, radiation or chemotherapy. Some forms of cancer don't lend themselves to surgery (for example, liver, brain, bone and blood), in which case chemotherapy – using drugs that are toxic to cancer cells – is employed. While these treatments can, and do, save lives, the trouble is that they often do so at a high cost: each treatment is traumatic and damages the body. Recent advances in such therapies have attempted to minimise the damage; for example, by developing chemotherapeutic drugs that target only cancer cells and don't damage healthy cells. Later in the book I'll be talking about nutrients that do exactly this.

In any event nutritional support is vital during these treatments – it can reduce side effects and speed up recovery (see Chapter 35).

Conventional cancer therapies, however, place remarkably little emphasis on eliminating the factors that cause cancer in the first place, or on boosting the body's natural defences to fight back and restore healthy cells.

What initiates cancer?

Cancer is the uncontrolled growth of cells. The key question is why do cells suddenly start growing and multiplying? There are many different kinds of cancers and no doubt many different answers to this question. However, in many cases, a major initiating factor is damage to the cell.

The outer membrane (or 'skin') of each cell contains sensors that tell it when to grow or multiply. If these sensors are damaged by an undesirable chemical, cancer can result. Each cell also contains instructions for its behaviour, and for the behaviour of future cells. These are contained within the genes, which are written in the DNA (the genetic blueprint material found in every single cell). If a chemical enters the body and damages the DNA, the cell can start to 'misbehave' by dividing and producing more errant cells.

Some of us also have dormant genes that, if awakened by a particular stimulus, can trigger cancer. These cancer-causing genes are called oncogenes and can be activated by a number of undesirable chemicals. Factors that can trigger cancer are called carcinogens and they are fully discussed in Chapter 4 as well as in Part 3.

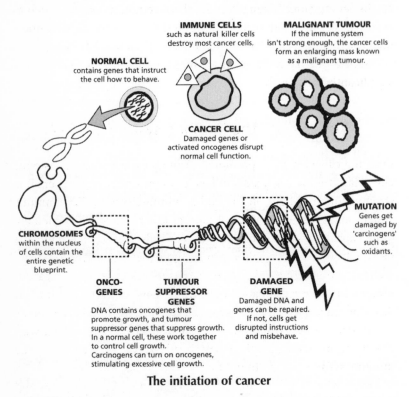

IMMUNE CELLS
such as natural killer cells destroy most cancer cells.

MALIGNANT TUMOUR
If the immune system isn't strong enough, the cancer cells form an enlarging mass known as a malignant tumour.

NORMAL CELL
contains genes that instruct the cell how to behave.

CANCER CELL
Damaged genes or activated oncogenes disrupt normal cell function.

MUTATION
Genes get damaged by 'carcinogens' such as oxidants.

CHROMOSOMES
within the nucleus of cells contain the entire genetic blueprint.

ONCO-GENES

TUMOUR SUPPRESSOR GENES

DAMAGED GENE
Damaged DNA and genes can be repaired. If not, cells get disrupted instructions and misbehave.

DNA contains oncogenes that promote growth, and tumour suppressor genes that suppress growth. In a normal cell, these work together to control cell growth.
Carcinogens can turn on oncogenes, stimulating excessive cell growth.

The initiation of cancer

What promotes cancer?

Although this whole process of undesirable chemicals altering cell function marks the beginning of the cancer process, this alone is not enough for a person to develop a malignant tumour. Indeed, such cellular changes are happening within us all the time, producing individual pre-cancerous cells that are found and destroyed by our immune system.

In order for the cancer cells to survive and take over, they must multiply and invade surrounding tissue. The mass must then develop its own defences and blood supply. A number of substances and circumstances can help or hinder the cancer's progression to this stage. Some chemicals, for example, do not initiate cancer but do encourage its progression. Having high levels of certain hormones, such as oestrogen, insulin and insulin-like growth factor (IGF-1), encourage the growth of cancer cells (more on this in Chapters 12 and 16).

Such hormonal imbalances are most common in people who are significantly overweight.

Why doesn't the immune system attack?

Even if a cancer mass is promoted through exposure to undesirable chemicals, the cancer mass still has to progress to a stage where it is strong enough to fight off the body's immune system. The immune system makes large numbers of natural killer (NK) cells, which are quite capable of destroying most cancer cells. But if, for example, a person drinks a lot of alcohol, which suppresses the immune system's ability to produce NK cells, then there is more likelihood of a cancer progressing. The combination of being very overweight, smoking and drinking is particularly bad news: the carcinogens in tobacco smoke can initiate cancer, while the hormonal imbalances associated with obesity promote the growth of cancer cells, and alcohol depresses the immune system's ability to fight it.

Even when a cancer mass has developed its own defences and blood supply, this alone is rarely fatal. Whether or not such a cancer mass goes into the metastatic phase (releasing mobile cancer cells that produce secondary cancers in other parts of the body) again depends on a person's chemistry. Some nutrients reduce the risk of metastasis, whereas other chemicals promote it.

In this book you will learn which nutrients, foods and lifestyle factors – including your mindset – can protect you against cancer, at every stage, and also which chemicals and lifestyle habits you need to avoid. You'll also learn how your body has the power to eliminate cancer cells and promote healthy cells that work together for the good of the whole – that's you.

CHAPTER 2

The Oxidant Factor

A big part of the cancer equation, and one reason for the rapid development of cancer in the 20th century, is our increased exposure to cancer-causing factors, especially those that directly damage our genes. These include:

- Tobacco smoke

- Exhaust fumes

- Industrial pollution

- Food and agricultural chemicals

- Burned, browned or fried food

- Excessive sun exposure

- Radiation

These, and many other factors, produce chemicals called oxidants (also known as 'free radicals' or 'free oxidising radicals'). Oxidants are a bit like the toxic exhaust of any burning process that involves oxygen. We even make oxidants in our bodies when the carbohydrate we eat 'burns' (to form energy) as it reacts with the oxygen we breathe in.

So, if you want to increase your risk of developing cancer, just stand in the main street of a polluted city, on a hot, sunny day, burning your skin, breathing in exhaust fumes, eating French fries and smoking a cigarette. Not many people do all these things at once, but many people's lifestyles do involve significant exposure to oxidants. (The effects of smoking, radiation and sun exposure are discussed in Part 3.)

Conversely, if you very rarely eat burned, browned or fried food, spend little time in traffic, live in an unpolluted environment, don't smoke, and avoid excessive exposure to strong sunlight, then your cancer risk will be lower.

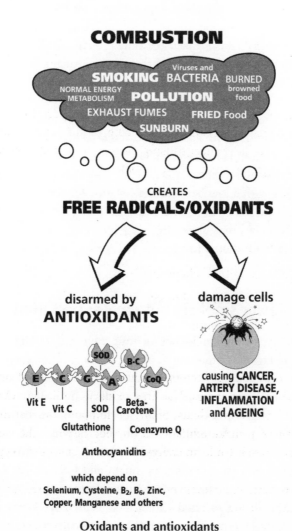

Oxidants and antioxidants

Antioxidant protection

There are two sides to the oxidant equation. Oxidants are on one side; on the other are antioxidants – chemicals that neutralise these harmful oxidants. There are literally hundreds of antioxidants, the best known of which are vitamins A, C and E. However, there are many others that you might not have heard of, such as polyphenols and salvestrols, found in fruits and vegetables. The evidence for the protective effect of taking in optimal amounts of these anti-cancer nutrients in your diet is substantial (this is discussed fully in Parts 2 and 4).

The power of antioxidants has been known for 30 years. One survey published in the *Lancet* medical journal in 1981 looked at the relationship between beta-carotene status and smoking. (Beta-carotene is the vegetable form of vitamin A.)[2] The researchers found that heavy smokers with a low beta-carotene status had a 6.5 per cent chance of developing lung cancer. On the other hand a heavy smoker with a high beta-carotene status had only a 0.8 per cent risk, as did a non-smoker with a low beta-carotene status. Finally, those who had a high beta-carotene status and who also didn't smoke had no risk. This study shows that increasing your intake of certain anti-cancer nutrients in your diet is just as important as limiting your intake of carcinogens. These nutrients are covered in detail in Part 4.

Fewer smokers but greater pollution

Although the overall incidence of lung cancer is falling in countries where cigarette smoking is on the decline, lung cancer among non-smokers is actually rising.[3] This is almost certainly because of increasing levels of air pollution, particularly from diesel fuel, says Professor Simon Wolff, a toxicologist. He points out that 'in rural China, where people tend to smoke very heavily and where air pollution is much less, the difference in lung cancer rates between smokers and non-smokers is very small, and lung cancer rates are about one-tenth of the lung cancer rates in industrialised countries'.[4] The traditional diet in rural China is substantially higher in anti-oxidants than the typical diet in industrialised countries.

Oxidant damage

We need to understand how oxidants do their damage in order to defend ourselves against cancer. Oxidants are unstable and dangerous because they have an uneven electrical charge (whereas a stable chemical has an even electrical charge). Oxidants are rather like amorous bachelors looking for a mate. To complete themselves, they steal electrons from cells, homing in on either the membrane of the cell or the DNA, because this is where the most 'double bonds' (atoms that are connected with two links) are found. These double bonds are particularly susceptible to oxidant damage.

Another source of double bonds is fat. The more unsaturated a fat, the more double bonds it contains. Polyunsaturated fats, such as sunflower oil, have plenty of double bonds, and if you use it for frying – which generates very high temperatures – these double bonds can get damaged. Eating fried foods therefore increases your intake of oxidants, which, in turn, can start to damage your cells.

Help from antioxidants

Antioxidants are real heroes. They mop up the dangerous oxidant 'sparks', but in the process, become oxidised and destabilise themselves. If, however, they then meet another oxidant they can be 'reloaded'. Like a team of bomb-disposal experts, antioxidants work together to defuse the dangerous chemical sparks called oxidants.

This synergistic partnership of antioxidants is important, as shown in the illustration overleaf. Key partnerships exist between different antioxidants, which become inactivated once they've disarmed an oxidant; for example:

- Vitamin E is recycled by vitamin C and coenzyme Q_{10}.

- Vitamin C is recycled by glutathione (one of the most important antioxidants of all – more about this in Chapters 6 and 7), carotenoids (in carrots), and lipoic acid.

- Glutathione is recycled by anthocyanidins (in berries) and resveratrol (see Chapter 25).

Antioxidants are team players

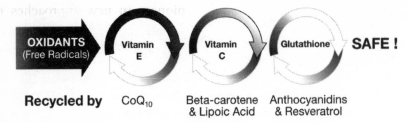

The synergistic action of nutrients in disarming a free radical

Vitamin E disarms a harmful free radical but becomes a radical in the process. It is recycled and turned back into an antioxidant by CoQ_{10}. Vitamin C then passes the free radical along to glutathione and then it is disarmed, making it safe. Vitamin C and glutathione are recycled by beta-carotene, lipoic acid, anthocyanidins and resveratrol.

The sum of the whole is far greater than the sum of the parts. So, having a high intake of both vitamins C and E, as well as glutathione and anthocyanidins, is much more protective than having a high intake of just one of these nutrients on its own. The body can only completely detoxify many harmful and potentially cancer-promoting substances if all these nutrients are present in the right amounts.

The synergy of nutrients is also vital because there are many different kinds of oxidants, each disarmed most effectively by a different kind of antioxidant. So, for all-round protection against all the oxidants that come your way, you need to take in a whole collection of antioxidants, including:

vitamin A	carotenoids
vitamin C	coenzyme Q_{10}
vitamin E	lipoic acid
selenium	polyphenols
glutathione	salvestrols
anthocyanidins	resveratrol

These nutrients are found in food and can also be taken in concentrated form as nutritional supplements, but unfortunately this is only part of the story.

In summary there are many cancer-causing chemicals that don't cause oxidation, so just avoiding oxidants and increasing your intake of antioxidants can offer only partial protection.

The next chapter looks at another factor: hormone-disrupting chemicals in our environment.

CHAPTER 3

Hormones in Havoc

Evidence is accumulating that the high incidence of cancer of the breast, cervix and ovaries in women, and of the prostate and testes in men, is related to disturbed regulation of our hormones. All of these body tissues are especially sensitive to the effects of hormones. The rapid increase in breast cancer (the most common cancer in women in the UK and US) and prostate cancer (the most common cancer in men in the UK and the US) has raised concerns about a number of chemicals in our foods, homes and medicines that may be adding to our risk of developing cancer, as well as the impact of modern living and eating on hormone levels.

Breast cancer incidence has increased by more than 50 per cent over the last 25 years. It now affects one in eight women in the UK at some time in their life (compared to one in 22 in the 1940s). Although breast cancer occurs mainly in women, men can get it too, with around 300 men each year being affected. Meanwhile, rates of prostate cancer have almost tripled over the last 30 years, and this disease now affects around one in 14 men at some point in their life.

The current approaches to breast cancer are not having much effect on this worrying trend, although advances in cancer treatment are increasing survival rates.

Hormone-disrupting chemicals

The fundamental question is: why are such cancers increasing and what can be done to reverse this? In one of the most extraordinary detective stories of our times (first documented in two excellent books, *Our Stolen Future*, by Theo Colborn, and *The Feminisation of Nature*, by Deborah Cadbury) leading scientists from many disciplines have come to the same conclusions: 'We've released chemicals throughout the world that are having fundamental effects on the reproductive system and immune system in wildlife and humans,' says Professor Louis Guillette from the University of Florida. 'We have unwittingly entered the ultimate Faustian bargain ... in return for all the benefits of our modern society, and all the amazing products of modern life, we have more testicular cancer and more breast cancer. We may also affect the ability of the species to reproduce,' says Devra Lee Davis, former deputy health-policy adviser to the American government.

They, and countless other scientists, came to the conclusion that a growing number of commonly occurring chemicals, found in our air, water and food, are disrupting hormone balances and acting as carcinogens: these include some pesticides, plastics, industrial compounds and pharmaceutical drugs (see Chapter 20 for more on these). But they also include 'natural' foods such as meat and milk that contain high levels of hormones such as oestrogen and other cell growth promoters. Of course, if you think about it, it isn't really natural to consume dairy products, which are designed for babies, as an adult. It's like breastfeeding at the age of 40 – from another species of animal! (See Chapter 12 for more on the link between milk and cancer.)

What the chemicals do in the body

Most of these chemicals mimic the role in the body of oestrogen, which is a hormone that stimulates the growth of hormone-sensitive tissue. They are classified as xenoestrogens (meaning oestrogenic compounds from outside, as opposed to inside, our bodies). When taken in on top of the natural oestrogen produced by both men and women, plus the added oestrogen and other cell growth promoters taken in from dairy products or by women on the Pill or HRT, these chemicals can 'over-oestrogenise' a person.

Too much oestrogen stimulates the excessive proliferation of hormone-sensitive tissue, thus increasing the risk of hormone-related cancers. However, the effect of these substances is not quite so linear. They may also alter genes or promote the expression of oncogenes (see Chapter 5). Essentially, they confuse the hormonal messages the body sends out, changing sexual and reproductive development. They are best thought of as hormone-disrupters, interfering with the body's ability to adapt and respond appropriately to its environment.

Pesticides

Researchers have been trying to measure the effects of global pollution by such chemicals for many years. In animal studies carried out more than 20 years ago, it was shown that exposure to certain pesticides induces breast cancer[5] and promotes the growth of tumours.[6] In Israel breast cancer mortality in pre-menopausal women dropped by 30 per cent following the implementation of regulations reducing levels of carcinogenic pesticides.[7] Furthermore, higher levels of DDT and PCBs have been found in human breast cancer tissue compared to healthy tissue.[8] Many other pesticides are known to be carcinogenic, although not necessarily by acting as hormone-disrupters (these are discussed more fully in Chapter 20). The average person who eats non-organic food will have up to a gallon of pesticides sprayed on the fruit and vegetables they consume each year. Because of this, the link between cancer and pesticide exposure definitely needs more research.

Plastics

Even more insidious is the potential effect of the hormone-disrupting chemicals found in plastics. One carcinogen found by chance is a component used in plastic to protect it from oxidation. Researchers studying breast cancer cells that had been placed in a plastic container couldn't understand why they were growing so prolifically, as if exposed to oestrogen. It turned out that nonylphenols were leaching from the plastic and having an oestrogenic effect.[9]

Since the first edition of this book, nonylphenols have been banned in the EU as a hazard to human and environmental safety,[10] although they are still permitted to be used in concentrations of less than 0.1 per cent in certain cases, which include cosmetic and personal-care products. Outside of the EU they are still used in detergents – classified as 'surfactants' – so check the products you buy. Previously, 18,000 tons of nonylphenols were produced each year in the UK, and some ended up in the water supply. It is this factor that is believed to have caused the infertility and feminising of fish in polluted rivers.

Evidence to date suggests it would seem prudent to limit the exposure of food to plastic, especially fatty foods, and to avoid foods that are heated in plastic, such as TV dinners. Buy non-PVC clingfilm, for example, but avoid using it to wrap cheese or fatty foods. Plastic packaging is used for most foods, including snacks, although less of it now contains the harmful chemicals mentioned above.

Card packaging

Even card packaging can contain toxins, and dioxins are one example, used to bleach paper and card. As well as being used as bleaching agents in other industrial chemical processes, they are used as pesticides in some countries. Although not oestrogen-mimickers, through some action that we don't yet understand, research has shown that they feminise male rodents both physically and behaviourally. Dioxins are a by-product of chlorine compounds. Like other organochlorines (see Chapter 20), they are non-biodegradable, and therefore tend to accumulate in the environment.

Chemical overload

Perhaps most concerning is the finding that 'acceptable' levels of a number of chemicals can, in combination, produce a vastly exaggerated oestrogen effect. As each new piece is fitted into the chemical jigsaw, the extent to which we may need to clean up the environment, industrial processing and the food chain becomes clearer.

Such worldwide increased exposure to these hormone disrupters is even more worrying in the light of the findings that a very small change in hormone exposure during foetal development sets a clock ticking for increased cancer risk in adulthood, as well as decreasing fertility. In other words, at its worst, over-exposure to these chemicals could be programming us for extinction.

Synthetic hormones, HRT and the Pill

Oestrogens make things grow. And too many oestrogens can promote hormone-sensitive cancers. One study showed that when oestrogen levels were increased in pre-menopausal women with breast lumps, the proliferation rate of breast epithelial cells (those lining the breast) increased by over 200 per cent – more than twice the normal rate. Oestrogen is usually kept in check by progesterone, another hormone produced by the ovaries, which has an anti-proliferation effect. According to the lead researcher, Dr Chang from the National Taiwan University Hospital in Taipei, if natural progesterone is given and the level in breast tissue is raised to normal physiological levels, cell multiplication rate falls to 15 per cent of that in women who have not been treated. So oestrogen promotes the proliferation of breast cancers, while progesterone is protective.[11]

The late Dr John Lee, a medical expert in female hormones, health campaigner and author of many books on the subject (see Recommended Reading), said this in the 1990s:

> The major cause of breast cancer is unopposed oestrogen and there are many factors that would lead to this. Stress, for

example, raises cortisol and competes with progesterone for receptor sites. Xenoestrogens from the environment have the ability to damage tissue and lead to an increased risk of cancer later in life. There are also clearly nutritional and genetic factors to consider. What is most concerning is that doctors continue to prescribe unopposed oestrogen to women.

He is, of course, referring to the widespread prescribing of synthetic hormones in contraceptive pills and HRT. The increasing use of synthetic hormones in medicine has been mirrored by the rise in hormone-related cancers. Fortunately, the practice of prescribing oestrogen-only HRT is now much rarer, as most doctors now recognise the risk.

The first synthetic oestrogen

There could be no more dramatic an example of the danger of altering our exposure to these powerful hormone-disrupters than DES, the first synthetic oestrogen, created by Dr Charles Dodds in 1938. Within 20 years, DES was being given to women and animals. For the latter it improved growth rates, while for women it apparently promised a trouble-free pregnancy and healthier offspring. Eventually, up to six million mothers and babies were exposed to it.

It wasn't until 1970 that the flaws surfaced. Girls whose mothers had been taking DES during pregnancy started to show genital development abnormalities and a substantial increase in cancer rates, especially vaginal cancer of a kind never seen before.[12] Then it was discovered that boys whose mothers had taken DES also had defects in the development of their sexual organs.[13] Many DES children died and many more were infertile.

Oestrogens today, and their effects

DES is no longer prescribed, but synthetic oestrogens and progestins are, and both are associated with increased cancer risk. Early trials of

HRT, which contained only oestrogen, showed a vastly increased risk of endometrial or womb cancer, because one of the jobs of oestrogen is to stimulate cell growth there, preparing the womb for a potential pregnancy. The increase ranged from 200 to 1,500 per cent, depending on how long you had been taking it; and your risk would still be significantly raised several years after you stopped taking it.[14] So progestin, a synthetic hormone, was added to the mix starting in the 1960s. The idea was that, by counteracting unopposed oestrogen, the womb lining would be protected from excess cell growth. Adding progestins to HRT did reduce the risk of endometrial cancer, although it didn't stop it.[15] (Progestins are the synthetic progesterone-like hormone, also called progestagens, which are quite different from the body's natural progesterone.)

HRT and breast cancer

The first major warning sign of a link between breast cancer and HRT came in 1989. A study by Dr L. Bergkvist and colleagues involving 23,000 Scandinavian women showed that if a woman is on HRT for longer than five years, she doubles her risk of breast cancer.[16] But it also revealed that adding progestins to cut down the womb cancer risk raised the risk of breast cancer. This was confirmed in a large-scale study, published in the *New England Journal of Medicine* in 1995, which showed that post-menopausal women in their sixties who had been on HRT for five or more years increased their risk of developing breast cancer by 71 per cent.[17] The longer you were on HRT, the greater the risk. Overall, there was a 32 per cent increased risk among women using oestrogen HRT, and a 41 per cent risk for those using oestrogen combined with synthetic progestin, compared to women who had never used hormones.

Other studies took place in 1997: one showed that women using combined oestrogen and cyclic progestin on a long-term basis had a higher risk of endometrial (uterine) cancer than those not on hormone replacement.[18] Another analysed the results of 51 clinical studies, involving over 160,000 women, and concluded that there was an increased risk of breast cancer in women using HRT, with the risk rising as the duration of use lengthened, and reducing once HRT was stopped.[19]

Evidence continued to accumulate year on year, but the real clincher came with the 'million women' trial in 2003. This trial, published in the *Lancet*, followed a million women aged 50 to 64, half of whom had used HRT.[20] It was found that those who had used oestrogen and progestin HRT doubled their risk of breast cancer.

The conclusion of Professor Valerie Beral from the UK Cancer Research Epidemiology Unit at Oxford, who was in charge of this study, was: 'Use of HRT by women aged 50 to 64 years in the UK over the past decade has resulted in an estimated 20,000 extra breast cancers, 15,000 associated with oestrogen-progestagen (progestin); the extra deaths cannot yet be reliably estimated.' This study predicted that stopping doctors prescribing HRT would result in a decrease in breast cancers, which is exactly what happened. Following this study in 2002, prescriptions for HRT slumped by over 50 per cent in both America and the UK. Research published in 2009 shows that breast cancer incidence has fallen in line with stopping HRT.[21] The result of this, according to a recent report in the *British Medical Journal*, is 1,500 fewer cases of breast cancer a year in the UK.

Ovarian cancers and oestrogen

Breast cancer isn't the only concern. A study in 1995, carried out by the Emery University School for Public Health, followed 240,000 women for eight years and found that the risk of ovarian cancer was 72 per cent higher in women given oestrogen.[22] An analysis of nine studies in 1998 also showed a higher risk among HRT users.[23]

Later studies regarding HRT use and ovarian cancer have been conflicting. An analysis of 15 studies in 2000 concluded that oestrogen therapy does not increase risk.[24] However, two years later a major study involving more than 44,000 women was published, and this showed that those who used oestrogen only – particularly for ten or more years – were at significantly increased risk of ovarian cancer, although the increased risk did not seem to apply to those women who used oestrogen and progestogen combined.[25] The jury is still out on this one.

Synthetic versus natural

The danger of using synthetic hormones doesn't just lie in the subtle differences in their chemical structure and effect, but also in the amounts given and their balance with other hormones. The amounts of hormones in a contraceptive pill or conventional HRT treatment can be many times higher than the body would naturally produce. Oestrogen produced by the body is balanced with progesterone but, if this balance is lost, oestrogen unopposed by progesterone becomes a health problem.

The late Dr John Lee pioneered the use of natural progesterone, which is identical to the progesterone produced in the body. Dr Lee treated over 4,000 women with a diagnosis of breast cancer, by giving them normal physiological doses of progesterone in a transdermal cream to counteract unopposed oestrogen. He said, 'Not one has had a recurrence. Of the tens of thousands of women using progesterone for other reasons not one has called to say they have breast cancer following the use of natural progesterone cream. Natural progesterone is completely safe, and beneficial to give to women with breast cancer.'[26] He also recommended eating a plant-based diet, excluding sources of oestrogens from meat and milk, and supplementing antioxidant nutrients, including vitamins C and E.

Testing for progesterone deficiency

If you are postmenopausal, or have menopausal symptoms or other menstrual irregularities, check your oestrogen and progesterone levels with a hormone saliva test (see Resources). If you are oestrogen or progesterone deficient, you can correct this with 'natural progesterone' HRT, although this is only available on prescription in the UK and I recommend that you only do this under the guidance of a doctor familiar with its use (for details, contact the Natural Progesterone Information Society; see Resources). Natural progesterone has none of the associated risks of HRT and your body can make its own oestrogen from progesterone.

The claim that progesterone may protect against breast cancer has been backed up by a large ongoing French study of 54,548 menopausal women, comparing what happens to those who take progesterone in their HRT with those who get progestin. The latest report has found that after eight years those on progestins have a raised risk of breast cancer, while those on progesterone don't.[27] As a result of this research there has been a change in prescribing in France away from progestins.

Other sources of oestrogen

Although men are not exposed to oestrogen compounds from taking the Pill and HRT, their oestrogen load may come from xenoestrogens, oestrogens in food and the small amount of oestradiol produced in a man's body. The fatter the man, the more oestrogen the body makes. These oestrogenic chemicals interfere with the male hormone testosterone, preventing it from being active. Also, older men do produce relatively more 'female' hormones later in life. The net effect is to 'oestrogenise' men, increasing the associated risks of getting prostate cancer and other hormone-related cancers.

Dietary oestrogens

We also take in oestrogens from 'natural' foods. Meat, for example, contains significant amounts of oestrogen, as does dairy produce, although the high levels in these foods may indicate that they aren't perhaps as 'natural' as we would like to believe. Until 2006, much of the meat in the EU came from animals whose feed contained added hormones. They were also fed a high-protein diet, which, combined with the hormones, artificially increased the animal's growth, thus producing more meat and therefore more profit. Wisely, this practice is now banned in the EU, although it still continues in the US. Other changes in farming practice now make it possible to milk cows continuously, even while they are pregnant. During pregnancy, the oestrogen concentrations in cow's milk goes up, but although calves may benefit from this extra oestrogen, we do not.

Meat and dairy products are also a storage site for non-degradable toxins, which accumulate along the food chain. Millions of tons of chemicals, such as non-biodegradable PCBs and DDT, have been released into the environment, contaminating the water and becoming absorbed by plants. Creatures then eat those plants or drink the water, and the contamination is passed on to the next level of the food chain. Traces of these non-degradable chemicals accumulate in the animal's fat, and when we eat meat, fish and fowl the chemicals accumulate in us.

Protection from plant oestrogens

Plants also contain natural, oestrogen-like compounds, known as phytoestrogens. These are found in a wide variety of foods, including soya, citrus fruits, wheat, liquorice, alfalfa, celery and fennel. The richest source is soya and its by-products, such as tofu and soya milk. However, unlike oestrogenic chemicals, such as PCBs, these phytoestrogens are associated with a reduced risk of cancer. A diet high in isoflavonoids, the active ingredient in soya, is associated with halving the risk of breast cancer in animals, and substantially reducing deaths from prostate cancer in men.[28] Even more encouraging are animal studies that show eating a small amount of isoflavones in early infancy results in a 60 per cent reduced risk of breast cancer later in life.[29]

The likely explanation for the protective effect of these oestrogen-like compounds is that they may block the action of other more toxic environmental oestrogens, perhaps by occupying the oestrogen receptor sites on cells. Since they are about a hundred times weaker in their oestrogen effect than xenoestrogens or the body's oestrogen, the net effect of eating foods rich in phytoestrogens seems to be to lower the body's oestrogen load and protect us against harmful hormone-disrupting chemicals.

Avoiding the hormone-disrupters

Why, you may ask, don't we just do the research to identify which chemicals are causing cancer and ban them? According to Dr Samuel Epstein, Professor of Occupational and Environmental Medicine at the School of Public Health, University of Illinois Medical Center, Chicago, much of the money for cancer research has been spent on looking for cures instead of ways to prevent exposure to the carcinogenic chemicals in the environment. It is a problem that must be addressed if we are to wage a genuine and successful war on cancer.[30]

His words are echoed by Professor Louis Guillette from the University of Florida: 'Should we change policy? Should we be upset? I think we should be fundamentally upset. I think we should be screaming in the streets.' Yet, the reality – until large-scale government action is taken – is that it isn't easy to eliminate all these substances because they are all around us: in our food, water, air and household products. There are, however, steps you can take to substantially reduce your own and your family's exposure (see Chapters 20 and 22).

Chemicals that have been shown to have oestrogenic effects

Here are some of the most common chemicals that are found in the environment or continue to be added to the household items we use and the food we eat:

* Alkylphenol: synthetic surfactants used in some detergents and cleaning products
* Atrazine: weedkiller
* 4-Methylbenzylidene camphor (4-MBC): sunscreen lotions
* Brominated flame retardants (BFRs): widely used in furniture
* Butylated hydroxyanisole (BHA): food preservative

cont ▶

- Bisphenol A: found in plastics, plasticisers, epoxy resin and used in container liners
- Dichlorodiphenyldichloroethylene: one of the breakdown products of DDT
- Dichlorodiphenyldichloroethylene dieldrin (DDT): insecticide
- Endosulfan: insecticide
- Erythrosine (E127): food colouring banned in Norway and the US
- Ethinylestradiol (combined oral contraceptive pill): released into the environment as an xenoestrogen
- Heptachlor: insecticide
- Lindane/hexachlorocyclohexane: insecticide
- Metalloestrogens: a class of inorganic xenoestrogens
- Methoxychlor: insecticide
- Nonylphenol and derivatives: industrial surfactants; emulsifiers for emulsion polymerisation; laboratory detergents; pesticides
- Polychlorinated biphenyls (PCBs): in electrical oils, lubricants, adhesives, paints
- Parabens: in lotions
- Phenosulfothiazine: a red dye
- Phthalates: plasticisers; DEHP: plasticiser for PVC
- Propyl gallate (E310): an antioxidant added to foods containing oils and fats

Although some of these chemicals have already been, or are in the process of being, phased out in certain countries, they may still be permitted for certain uses in other parts of the world, and therefore continue to accumulate in the environment and can continue to exert their effects.

Many of the above chemicals not only disrupt hormones but are also carcinogenic (cancer-causing). Pesticides, for example, have been linked to some cancers in certain populations. However, although some hormone-disrupters are carcinogens, not all carcinogens are hormone-disruptors, as you'll see in the next chapter.

CHAPTER 4

Toxic Living – Carcinogens Identified

W e live in a chemical world. Without realising it, we are all exposed to over 10,000 man-made chemicals, an increasing number of which are being identified as carcinogens – that is, potentially cancer-causing. The American Chemical Society has catalogued over ten million man-made chemicals and it is becoming increasingly clear that only a minority of these substances are ever thoroughly tested by independent scientists. There are about 3,500 chemical food additives in addition to chemicals sprayed on our food. We eat, on average, 7.25kg (16lb) in a year – that's if you don't eat organic, additive-free food. There's a similar quantity of chemicals in our homes – in household products, toiletries and detergents – and many more in our environment, contaminating our air, water and food. The US Environmental Protection Agency estimated that in 1991 US industries discharged 3.6 billion pounds of chemicals, including a wide range of carcinogens, into the environment.

Few, if any, of these man-made chemicals have been thoroughly investigated for their individual or combined long-term effects on health. Many chemicals to which we are exposed greatly multiply the toxic effects of others, rendering an otherwise 'safe' exposure unsafe.[31] According to a report published in 1971 by the Massachusetts Institute of Technology (MIT), 'Man's Impact on the Global Environment',

29

'Synergistic effects among chemical pollutants are more often present than not.' For example, the liver damage caused by small amounts of the solvent carbon tetrachloride is greatly increased by a small amount of DDT, and its effects are increased a hundredfold if the common drug phenobarbital is added to the cocktail.

Pollution

Dr Samuel Epstein of the University of Illinois School of Public Health, Chicago, is also Chairman of the Cancer Prevention Coalition. He believes the impact of our massively increased exposure to carcinogenic chemicals is greatly downplayed by the cancer institutions, many of which have links with the pharmaceutical and chemical industries. He believes our failure to reverse the cancer epidemic is a direct consequence of political decisions, which have allowed only a fraction of cancer research to investigate true causes and means of prevention. The majority of funds have instead been channelled towards developing a 'cure', in the form of highly profitable medical treatments. Dr Epstein's research suggests that the prevention spotlight has been solely focused on diet and smoking, while allowing the chemical industries to continue making profits and keep polluting our environment. Prevention has been interpreted to mean early detection, followed by chemotherapy, surgery or radiation, rather than true prevention, which means identifying the cause of cancer and eliminating it in the first place.

There are enough holes in cancer statistics to support Epstein's views. Take lung cancer, for example. Although no one questions that smoking is a major causative factor for lung cancer, this doesn't explain how the incidence in non-smokers has doubled over recent decades and is still on the increase. Pollution, especially exhaust fumes and occupational exposure, is almost certainly playing a role. The National Institute for Occupational Safety and Health has estimated that approximately 11 million workers in the US are exposed to occupational carcinogens. The figure in the UK is likely to be in the order of two million.

Pesticides

One group of workers at risk are farmers, even though they are usually considered to be healthier, tend to smoke less, have generally healthier diets and get plenty of exercise. Yet, in the last several decades, farmers have experienced higher than average rates of leukaemia, non-Hodgkin's lymphoma and cancers of the brain and prostate. In animal studies these cancers have been linked to pesticide exposure. (These are discussed more fully in Chapter 20.)

Low-level radiation

The effect of low-level radiation is a factor that is often downplayed. There is no question that radiation is a carcinogen. Rather, the question is, what level of exposure makes a difference and what part is radiation playing in the cancer equation? Since the time lag between carcinogen exposure and cancer can be 15 to 20 years, the almost worldwide increase in cancer incidence in the mid-1970s could point to the release of a new carcinogen between 1955 and 1960. This coincides with the start of nuclear bomb testing. At the peak of testing, concerns were raised about the level of radioactive strontium-90 in milk. (The consumption of milk, potentially contaminated with strontium-90 from fallout on pastures, tends to be highest among nursing mothers.)

According to Dr Chris Busby of the Low-Level Radiation Campaign, 'Nursing mothers exposed at the peak of testing, who received the largest dose from strontium-90, had the largest increase in breast cancer.' He believes that low-level radiation exposure may also explain why areas in the UK with the highest rainfall, where nuclear fallout would be expected to be higher, first began to show increases in cancer incidence. For example, in 1987 the rate for all cancers was 54 per cent higher in Wales than in East Anglia.

Radiation doesn't just come from man-made sources, such as nuclear power generation and medical X-rays. We are all exposed to radiation from the sun and deep space. There are even naturally occurring radioactive materials in our air, food and water. The average person in the UK receives about 87 per cent of their annual radiation dose from natural sources and 11.5 per cent from medical X-rays. The remaining 1.5 per cent comes from artificial non-medical sources, like nuclear power generation – unless something goes wrong, as it did at Chernobyl. (Radiation is discussed more fully in Chapter 18.)

Mobile phones

Although the birth of the nuclear industry added a new and powerful carcinogen – ionising radiation – the growth of the telecommunications industry exposes all of us to non-ionising radiation from the signals of TVs, radios and, especially, mobile phones; and there are microwave ovens too. While assumed to be harmless, evidence is continuing to grow that exposure to certain types of non-ionising radiation, especially mobile phones, may be adding to our risk of getting cancer. (You'll find more information on mobile phones in Chapter 18.)

Radon gas

One of the largest 'natural' sources of radiation is radon gas; and most human exposure to this occurs indoors. Radon gas is produced by uranium as it decays to become lead. Uranium and radium are found naturally in rocks and soil and also in building materials such as wood, bricks and concrete. When the decaying products (contained in small dust particles) are inhaled, the radioactive particles settle in the lungs and irradiate intensely at close range for many years.

In the open air any radon is mixed and diluted with air and quickly dispersed. Indoors, however, radon particles released from building materials, and from the ground, are inhaled by the occupants.

Surveys carried out in the UK suggest that residents in some parts of the country are at greater risk than others. The south-west seems to be the most affected area, but other local 'hot spots' have been identified. Areas with high levels of granite are the most affected. In some cases the radiation dose from radon accounts for over 50 per cent of total natural radiation. At this level it is suggested that it could be responsible for about 500 deaths from cancer per year. If you live in an area with high levels of granite, contact your local environmental health officer to find out what your radon exposure is likely to be. When radon levels are high it is better to use certain building materials than others. Adequate ventilation under floorboards is also important, to remove the radioactive compounds before they can build up to significant levels.

Food carcinogens

Not all carcinogens are man-made. Many carcinogenic chemicals occur in nature and come to us through natural food. These include psoralens, found in parsnips and celery, mycotoxins from moulds found in cheese, milk and bread, and aflatoxins sometimes found in peanuts. In rare cases, when dietary consumption of a natural carcinogen has been excessive, high incidences of cancer have resulted. This occurred in a rural area of China, where the combination of widespread selenium deficiency due to poor soil levels, and the consumption of a type of pickled cabbage (found to be high in the carcinogen nitrosamine), resulted in a high incidence of oesophageal cancer. This was effectively eliminated by enriching the soil with selenium and staying off the pickled cabbage.

However, it is surely beyond the bounds of possibility to suggest that the massive escalation of cancer over the past 30 years is solely a result of people eating more blue cheese or parsnips. Having said that, it is wise to limit consumption of foods potentially high in natural carcinogens by not eating them daily, and probably not more than two or three times a week.

How we process foods and what we add to them is of greater concern. Some permitted food additives are carcinogenic, depending on the dose and whether they are combined with certain other chemicals. These include butylated hydroxyanisole (E320), which interacts with nitrates to form chemicals known to cause changes in the DNA of cells, and potassium nitrate (E249), which is used as a preservative in cured and canned meats. There are also some permitted food additives that are suspect, such as saccharin, which the International Agency for Research on Cancer believes is possibly carcinogenic to humans.

Acrylamide: the crispy carcinogen

Any fried, burned or browned food – which means the food has been oxidised – adds to the carcinogenic load of the meal. This applies to a lot of fast food such as French fries, charred burgers, fried fish and crispy pizzas – the staple diet of the younger generation. Since 2003 we've known about another cancer-promoting substance, acrylamide, which is generated in foods cooked at high temperatures, with or without fat. Although the safe limit set for acrylamide is 10 parts per billion (ppb), some foods have been found to contain more than 100 times this amount! Fast-food-chain chips, crisps, taco shells and breakfast cereals are the worst. Potato chips (crisps) averaged 1,250 and Pringles 1,480. However, even home-cooked chips were found to be high.

A recent review of research into acrylamides by the European Food Safety Authority concludes that the risk still remains. A recent study from the Netherlands reported that increased dietary intakes of acrylamide could raise the risk of kidney cancer by 59 per cent.[32] Five thousand participants, aged between 55 and 69, took part in the research, one of a number of studies showing significant increases in kidney cancer risk, but no change in prostate or bladder cancer risk.

Acrylamide is produced by frying, barbecuing, baking and even microwaving. So, the honest answer is that anything crispy, browned or burned, or cooked or processed using high heat, may be bad for you. The bottom line is to eat more raw foods and steam-fry (page 284) or boil food, rather than use high-heat cooking.

As you will have seen, there is no doubt that a significant contributor to cancer is our increased exposure to carcinogens. Some of these act as oxidants and some as hormone-disrupters, while others damage genes and alter cell behaviour. We can avoid or, at least, substantially reduce our exposure to many of them. I'll show you how in Chapter 22.

CHAPTER 5

In the Genes?

Cancer is a gene-related disease. The changes that occur in cells seem to be the direct result of mutations or changes to genetic instructions. The genes are like the software that tells the molecules in your body – the hardware components – how to organise themselves. Genes interact with the environment: when that interaction goes seriously wrong, cancer results. Genes and environment are interdependent, like the chicken and the egg.

Some scientists argue that genes play a more significant role in cancer than environmental factors, such as food, chemical carcinogens and smoking. But if cancer is primarily genetic, why did it emerge as a major cause of death only with industrialisation? There are two possible answers. One is that there have always been people who were genetically predisposed to cancer but that the gene is only 'activated' by exposure to carcinogens. The other is that genetic predisposition to cancer plays a very small part in the overall picture. Both are true.

Carcinogens affect defective genes

Some people carry defective genes that cause cells to misbehave. These are called oncogenes. Two oncogenes that increase the risk of breast cancer are BRCA1 and BRCA2, estimated to be carried by one in 200 women. A small percentage of women with breast cancer have, as a contributory factor, the inheritance of such oncogenes.

It is, however, unlikely that just having the oncogene is enough to trigger breast cancer. One survey of women with the BRCA1 gene found that they were actually no more likely to die of the cancer than women with the disease who did not have this gene. The researchers suggested that, by making certain dietary and lifestyle choices, women carrying the gene could substantially reduce their risk of developing cancer.[33] This is because most oncogenes release their disruptive instructions only when activated by carcinogens.

To illustrate how this works, consider the example of the chemical nonylphenol found in paints, detergents, lubricating oils, toiletries, spermicidal foams, agrochemicals and many other products.

Inside our cells are receptors for hormones (see the illustration below). The hormone fits like a 'key' into the receptor 'lock'. If the key fits, specific genes are activated, starting a particular biological

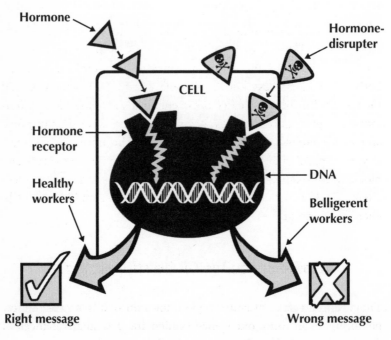

How hormones and chemicals affect genes

programme. 'Fake' hormones – or substances that can act like hormones (such as nonylphenols) – are like wonky keys. They can activate genes, but not necessarily the right ones, perhaps triggering an oncogene; so that they change the way our biology works. Nonylphenol is known as an 'oestrogen-mimicker' and, like oestrogen itself, it can change the programming of the body's biochemistry, depending on how much there is in the body and what else the cells are exposed to.

Nutrition can provide a solution

The soya bean also contains an oestrogen-like molecule. However, in this case, it seems to bind to oestrogen receptors and stop harmful substances like nonylphenols from perverting the course of genetic expression. So, if anything, it helps to balance hormones; whereas substances like nonylphenols – fortunately now banned in the EU – disturb normal hormone balance.

These oestrogen-mimickers are thought to disrupt the body's biochemistry because of their ability to lock onto hormone receptor sites. This alters the ability of genes to communicate with the body's cells (a process known as gene expression), which is vital for our health. In some cases these chemicals actually block a hormone receptor; in other cases they act as if they were the hormone; and in yet other cases they simply disrupt the hormone message. If you think of this hormone–hormone receptor–gene expression–biochemical response sequence as 'communication', what these chemicals do is turn the sound up or down and scramble your cells' chemical messages.

Could cancer genes be suppressed?

This information is, of course, good news, in that it means the few people who do carry oncogenes (which increase their chances of developing cancer) can counteract this by avoiding carcinogens and increasing their intake of cancer-protective nutrients to suppress the activation of these genes. Such testing, both to determine whether a person has inherited certain oncogenes and whether or not those oncogenes have been activated, is available in the UK (see Resources). Being able to test for cancer genes, and finding out whether or not those genes are active, is helpful, because it will enable more specific and personalised prevention strategies to be developed.[34] In his pioneering book *Genetic Nutritioneering*, biochemist Dr Jeffrey Bland explains how such genetic profiling is helping scientists develop more effective cancer-prevention strategies.

For example, there is a strain of mice predisposed to develop skin cancer due to an inherited gene, provided they are exposed to UVB radiation. However, if their diet includes the herb milk thistle, a rich source of the antioxidant silymarin, they don't develop skin cancer.[35] In this case UVB radiation is the triggering carcinogen and silymarin the antidote.

Gene therapy

Of course, the biotech industry have other plans in mind, as their solution is to manipulate the defective gene with gene therapy. This, of course, carries unknown risks and is certainly more expensive than nutrition solutions.

A great example of this dilemma was the discovery by researchers at the Imperial Cancer Research Fund of a specific oncogene in mice that resulted in them being unable to detoxify smoke. These genetically susceptible mice had a higher risk of developing cancer because the gene in question is partially responsible for making the antioxidant enzyme glutathione transferase. According to newspaper reports, a gene pill for people with this defective gene may be available in a few years. Yet the body's ability to make more glutathione transferase is dependent on the protein glutathione and the mineral selenium – which are both widely deficient among British people. An alternative to gene manipulation would be to ensure an optimal intake of these nutrients.

The role of our environment

One major study looked at the medical records of 44,788 pairs of identical twins – siblings with the same genes – and found the risk of both getting any one of 28 different kinds of cancer was very small: between 11 and 18 per cent. The researchers concluded that 'the overwhelming contributor to the causation of cancer was the environment',[36] in other words, what you eat and how you live.

As we have seen, genetic predisposition to cancer plays a small role in the major cancers of the 21st century. In any event, they are likely to require activation by avoidable carcinogens and can be effectively left 'dormant' by ensuring optimal intakes of key nutrients. Part 4 explains exactly how to do this.

CHAPTER 6

How Strong Are Your Immune Defences?

As well as being a disease of the genes, cancer is an immune disease. It is the immune system's job to hunt around the body, identify pre-cancerous cells and put them out of action. This happens in each of us every single day.

However, if a person's immune defences are weak, pre-cancerous cells can multiply, possibly resulting in some form of cancer. An example of this is HIV infection. The virus responsible for AIDS selectively destroys immune cells, leaving the body without its usual defences. The incidence of one type of cancer, Karposi's sarcoma, is consequently high in people with AIDS.

Until recently, the accepted method of dealing with immune-related diseases was always to kill the invader – be it a bacteria, virus or cancer cell. This approach is, however, becoming less popular because of the high cost of combative drugs.

An alternative strategy is to support the body's own immune system. A new class of cancer drug works on this basis: monoclonal antibodies, for example, target cancer cells for non-Hodgkin's lymphoma, tagging them so that the body's own immune system sees them clearly and moves in for the kill.

A natural boost

You can also boost your immune system naturally. The immune system depends on a whole host of nutrients, and supplementing these has been proven to enhance immunity. The approach of also boosting immunity, rather than just focusing on killing the invader, is likely to prove much more effective. Our immune systems are showing signs that they may be weakening generally, as the rise in infections shows. After all, we achieved vast improvements in sanitation in the Western world in the 20th century, yet, in the 20 years since 1989, the medical profession has doled out billions of antibiotic, anti-viral and anti-fungal medicines. If the invader-killing approach was working you'd expect fewer overall deaths from infections. In fact exactly the opposite has occurred.

In both the US and the UK the number of infections of all kinds has increased dramatically. A survey of all deaths in the US between 1980 and 1992 revealed an alarming 58 per cent rise in deaths from infectious diseases.[37] A six-fold increase occurred in those between the ages of 25 and 44. This is only partly due to the increased number of deaths from HIV infection. Deaths from respiratory infections increased by 20 per cent. And the same trends can be seen in Britain.[38]

According to Spence Galbraith, former director of the Communicable Diseases Surveillance Centre,[39] 'The rate of change of human infection appears to be increasing. It is now recognised that it can only be a matter of time until the next microbial menace to our species emerges amongst us.' Swine flu is a case in point. Coupled with the increased risk of cancer, this global trend suggests that our immune defences aren't as strong as they should be.

How does your immune system work?

Before discussing ways of boosting the immune system, we need a brief description of the 'immune army' and its role.

Immunological battles can occur anywhere in the body – against invading organisms or against our own rebellious cells (as in cancer). To fight off these enemies, we have a fixed defence framework, called the lymphatic system (shown in the illustration below), which works alongside other parts of the body, such as the bone marrow, thymus and spleen. The complex workings of the immune system are largely controlled by the pituitary and adrenal glands.

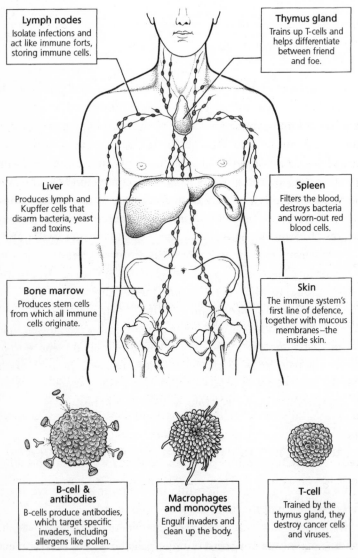

Lymph nodes
Isolate infections and act like immune forts, storing immune cells.

Thymus gland
Trains up T-cells and helps differentiate between friend and foe.

Liver
Produces lymph and Kupffer cells that disarm bacteria, yeast and toxins.

Spleen
Filters the blood, destroys bacteria and worn-out red blood cells.

Bone marrow
Produces stem cells from which all immune cells originate.

Skin
The immune system's first line of defence, together with mucous membranes – the inside skin.

B-cell & antibodies
B-cells produce antibodies, which target specific invaders, including allergens like pollen.

Macrophages and monocytes
Engulf invaders and clean up the body.

T-cell
Trained by the thymus gland, they destroy cancer cells and viruses.

The immune system

What happens in the blood?

The blood plays a vital role in our defences. Made up of a clear yellow fluid (called plasma) and blood cells, which are suspended in the fluid, our blood provides us with a mobile fighting force of white blood cells (or leukocytes), which are our main immune soldiers. When our systems are in good working order, we can produce around 2,000 new immune cells every second. These white blood cells are present in lymph as well as in the blood.

There are three main types of white blood cell: granulocytes, monocytes and lymphocytes.

Granulocytes and monocytes Most of the granulocytes are phagocytic (which means that they gobble up any foreign bacteria they come across). Monocytes or macrophages perform a crucial 'cleaning' role, eating anything that is rubbish or foreign, and cleaning our blood, tissues and lymph. They are also major 'armament factories', capable of making at least 40 different enzymes and immune proteins needed to destroy enemies.

Lymphocytes are the most competent and versatile group of cells for getting rid of 'unwanted guests'. Some of them have a memory system, so that they recognise a bug that has previously attacked the body, and thus trigger the immune system to fight back straight away. Lymphocytes also have a special method of dividing rapidly when they are under attack, producing reinforcements almost immediately. This rapid division is very nutrient-dependent; for example, vitamin C levels are crucial. The three types of lymphocytes are T-cells, B-cells and natural killer (NK) cells. The natural killer cells are particularly important, as they seek and destroy cancer cells.

T-cells regulate the immune system and decide whether it should go into battle or withdraw. They provide the initial response to viruses and tumour cells. But it takes three or four days after recognition of these for the T-cells to get their act together and attack.

B-cells deal mainly with bacteria and viruses that have been encountered before. A B-cell takes an invading bug into the tissues, where

43

it ascertains its exact size and shape. It then tailor-makes a protein 'straitjacket' (called an antibody) that will fit that bug and no other. Finally, it gets a production line going to manufacture thousands more of these antibodies, which are released back into the body. The antibodies seek out their targets like mini guided missiles and attach themselves to the bacteria. The invader becomes harmless and is held until the macrophages come along to devour it.

Boosting your immune system

The idea that people may be prone to cancer partly because of immune deficiency is largely uncharted territory as far as cancer research is concerned. However, we do know which nutrients boost immunity (the ones that tend to be low in those who succumb to cancer) and which nutrients aid recovery. This whole area of optimum nutrition and its role in boosting immunity and preventing cancer is covered in detail in Part 2. But, at this stage, we can say that deficiencies in the following nutrients increase a person's risk of developing this disease (for dosage levels see Chapter 34):

Vitamin A is especially important because it helps to maintain the integrity of the digestive tract, lungs and all cell membranes, preventing foreign agents from entering the body, and preventing viruses from entering cells. In addition, vitamin A and beta-carotene (its vegetable form) are potent antioxidants. Many foreign agents produce free oxidising radicals (oxidants) as part of their defence system. Macrophages also produce free radicals to destroy invaders. A high intake of antioxidant nutrients helps to protect immune cells from these harmful weapons.

Vitamins B_5, B_6, B_{12} and folic acid are all important to the immune system. The production of antibodies and the function of T-lymphocytes depend on B_6, so it is essential when fighting cancer cells. Vitamin B_{12} and folic acid are also important for the same reasons. Pantothenic acid (B_5) helps macrophages and NK cells do their job, while deficiency is associated with inhibition of T-cell and antibody production.

Vitamin C is unquestionably the most vital immune-boosting nutrient, with more than a dozen proven immune-boosting roles (see Chapter 26) – including production of T-cells, which destroy cancer cells.

Vitamin E is another important all-rounder. It improves B- and T-cell function and is a powerful antioxidant. Its immune-boosting properties increase when given in conjunction with selenium.

Selenium, manganese, copper and zinc are all involved in anti-oxidation and have all been shown to enhance immunity. Of these, selenium and zinc are the most important. Zinc is critical for immune cell production and the function of B- and T-cells, which tag and destroy cancer. Selenium boosts immunity and works synergistically with vitamin E.

Calcium is needed for the immune cells to produce enzymes that will knock out cancer cells.

Cysteine is very important for the immune system, mainly because it is turned into glutathione (an essential antioxidant) in the body. When we are exposed to toxins, provided there is sufficient cysteine present, the body can increase its levels of glutathione to detoxify them. High cysteine levels are associated with longevity and reduced cancer risk. In chronic infections such as AIDS, depletion of glutathione is a major concern. Glutathione is vital for macrophages to make the chemicals they need to kill invaders, for lymphocyte production and for red-blood-cell membranes. It is also critical for the function of NK cells. Good sources of cysteine are meat, eggs, soya, quinoa (a grain that cooks like rice), seeds, nuts, onions and garlic. It can be supplemented as N-acetyl-cysteine.

Other antioxidants

There are many other important antioxidants not classified as essential vitamins, minerals or amino acids. Some, however, have a major role in boosting the immune system and protecting against cancer.

Of particular importance are anthocyanidins, especially resveratrol, which give berries, grapes and beetroot their red/blue colour; co-enzyme Q_{10} which helps 'recycle' (retain for further use) vitamin E and protects cells from harmful oxidants; lipoic acid, which helps recycle vitamin C; and carotenoids, substances related to beta-carotene such as lutein and lycopene, especially rich in cooked tomatoes. Similar to vitamin E (called tocopherol) are tocotrienols, also found in seeds and nuts. As more and more active chemicals are found in natural foods, it is becoming increasingly clear that food is the best medicine of all.

Although some people have attributed their recovery from cancer to dietary changes, nutritional therapy is never claimed to 'cure' cancer. Rather, it can create the best possible conditions within the body for its own anti-cancer mechanisms (primarily the immune system) to restore health. In a healthy individual, cancer is kept at bay by the immune system, which can be very powerful, and is responsible for the natural remissions that can occur in this disease.

It is also possible to stimulate the immune system by means of the appropriate mental attitude (see Chapter 23). Conversely, emotional factors (see Chapter 9), such as long-term depression or grief, also suppress the immune system and thus weaken a person's defence against cancer and other diseases.

Viruses and cancer

Some rather rare viruses can trigger cancer, although they don't appear to do it on their own; for example, Karposi's sarcoma (a cancer that AIDS patients are more likely to develop) is probably not so much caused by the HIV virus itself but, rather, results from the HIV virus weakening a person's immune system. The papilloma virus is implicated in the majority of cases of cervical cancer – a condition that is also more prevalent among women with many sexual partners. It is not, however, the only cause of the disease. A few other rare viral infections have been linked to rare types of cancer, but again only as part of a larger causative picture. Suffice to say that, in the vast majority of cancers, there is no evidence to suggest that viruses are responsible. In any event, following the advice in this book will help to strengthen your immune system and, in so doing, minimise the harmful effects of viruses.

CHAPTER 7

Why Your Liver is Your Best Friend

One of your key lines of defence is your body's ability to detoxify harmful chemicals. From a chemical perspective, much of what goes on in the body involves substances being broken down, built up and turned from one thing into another. A good 80 per cent of this work involves detoxifying potentially harmful substances. This is largely done by the liver, which represents a clearing house able to recognise millions of potentially harmful chemicals and transform them into something harmless or prepare them for elimination. This often means turning a fat-based toxin into something water-soluble that can be eliminated in the urine. The liver is the chemical 'brain' of the body: recycling, regenerating and detoxifying in order to maintain your health. In this chapter, I'll explain why the liver is such a vital part of the immune system and why your liver really is your best friend.

Packing up and throwing away the toxins

Not only do we take in many toxic chemicals, but the body also produces its own. As we process food – turning it into energy or building materials – toxic substances are produced and processed, ready for elimination. This ability to detoxify gives us built-in protection from a certain degree of exposure to toxic substances. It probably explains why mankind has been able to eat natural foods, with their inherent levels of toxic substances, without developing cancer. However, the more toxic substances we are exposed to, the harder the body has to work at detoxifying.

One of the main ways the body neutralises harmful chemicals and carcinogens is to 'package' them ready for export. By sticking harmless molecules onto poisons (in a process called 'conjugation') toxins can be eliminated from the body without doing damage. Of all the building activity that goes on in the body, no less than two-thirds is spent 'conjugating' toxins ready for elimination.

A healthy liver is essential

If your liver detoxification potential is compromised, either as a result of over-exposure to toxins (the most common being excess alcohol and sugar) or due to an underlying imbalance, this makes you more sensitive to carcinogens. Indeed, one of the key genes thought to predispose a person to cancer is responsible for making a key detoxifying enzyme called glutathione transferase.

In mice, if you knock out this gene – thus lowering the body's levels of this enzyme – and then expose the subjects to cigarette smoke, they will rapidly develop lung cancer. While the geneticists scramble to produce a treatment to correct a defective gene, we can already improve the body's levels of glutathione transferase simply by ensuring an adequate intake of glutathione (or its precursor, N-acetyl-cysteine) and selenium, which helps the enzyme to work.

Of course, glutathione transferase is only one of many enzymes involved in detoxification. The five main chemical pathways by which the body detoxifies harmful substances are shown in the illustration How the liver detoxifies, on page 51. As you will see later, these are completely dependent on a wide range of nutrients, including vitamins, minerals, amino acids and 'phytonutrients' found in foods such as garlic or cruciferous vegetables like broccoli.

Liver detoxification is a two-step dance

The ability of the liver to detoxify has two distinct phases. You can think of Phase 1 as the preparation phase, where toxins are acted on by a series of enzymes (called P450). This phase converts toxins into a form that can be disarmed. Often, however, this process itself can produce unwanted by-products or 'reactive intermediates' such as free radicals that could actually produce even more toxins. To avoid this Phase-1 side effect there is a whole series of nutrients, particularly antioxidants, that you need to support your liver.

Detox nutrients – the Phase-1 heroes

The first phase of liver detoxification (the grey area above the line in the illustration opposite), which involves the P450 family of enzymes, mainly depends on having a great supply of antioxidant nutrients. These include:

- Glutathione and/or N-acetyl-cysteine[40] – found in onions and garlic
- Coenzyme Q_{10}[41] – found in oily fish, spinach, raw seeds and nuts
- Vitamin C[42] – found in broccoli, peppers, citrus fruit and berries
- Vitamin E[43] – found in raw seeds, nuts and fish
- Selenium[44] – found in raw seeds, nuts and fish
- Beta-carotene[45] – found in carrots, peaches, watermelon, sweet potato and butternut squash

Working together

These antioxidants are team players. You need all of them for your detox potential to be optimum. You may have seen newspaper headlines claiming that some recent research shows antioxidants confer no benefits. This is because the antioxidants have been tested alone, whereas in fact they work best in synergy with other antioxidants; for example, in one study, beta-carotene given on its own to smokers

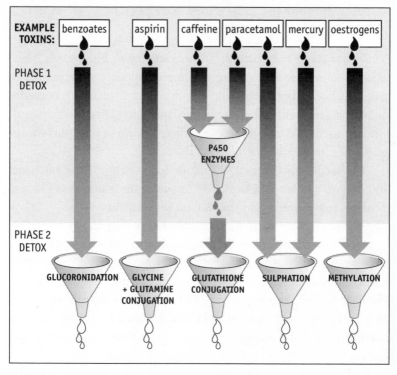

EXAMPLE TOXINS: benzoates | aspirin | caffeine | paracetamol | mercury | oestrogens

PHASE 1 DETOX

P450 ENZYMES

PHASE 2 DETOX

GLUCORONIDATION | GLYCINE + GLUTAMINE CONJUGATION | GLUTATHIONE CONJUGATION | SULPHATION | METHYLATION

How the liver detoxifies

had slightly increased their risk of cancer, but it reduced the risk if given in combination with other antioxidants.[46] Vitamin E generally reduces your risk of heart disease as part of a multivitamin, but not if you take a large amount on its own with cholesterol-lowering statin drugs.[47] This is because cholesterol-lowering statin drugs knock out coenzyme Q_{10} (CoQ_{10}), another natural antioxidant, which is vital for 'reloading' vitamin E to detoxify another oxidant. Without enough CoQ_{10} vitamin E becomes an oxidant – a toxin in its own right. (See illustration The synergistic action of nutrients in disarming a free radical, on page 14, to see how antioxidants work together.)

There are also various phytonutrients (substances from plants that have nutritional value) and herbs that can help. These include:

DIM (di-indolylmethane) A substance in cruciferous vegetables, such as broccoli, that helps detoxify excess oestrogens and hormone-disrupting chemicals such as PCBs and dioxins, as well as some herbicides and pesticides.[48]

Bioflavonoids[49] These include anthocyanidins in blueberries,[50] resveratrol in red grapes,[51] quercetin in red onions,[52] polyphenols in green tea[53] and the herb milk thistle, which contains a powerful detoxifying nutrient called silymarin that protects liver cells from all kinds of toxins.[54] Most of these have been shown to have anti-cancer properties, especially in protecting the liver.[55]

The recipes in Chapter 33 include foods rich in these nutrients and, as you will see in Chapter 34, many of these nutrients are also available in concentrated form as food supplements.

At Phase 2 these reactive intermediates are rendered non-toxic. This happens by enzymes linking the toxin to another molecule that makes it more water-soluble and less toxic. This is the process called 'conjugation' where the toxin is 'married' to a key detoxifying nutrient. For example, the illustration on page 51 shows you how your body detoxifies paracetamol (acetaminophen), aspirin and caffeine. (You'll see on page 54 how a simple urine test that involves taking a measured amount of caffeine, paracetamol and aspirin can determine your liver's detox capacity.)

The body processes toxins in the liver using different chemical pathways. These different pathways (for example, glutathione conjugation or sulphation) need different nutrients to work properly.

Detox nutrients – the Phase-2 heroes

In Phase 2 the liver detoxifies substances by attaching things on to them so that they are ready to be eliminated from the body in the process called conjugation described above. There are five main ways in which the liver detoxifies.

Glucoronidation is possibly the most important detox pathway of all, dependent on calcium-d-glucarate, which is found in apples, Brussels sprouts, broccoli, cabbage and beansprouts.[56]

Glycine and glutamine conjugation These are amino acids found in root vegetables and sprouts.

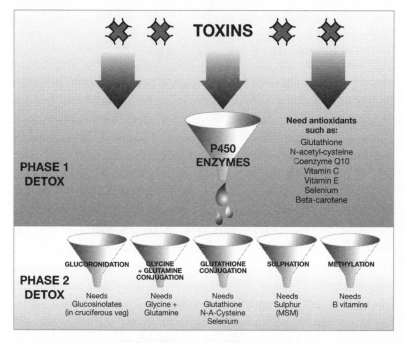

The key nutrients your liver needs

Your liver cleans up and detoxifies the blood in two stages. Phase 1 involves enzymes dependent on antioxidant nutrients. Phase 2 requires certain amino acids, vitamins, minerals and antioxidants. Optimising your intake of these nutrients supports 100 per cent healthy liver function.

Glutathione conjugation This pathway depends on a good supply of glutathione, an amino-acid complex made from three amino acids (glycine, cysteine and glutamic acid). Onions and garlic are a good source. Root vegetables are also rich in glycine. The mineral selenium also helps glutathione to work. Glutathione can be made in the body from N-acetyl-cysteine (NAC), a substance that is usually given in cases of paracetamol overdose to trigger the liver into detoxifying.[57] Glutathione is recycled by anthocyanidins in berries as well as alpha lipoic acid,[58] so supplementing with both anthocyanidins (blueberries are particularly rich in these) and glutathione plus alpha lipoic acid, is much more powerful. Glutathione is one of the most potent anti-cancer nutrients.

Sulphation depends on the sulphur-containing amino acids, found in onions, garlic and eggs. There's a type of sulphur you can supplement, called MSM, which helps the body detoxify.

Methylation This is a key detoxifying process that depends on B vitamins, especially folic acid (in greens and beans), vitamin B_{12} (animal source only), B_6, as well as tri-methyl-glycine (TMG), once again found in root vegetables. As you'll see in Chapter 8, being good at methylation is a key to protecting yourself from cancer.

How to find out if your liver is firing on all cylinders

There is a simple test that you can do to find out if your liver function is up to scratch. It measures two enzymes called AST and ALT. Your GP can run this test or, alternatively, you can do it yourself with a home-test kit called LiverCheck (see www.yorktest.com). Although this test will tell you whether you have liver dysfunction or not, it won't tell you exactly which pathways or processes need your attention.

To find this out there's another test called the Liver Detoxification Capacity Profile, which involves a test kit that you order by post. It's best to do this through a nutritional therapist who can explain the results and work out what you need to do.

The test involves you swallowing a measured amount of caffeine, paracetamol and aspirin in a pill. You then collect your urine sample (the kit provides a container) and you'll get a report that looks like the illustration on the facing page.

Looking at the profile report

As I described earlier, Phase 1 is where toxins are worked on by P450 enzymes to prepare them for Phase 2. This person's Phase 1 is just within normal range but is verging on sluggish, so they would benefit from the vitamins and minerals that would help boost Phase-1 detoxification (see page 50).

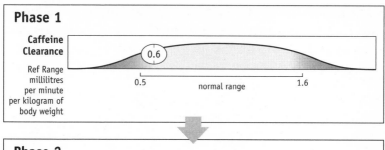

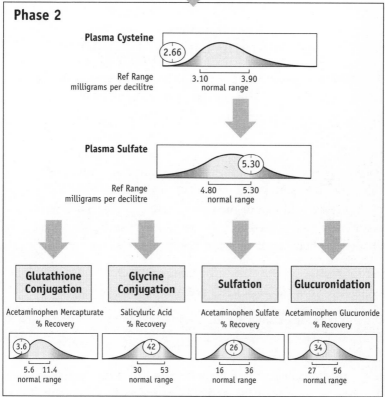

A typical detox capacity profile report

Phase 2 is where toxins from Phase 1 are 'conjugated' to make them non-toxic. This person has extremely low plasma cysteine, which is used to make glutathione for glutathione conjugation. Consequently, you can see that glutathione conjugation is also below normal range. They would benefit from eating more onions and garlic, nuts and seeds for selenium (to help manufacture the glutathione enzymes) and supplementing NAC or glutathione (as well as eating berries to improve their utilisation). This person's plasma sulphate is high, and consequently sulphation is working normally. Glycine conjugation and glucuronidation are similarly normal.

If you'd like to be guided by tests like this, see Resources to order a test kit. It gives you the option to retest yourself to see how you've improved your liver detox function.

Maintaining the right balance

The final key factor in supporting the detoxification pathways is maintaining the right acid–alkaline balance in the body. The correct balance is one that is not too acid. When foods are metabolised by the body, a residue is left that can alter the body's acidity and alkalinity. Depending on the chemical composition of the metabolised foods ('ash') the food is called acid-forming or alkaline-forming. However, this is not the same as the immediate acidity of a food. Oranges, for example, are acid due to their citric acid content, but citric acid is completely metabolised and the net effect of eating an orange is to alkalise the body, so oranges are classified as alkaline-forming.

What should we be aiming for?

Protein is made of amino acids, and is acid-forming. Foods such as fruits and vegetables are high in potassium and magnesium. These foods, as well as seeds and nuts, are high in calcium. They have a more alkaline effect on the body because the minerals they contain are alkaline. Your body can and does compensate, keeping the blood at the right pH; however, excessively high acid-forming diets are not good for you. By eating plenty of fresh fruit and vegetables on a daily basis, you will ensure that your diet is more alkaline-forming. Roughly 80 per cent of our diet should come from alkaline-forming foods, and 20 per cent from acid-forming foods. The table opposite shows which foods are which. This is not a comprehensive list of all foods because not all foods have been analysed, but it gives you a pretty good idea.[59]

Acid, neutral and alkaline foods

High acid	Medium acid	Neutral	Medium alkaline	High alkaline
	Brazil nuts			Almonds
	Walnuts			Coconut
Edam	Cheddar cheese	Butter		Milk
Eggs	Stilton cheese	Margarine		
			Avocados	
Mayonnaise			Beetroot	Beans
		Coffee	Carrots	Cabbage
Fish	Herrings	Tea	Potatoes	Celery
Shellfish	Mackerel	Sugar	Spinach	Lentils
				Lettuce
Bacon	Rye			Mushrooms
Beef	Oats			Onions
Chicken	Wheat			Root vegetables
Liver	Rice			Tomatoes
Lamb			Dried fruit	
Veal	Plums		Rhubarb	Apricots
	Cranberries			Apples
	Olives			Bananas
				Berries
				Cherries
				Figs
				Grapefruit
				Grapes
				Lemons
				Melons
				Oranges
				Peaches
				Pears
				Raspberries
				Tangerines
				Prunes

Acid ⟵   ⟶ Alkaline

Heal your digestive tract – and take a load off your liver

Whereas your liver does most of the detoxing, effectively filtering and cleansing the blood of toxic material, your digestive tract is the gateway between the food you eat and your bloodstream. It is actually the first line of detoxification, with the gut bacteria helping to neutralise unwanted microorganisms, while the digestive enzymes help to break down food into the right pieces to enter your body.

The digestive tract, which represents a surface area the size of a tennis court, can be healthy or unhealthy. If it is unhealthy it will become more permeable, which means that larger food particles not on the 'guest list', so to speak, will get into the bloodstream; this is called leaky gut syndrome. Whole food proteins, rather than their constituent amino acids, will gatecrash into your bloodstream, and your body's policemen – antibodies – will attack, forming what is known as an 'immune complex'. This is then treated by the body as a toxin and forms the basis of most food allergies and sensitivities, which have a detrimental effect on our overall health.

So, one immediate way to help detox your body is to improve the integrity of your digestive tract. You can actually test the 'intestinal permeability' of your digestive tract (see page 386), but for now I'm going to recommend something much simpler: a teaspoon of glutamine powder.

The G factor – your gut's best friend

Although most of your body's organs are fuelled by glucose, your digestive tract is a different story. It's a vast and highly active interface between your body and the outside world, and it needs a lot of fuel to work properly day in and day out. It runs on an amino acid called glutamine – thus sparing the glucose from your food for your brain, heart and liver.

Not only does glutamine power your gut, it heals it as well. It can also neutralise over-acidity. The cells that make up the inner lining of your digestive tract replace themselves every four days and are your most critical line of defence against developing food allergies or getting infections. As your 'inner skin', your gut takes lots of hits: alcohol, non-steroidal anti-inflammatory drug painkillers (NSAIDs) such as aspirin or ibuprofen, antibiotics, coffee and fried food are some common gastrointestinal irritants. In Japan, people taking NSAIDs for pain and inflammation are also often instructed to take 2,000mg of glutamine 30 minutes beforehand to prevent stomach bleeding and ulceration.

Heal the gut

Many people suffer from digestive problems and possibly food allergies. Our top tip (besides avoiding allergenic foods) is to take glutamine, together with digestive enzymes and a probiotic supplement (see Resources, page 381). Glutamine is the preferred food of the cells lining the intestine, so I recommend one or two heaped teaspoons (that's 4,000 to 8,000mg) of glutamine powder taken last thing at night, diluted in a glass of water. This will help your gut to heal and rejuvenate. Glutamine depletion is extremely common in people with cancer.

Under normal circumstances, most of the glutamine in your food gets used up as fuel for your gastrointestinal tract. However, about 5 per cent of it is used to make glutathione, the liver's most powerful antioxidant.

Build up your glutathione levels from food

Glutathione, as we saw earlier, is made from three amino acids: glycine, cysteine and glutamic acid or glutamine. Think of them as the Three Musketeers. Glutamine is found in protein foods such as beans, fish, chicken and eggs, as well as in vegetables such as cabbage, spinach, beetroot and tomatoes. Cysteine is a sulphur-containing amino acid found in onions, garlic and eggs. And glycine is found plentifully in root vegetables. By getting more of each of these amino acids, you are providing yourself with the building blocks for glutathione, which boosts your liver and protects every single cell in your body from the dangerous oxidising chemicals: free radicals. It is certainly one of the most important anti-cancer nutrients. Upping your glutathione levels can be achieved by eating these foods and by supplementing glutathione and/or its precursors, N-acetyl-cysteine (NAC) and glutamine.

So that's the end of your whistle-stop tour of how your body detoxifies. If you want to dig deeper, and tune up your liver, read my book *9-Day Liver Detox*, co-authored with Fiona McDonald Joyce, which gives daily menus and recipes for you to follow.

CHAPTER 8

The Homocysteine Connection

I n recent years I've been explaining why the homocysteine level in your blood is your greatest single health statistic. Your homocysteine level is a better indicator of whether you will live a long and healthy life, or die young, than your blood pressure, your cholesterol level, or even your weight. In this chapter I will explain why your homocysteine level is linked to the cancer process and predicts your risk, and I will show you how to reduce your risk using simple dietary and lifestyle changes.

What is homocysteine?

Homocysteine is a type of protein produced in the body from the amino acid methionine, which is found in normal dietary protein. Ideally it should be present in very low quantities in the blood. Homocysteine in itself isn't bad news, as your body naturally turns it into one of two beneficial substances, glutathione and SAMe (s-adenosyl methione), providing there are enough B vitamins and other nutrients in the body to handle it. Glutathione, as I explained in Chapters 2, 6 and 7, is the body's most important antioxidant and vital for your immunity and liver function. SAMe, an amino acid, is a very important type of

61

'intelligent' nutrient for both brain and body, participating in over 40 essential biochemical reactions. In the illustration opposite you will see that the enzymes that turn homocysteine into either glutathione or SAMe require B vitamins and other vital nutrients. So, if you don't have an optimal amount of these nutrients in your diet, homocysteine can accumulate, increasing your risk of over 50 diseases, including certain cancers. The good news is that, with the right nutrients, this important risk factor can be reversed.

Methylation: keeping your body working efficiently

So why does the body make homocysteine and what does a high level tell us? It's all to do with a fundamental process upon which your life depends. It's called methylation, and it happens over a billion times a second. Every second there are hundreds of thousands of adjustments made in your body to keep you healthy and alive; for example, when your body is under stress, the body makes more adrenalin to keep you going. When you go to bed, the body releases melatonin to help you sleep. When you've got a cold or flu the body makes more glutathione, which turns your immune cells into cold-busting warriors. It's like one big dance, with biochemicals in your body passing 'methyl groups' (made of one carbon and three hydrogen atoms) from one partner to another.

These methyl groups are also being continually added to and subtracted from our DNA. When not enough methylation is going on, our DNA cannot properly repair itself, which puts us at higher risk of cancer. However, with cancer it is important to realise that problems can also arise when there is too much methylation.[60] Although this situation is rarer, it is very important to be tested first (see page 71) before you consider supplementing high doses of these nutrients.

We all make homocysteine from eating protein. Normally, it is quickly turned into SAMe or glutathione – two essential and health-promoting substances in the body. But if you lack enough of certain nutrients, such as B_2, B_6, B_{12}, folic acid, zinc or tri-methyl-glycine (TMG), you may end up accumulating toxic homocysteine.

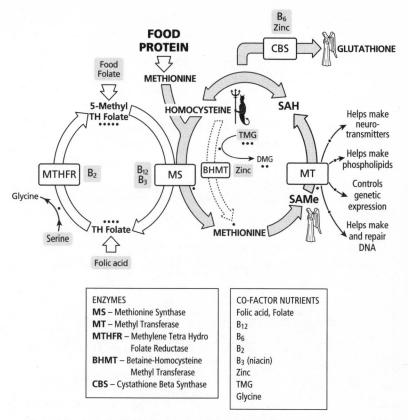

The homocysteine pathway

How to cut your cancer risk by a third

So, how is homocysteine linked to cancer? Cancer is triggered in large part by damage to DNA, as explained in Chapter 1, and having a high homocysteine level means your DNA is more vulnerable to damage, and poorly repaired once damaged. At the other end of the scale, homocysteine levels have been found to be a good indicator of whether cancer therapies are working. The homocysteine level rises when tumours grow, and falls when they shrink. Low homocysteine is likely

cont ▶

63

to reduce your risk of cancer by a third, as shown by a comprehensive research study at the University of Bergen in Norway, published in 2001 in the *American Journal of Clinical Nutrition*.[61] The study showed that, with every five-point decrease in your homocysteine level (H score), you will gain:

* A 26 per cent reduced risk of death from cancer
* A 49 per cent reduced risk of death from all causes
* A 50 per cent reduced risk of cardiovascular death (such as heart attacks and sudden death)
* A 104 per cent reduced risk of death from any causes other than cancer or heart disease.

They measured the homocysteine levels of 4,766 men and women aged 65 to 67 back in 1992, and then recorded any deaths over the next five years, during which 162 men and 97 women died. They then looked at the risk of death in relation to their homocysteine levels. Remarkably, they not only reconfirmed the relationship between heart attacks, strokes and high homocysteine, but also found that 'a strong relation was found between homocysteine and all causes of mortality'. In other words, homocysteine is an accurate predictor of how long you are going to live, whatever the eventual cause of death may be!

The importance of glutathione

As we saw in Chapter 2, the more antioxidants your immune army has available, the stronger it becomes and the more able to stop the damage wreaked by invaders, such as viruses, bacteria or rogue cancer cells. The most important and powerful antioxidant of all is glutathione, an essential sulphur-containing compound that lives inside your immune cells – in fact every cell – acting much like a benevolent police force. Oxidants also get produced when cells break down glucose to make energy, and glutathione helps mop up the cell's own 'exhaust fumes'.

Glutathione is also essential in detoxifying the body and helping repair damaged DNA. So if you have a high H score, and therefore low glutathione, you will increase your risk of getting many kinds of cancer, and of premature cell death. Just about every cancer known is linked to glutathione deficiency, and many are linked to high homocysteine. Glutathione, along with SAMe, is your liver's best friend, too. Any insult to the body – smoking, drinking, allergens, viruses, chemicals or drugs (both illegal and prescribed) – increases your need for glutathione and dramatically raises your homocysteine level.

You may have a glutathione deficiency if you have smoker's cough, chronic bronchitis, asthmatic coughing and wheezing, difficulty concentrating, frequent headaches, food allergies and cravings, joint pain, muscle pain, frequent tiredness, irritability and mood swings, or recurrent colds and other infections.

So how do you boost your glutathione?

One excellent way is to lower your homocysteine to a safe range. As you can see in the illustration The homocysteine pathway, on page 63, if you have a high homocysteine level, you are not making enough glutathione. You can raise your glutathione levels with the correct intake of B vitamins, zinc and nutrients, such as TMG and SAMe, from both diet and supplements. (TMG and SAMe contain methyl groups, thus helping methylation; see illustration The methyl donors, page 74.)

How high homocysteine and faulty methylation cause abnormal cell growth

If oxidation is one of the prime ways DNA becomes damaged, high homocysteine and associated abnormal methylation is another. DNA is always being damaged, often by oxidants, and therefore needs to be constantly repaired. It also needs to be copied, encoding new cells that we make at an extraordinary rate of tens of millions per minute. Methylation controls both the synthesis and the repair of DNA, putting homocysteine, and the key homocysteine-lowering nutrients, such as vitamin B_{12}, folate, vitamins B_6, B_2 and TMG, smack in the middle of the whole cancer process.

Any failure to do the right thing with methyl groups could conceivably increase the risk of abnormal cell growth. There are a number of nutrients involved, including methyl donors such as TMG, and the nutrients needed for the methylation to proceed, mainly the B vitamins. Any lack of these B vitamins is already well established to increase the risk of certain cancers.

High homocysteine predicts cancer

Does a high H score increase your risk of cancer? This is a key question and one that is only starting to be explored. As with heart disease, having accurate markers for cancer helps in the diagnosis, prevention and treatment. Such markers not only identify someone at risk but can also encourage immediate preventive steps and even measure the success of a cancer treatment.

Dr Wu and colleagues at the University of Utah's Health Science Center wondered whether homocysteine might act as a tumour marker, so they decided to measure homocysteine along with other known tumour markers in cancer patients undergoing treatment.[62] They found that when the other tumour markers went up, the homocysteine went up, and when the tumour markers went down, the homocysteine went down. They also observed that homocysteine proved to be a better marker than the other more conventional indicators. Remarkably, homocysteine also predicted much more accurately whether cancer therapy was going successfully or not. If the cancer was growing larger and therefore not responding to therapy, homocysteine increased at the same time; if the cancer was growing smaller with therapy, homocysteine levels decreased. Among the tumour markers, only homocysteine revealed the success of cancer therapy in this way. Although it's in the early days of research, this study certainly indicates that homocysteine levels may prove to be a very useful indicator of the existence of cancer as well as the success or failure of cancer therapies.

Homocysteine, leukaemia and dysplasia

Most people have heard of leukaemia, a cancer of the bone marrow in which the number of white blood cells in the blood greatly increases. There are also a number of similar but lesser-known (and often less severe) conditions that originate in the bone marrow where the body's cells are made – and all are called bone marrow myelodysplasias. Dysplasia means that the cells are malformed as if overgrowing – and this can occur not only in the bone marrow but in any area of the body.

Leukaemia affects about 40,000 people, mainly children, in the US and about 6,000 in the UK each year. The number with dysplasia is even higher. These conditions appear to be more genetic than environmental.

Research at the Department of Medical Science at the University of Milan in Italy found that 42 per cent of those with myelodysplasias have high H scores.[63]

Another form of dysplasia is cervical dysplasia, a pre-cancerous lesion of the vaginal cervix. Once again, research has found that the more severe the dysplasia, the higher the homocysteine levels.[64] Conversely, the higher the folate and B_{12} levels, the less severe the dysplasia. These, of course, are the vitamins that lower high homocysteine levels.

So if you have a family history of cancer or dysplasia, have developed one of these conditions or are fearful you may, getting your homocysteine tested and following an appropriate diet and supplement programme to reduce it to safe levels is your first priority. This not only helps prevent cervical dysplasia but it also helps to reverse the condition if you have it. (See Eight ways to lower your homocysteine and The best homocysteine-lowering supplements on page 75).

Homocysteine and colon cancer

It is well known that colon cancer risk is strongly linked to a poor diet – diets high in cooked, especially burned, meat and low in fibre, fruit and vegetables – and that diets high in folate, a key nutrient in vegetables, is highly protective.[65] This is also true for breast cancer (see page 70). Could this be because the absence of folate means higher homocysteine and more methylation, oxidation and glutathione problems, leading to DNA damage? The cancer/homocysteine link gets even more interesting due to the discovery of two different defective genes that cause methylation problems. These genes provide the instructions that make enzymes that convert potentially toxic homocysteine into useful substances. One is the cystathionine beta-synthase enzyme (CBS) that turns homocysteine into cystathionine and then on to glutathione. The other is the MTHFR enzyme that works with folic acid and B_{12} to improve methylation. The MTHFR enzyme doesn't work as well in some people (approximately one in ten) due to an inherited genetic mutation. For these individuals to stay healthy, higher intakes of homocysteine-lowering nutrients are needed, especially 'methyl' folic acid or methylcobalamin (B_{12}).

Researchers in the Department of Surgery at the University of Western Australia wondered whether there might be a connection between inheriting the damaged MTHFR gene, homocysteine and colon cancer. So they checked for this genetic mutation in over 500 patients with colon cancer and found that, especially in older patients, the abnormal gene and elevated homocysteine were often present.[66]

Both genetic mutations, interestingly enough, also seem to need more vitamin B_2 (riboflavin) in order to work optimally in keeping homocysteine low. This means that the combination of a damaged gene, plus low folate and low B_{12}, which is very common in older people, and possibly low vitamin B_2, leads to a high risk of disease and ill health. How do you know if you have this genetic defect? You can get it tested (see Resources). However, since the net consequence would be raised homocysteine you can cut to the chase and test your homocysteine level. If high, the right combination of nutrients, which should also include B$_2$, zinc and TMG, at the correct levels, can lower your H score and therefore reduce your cancer risk.

Folic acid – the good, the bad and the likely

Although many studies have reported that higher intakes of folate (from the diet) may reduce the risk of colorectal cancer by 40 to 60 per cent, when it comes to supplementing folic acid (the supplement form of folate), there is a need to be more cautious.

Folic acid was one of the first vitamins that the government recommended we supplement – pregnant women are told to supplement 400mcg per day to reduce the risk of neural tube defects (NTDs). Recommended intakes are usually between 200mcg and 800mcg.

Although the debate regarding food fortification in the UK continues, the US government decided to fortify food with folic acid in 1996, with Canada following suit in 1998. Since then, NTDs in the States have dropped by more than 20 per cent. What's worrying, however, is that since 1996 in the US, and 1998 in Canada, absolute rates of colorectal cancer have increased.[67] In support of this, a large Swedish study found that people with a high level of folate in their blood had a significantly increased risk of colorectal cancer.[68]

I believe there are two reasons for this. One is that enough folic acid is good for you and too much is bad for you, especially if you don't have enough B$_{12}$. Folic acid is normally converted in the body to the naturally circulating form of folate (the kind that comes from food). However, some experts believe that high levels of folic acid are unable to be converted, especially in the absence of other co-factor nutrients, and therefore 'overwhelm' the body's natural mechanisms.[69]

The second appears to be that folic acid, certainly in isolation, while being very good at stopping normal cells becoming cancer cells, seems to encourage the growth of pre-cancerous cells, called adenomas, in the gut. About one in five middle-aged people have pre-cancerous cells in

cont ▶

their colon, and most middle-aged men have them in their prostate too. For these people, too much folic acid, especially in combination with a bad diet, could be bad news.

A study just published in the *Journal of the American Medical Association* certainly seems to support the view that taking high-dose folic acid (above 350mcg) if you have cancer or a pre-cancerous condition is not a good idea. Researchers followed up group of Norwegian people with cardiovascular disease, who were given either folic acid (800mcg) with vitamin B_{12} and some with B_6, versus placebo, over six years.[70] They found that 10 per cent of those receiving folic acid were diagnosed with cancer, compared to 8.4 per cent in the group given the placebo. However, most of the increased cancer risk was due to deaths from lung cancer (not colorectal cancer, as was predicted), primarily among smokers and those with a variation in a particular gene (found in about 10 per cent of the population). However, if you don't smoke, don't have cardiovascular disease and don't have this gene variation, this small potential increase in risk may not apply to you.

I advise supplementing up to 400mcg a day even if you are not pregnant, but together with B_6, B_{12} and zinc, and to keep eating greens, beans and fruit. But don't take more unless your homocysteine level is high and you want to lower it.

Homocysteine and breast cancer

The same risk combination (a damaged gene, plus low folate, B_{12} and vitamin B_2) holds for breast cancer, too. And a high intake of folate is also associated with a reduction in risk.[71] Swedish researchers looked at the folate intake of 11,699 postmenopausal women. The women who consumed an average of 456mcg of folate per day from whole foods had a 44 per cent lower risk of breast cancer than women in the lowest average-intake group (160mcg of folate per day). However, another study found that high levels of folate (more than 853mcg per day) were potentially harmful rather than beneficial. The likely explanations for this are as explained above.

Just as for colon cancer, a particular gene mutation, this time called COMT, leads to high homocysteine and methylation problems. So, once again, researchers wondered whether women with breast cancer might have methylation problems as reflected by high homocysteine levels, in part due to this genetic risk factor. To date, research has shown that people with this gene mutation do indeed have raised homocysteine levels, but as yet no strong association between homocysteine and breast cancer has been found.[72] However, once you know your H score, no matter what your genetic make-up, you can lower it and reduce your risk of breast cancer, or any disease associated with high homocysteine, with the right diet and supplements (see below).

The cancer marker of tomorrow?

It is highly likely that, as the spotlight focuses on homocysteine as the marker for methylation problems, and methylation problems are seen as part of the root cause of many cancers, that we'll start to see an association between homocysteine and many different types of cancer.

For now, we can only say that there is reasonable evidence that having a high homocysteine level increases cancer risk, especially colon cancer, skin, leukaemia and the dysplasias, including cervical dysplasia. And there is good reason to believe that a homocysteine-lowering diet and supplement programme, explained at the end of this chapter, will do much to cut cancer risk, probably by at least a third.

All of this suggests that measuring homocysteine may well help to alert us to existing problems that could lead to cancer, so that we can look at ways where we might be able to alleviate those problems and perhaps prevent cancer from occurring or progressing. As I mentioned earlier, it is *vital* to measure, as homocysteine levels can be both high and low in cancer sufferers.

Measuring your homocysteine

Your homocysteine level is easy to measure at home (See Resources). Your doctor can also test you, although few do. Homocysteine is measured in mmol/l. We used to think a 'high' level was above 15 units (mmol/l). This is what increases your risk of a heart attack and doubles your Alzheimer's risk. Up to 30 per cent of people with a history of heart disease have a homocysteine level above 14 units. A level above 10 is associated with increased cancer risk. The average level in Britain is 10.5. However, most experts believe that a level below 6 units is ideal.

Basically, there's no official safe level and no guarantee that your diet and the supplements you are currently taking are keeping homocysteine at bay. If you have any of the associated risk factors below it's especially important to get tested.

High homocysteine risk factors

These include:

- Genetic inheritance – meaning a family history of heart disease, strokes, cancer, Alzheimer's disease, schizophrenia or diabetes
- Folate intake of less than 800mcg/day (the average intake from food is 200–250mcg; 800mcg is the equivalent of eating 1.2kg (2½lb) of strawberries)
- Increasing age (homocysteine levels increase with age; I recommend your level should be about one-tenth of your age)
- Male sex
- Oestrogen deficiency
- Excessive alcohol, coffee or tea intake
- Smoking
- Lack of exercise
- Hostility and repressed anger
- Inflammatory bowel diseases (coeliac, Crohn's, ulcerative colitis)
- *H. pylori*-generated ulcers
- Pregnancy

- Being a strict vegetarian or vegan

- High-fat diet with excessive red meat, high-fat dairy intake

The good news is that, whatever your homocysteine level is, you can lower it with the right combination of nutrients and dietary changes, together with lifestyle changes designed to reduce your risk.

The current vogue is to recommend folic acid. However, this alone is far less effective than the right nutrients in combination. The amount you need also depends on your current homocysteine level (see chart below for guidelines). One study found that homocysteine scores reduced by 17 per cent on high-dose folic acid alone, 19 per cent on vitamin B_{12} alone; 57 per cent on folic acid plus B_{12}; and 60 per cent on folic acid, B_{12} and B_6.[73] All this was achieved in three weeks!

However, even better results would have been achieved by including tri-methyl-glycine (TMG). TMG is the best 'methyl donor' to supplement, better than SAMe. This is because 'tri' means it has *three* 'methyl groups' and it can immediately donate one to homocysteine, thus detoxifying it (see illustration below).

In a study in New Zealand, the homocysteine scores of patients with chronic kidney failure and very high homocysteine levels were reduced by a further 18 per cent when 4g of TMG was given, along with 50mg of B_6 and 5,000mcg of folate, compared with levels of patients taking just B_6 and folate.[74] Some companies produce combinations of these nutrients (see Resources, page 381), which are the most cost-effective supplements for restoring a healthy homocysteine level.

Lower your homocysteine score

The combination of the diet and supplements recommended on page 75 has the potential to halve your homocysteine score in weeks. However, if you have cancer you should not take these supplements unless guided by a nutritional therapist or doctor (see the caution on page 76). The goal is to bring your score to below 6. Mine is 4.5. Your homocysteine score is probably the best objective measure of whether you are achieving optimum nutrition.

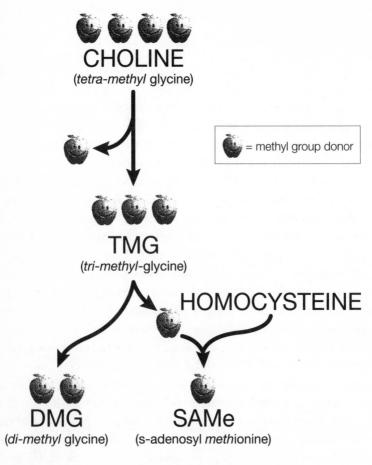

The methyl donors

The body needs 'methyl groups' (made of one carbon and three hydrogen atoms). Choline, found in eggs and in lecithin, contains these, as does TMG (also called betaine), found in sugar beet and other vegetables. TMG is the best source, because it can donate one methyl group (DMG) and turn toxic homocysteine into SAMe, the body's best methyl-group carrier.

Eight ways to lower your homocysteine

1 Eat less fatty meat, and more fish and vegetable protein (beans, lentils, nuts and seeds)
2 Eat your greens
3 Have a clove of garlic a day
4 Cut back on coffee
5 Limit your alcohol intake
6 Reduce your stress
7 Stop smoking
8 Supplement homocysteine-lowering nutrients every day

The best homocysteine-lowering supplements

These are guidelines for the amount of homocysteine-lowering nutrients to supplement depending on the level of homocysteine in your blood after testing. If your level is below 6, a high-strength multivitamin should do the trick. If your homocysteine is above 6, it is best to supplement a homocysteine formula – shown here as a number of tablets spread throughout the day – to lower your level to below 6. If you're supplementing these nutrients separately, you can also do that using the guide below.

Homocysteine-lowering supplements and dosages

Nutrient	No risk	Low risk	High risk	Very high risk
	below 6	7–9	10–15	above 16
Folic acid	200mcg	400mcg	800mcg	1,000mcg
B_{12}	10mcg	250mcg	500mcg	1,000mcg
B_6	25mg	50mg	75mg	100mg
B_2	10mg	15mg	20mg	50mg
Zinc	5mg	10mg	15mg	20mg
TMG	500mg	750mg	1–1.5g	3–6g
NAC	250mg	500mg	750mg	1,000mg

Note Since B vitamins tend to increase alertness, it is a good idea to take homocysteine supplements in the morning rather than at night.

The next step

Test your homocysteine level. You can do this using a home test kit (see Resources). The most powerful and quickest way to restore a normal H score to below 6 units, is to supplement specific homocysteine-lowering nutrients, which are easily available in homocysteine nutrient formulas. This should provide vitamin B_6 (25 to 100mg), B_{12} (10 to 1,000mcg), and folic acid (200 to 1,000mcg) a day or, better still, take an all-round homocysteine-lowering formula containing TMG and B_2 as well. Also supplement N-acetyl-cysteine (NAC) (250 to 1,000mg a day). A good homocysteine-lowering formula should include a special form of B_{12}, methylcobalamin, which works best. Use the chart above as your guide, depending on your homocysteine level.

Also eat whole foods rich in B vitamins – whole grains, beans, nuts, seeds, fruits and vegetables. Folic acid is particularly abundant in green vegetables, beans, lentils, nuts and seeds, whereas B_{12} is found only in animal foods – meat, fish, eggs and dairy produce.

The best foods for 'methyl donation' are liver, beef, egg yolk (for choline); and beans, peas, prawns, fish, eggs and especially liver (for TMG, sometimes called betaine).

If you do take large amounts of homocysteine-lowering nutrients to correct high homocysteine, don't keep taking them for ever. Recheck your homocysteine score after three months and adjust your supplements accordingly.

Dig deeper by reading my book, co-authored with Dr James Braly, *The H Factor*.

CAUTION

While there is evidence to suggest that methyl supplementation will help prevent cancer, we don't know what methyl supplementation will do in people who already have cancer. So, until you have tested your homocysteine level, I would not recommend them. Even after testing, it is important to get advice from a nutritional therapist or nutritionally trained doctor before taking these supplements in high doses.

CHAPTER 9

How Stress and Negative Emotions Leave You Vulnerable

Over the last three decades, many researchers have attempted to discover whether stress, suppressed anger and/or other 'negative' emotions can cause cancer. There continues to be mixed opinions about the extent to which the mind can influence the body. Some say that feelings and thoughts neither cause nor cure cancer, but, at the other end of the spectrum, is the notion that people can cure themselves of many diseases by making themselves happy or thinking positively. However, it can sometimes be unproductive, or even harmful, to make people think that they are somehow responsible for their illness.[75] As we will explore in this chapter, evidence has shown that because the body and mind are seamlessly integrated, the truth probably lies somewhere in between.

Being in touch with our emotions

Lydia Temoshok is a psychologist and author of many books on the subject of emotions and health, including *The Type C Connection*. In the 1980s, studies carried out by her showed that cancer patients who kept emotions such as anger under the surface, remaining ignorant of their existence, had slower recovery rates than those who were more expressive. A trait that was common to these patients was self-denial, stemming from a lack of awareness of their own basic emotional needs. In contrast, those people who were in touch with their emotions had stronger immune systems and their tumours were smaller.

In addition, various researchers, including David Spiegel of Stanford University in California, have shown convincingly that being able to express emotions such as anger and grief can improve cancer patients' survival rates.

In his book *Love, Medicine and Miracles* (see Recommended Reading), Dr Bernie Siegel suggests that certain personality types are more prone to cancer: people who do not easily form close bonds or love relationships; those who internalise or deny their feelings; and those who do not easily express negative emotions such as anger or frustration. On the other hand, people who are active and assertive, who avoid people-pleasing and who have an underlying high sense of self-esteem are less likely to experience unresolved loss or a sense of helplessness or hopelessness – which can weaken the immune system.

Stress affects the immune system

It is well known that cancer is frequently diagnosed in people who have suffered a major loss or traumatic event within the previous two years. Cancers normally appear to have a long 'incubation' period – usually manifesting ten to 40 years after initial exposure to a carcinogen, as in the case of exposure to cigarette smoke and asbestos. Yet, in the case of stress or loss, the time frame appears to be much shorter.

From what we know about the effects of stress and loss on the immune system, it is highly likely that, in people who succumb to cancer, the process had already begun before the stressful event. The stress then dramatically weakened the immune system, allowing the process to speed up rapidly.

We all need some stimulation or we slide into apathy. Indeed, boredom can be stressful in itself. For many of us, however, 'overstimulation', leading to excessive stress, is the problem. We all have different abilities to cope with different circumstances, and each person has an optimal stress level, at which they can function well. Most of us find a certain amount of stress is useful to spur us on towards producing good work or achieving something we aim for. However, extreme stress that becomes a daily part of life is not good for us.

In order to avoid excessive stress, we need to understand its symptoms and causes. Stress – that is, anger, fear, excitement and frustration – stimulates the adrenal glands. Certain chemical substances, when taken in excess, also cause the same reaction; these include refined sugar, alcohol, tea and coffee (we discuss these in Chapters 16 and 17).

The mechanisms of stress and the bodily systems it affects

Stress affects us on several levels: physical, mental, emotional and spiritual. We are creatures built for short intense bouts of stress rather than the prolonged stress that many of us encounter every day. Stress in the 21st century tends to be longer in duration, and often includes worries over family relationships, money, exams, missed deadlines or even things we can't do anything about, such as traffic jams.

The stress reaction is a physical one, for the reason that, when primitive humans had feelings of stress, the cause was likely to be physical danger. The body's reactions prepared them to run away fast, or to turn and fight.

The effect stress has on hormones

Stress encourages the production and circulation of hormones, which are released by the adrenal glands – small glands that sit on top of the kidneys. When our adrenal glands are functioning normally, we feel well, have adequate amounts of energy, good immunity against infections, no water retention, and are fairly relaxed and easy-going.

However, stress causes the adrenal glands to release adrenalin, which produces a 'high' almost like a drug. They also release cortisone. These two hormones gear the whole body for action: digestion shuts down; glucose is released into the bloodstream to fuel the nerves and muscles; breathing, heart rate and blood pressure all increase, ready to deliver oxygen to the cells to burn the fuel and make energy. This response, known as 'fight or flight', has helped to keep us alive through the evolution of humankind. In a small number of situations today, it still serves the same purpose.

However, the majority of our day-to-day stresses are not life threatening, although the response of our adrenal glands remains the same. In the absence of a 'fight' or the need for 'flight' the body causes the effects described above unnecessarily, and because of the chronic nature of today's stressful life, the reaction is often ongoing.

Illnesses often occur after bouts of stress

The continual release of adrenalin and cortisol, in turn, inhibit the immune response by lowering levels of the important white cells. Depression, stress, anxiety, hostility and fatigue all result in poorer function of the immune T-cells.[76] Those who suffer with cold sores (caused by the herpes virus) will know that they often flare up during, of after, a period of stress. You are also more likely to get a cold during a period of high stress. One study concluded that 'the combination of anger and chronic stress can result in reduced immune function',[77] and researchers at Ohio State University College of Medicine and Comprehensive Cancer Center reported impaired DNA repair in highly distressed people who have difficulty coping with problems.[78]

How stress affects the gut

Stress also dramatically suppresses the immune defences in the digestive tract – a major entry route for carcinogens into the body. This is highly significant because about three-quarters of all our immune cells are situated there. Our first line of defence is a substance called secretory immunoglobulin A (SIgA). Prolonged stress lowers our levels of this substance, leaving us more vulnerable to the effects of carcinogens in the digestive tract. This may explain why the risk of colorectal cancer becomes greater after a period of high stress.[79]

Much of what we know about stress today was discovered in the 1930s by Dr Hans Selye, an endocrinologist and stress expert. In studies he conducted on rats, they were chased regularly and then given injections. It became apparent that even when the rats were not receiving the injections, the fear and anticipation of an injection was causing them to develop ulcers. This showed that the stress response can eventually become more damaging than the stressor itself. Although it is now known that stress isn't the only cause of stomach ulcers (most stomach ulcers in humans are caused by infection from a bacteria called *Helicobacter pylori*, or *H. pylori* for short), stress is still believed to be a contributing factor in that it promotes *H. pylori* infection in susceptible individuals.

The three stages of stress

Dr Selye described three 'stages' of stress. The first is the 'fight or flight' response. The second stage is called the 'resistance stage', which can see our bodies through a stressful episode before our bodies return to normal. This works if the source of the stress is something short term, like exam pressure or a work deadline, for example. Unfortunately, our bodies still respond today as if our stresses are physical, flooding the body with hormones to help us 'fight' or 'take flight'. If there is no resulting 'fight or flight', or exercise, to help 'disperse' the hormones, these hormones continue to be released, damaging our bodies. This is when the body moves into a third stage, the 'exhaustion stage'. At this point, all of the body's resources are eventually depleted and the body is unable to maintain normal function. If the source of stress still remains and this stage is extended, long-term damage may result. This is when stress becomes chronic and is termed 'bad' stress.

Previously I talked about how stress can lead to ulcers; Robert Sapolsky, in his book *Why Zebras Don't Get Ulcers*, explains that there is a big difference between humans and animals. Animals also have a 'fight or flight' response to danger, but under natural conditions only humans struggle to turn this response off. These prolonged bouts of emotional disturbances result in ulcers, exhaustion and other factors that severely damage our health. When we worry or experience stress, our body turns on the same physiological responses as an animal would (the zebra being chased by a lion, for example,) but we do not resolve the conflict in the same way: through fighting or fleeing. What is more, our responses are often switched on for months on end, while we worry about recessions, mortgages, relationships, and so on, far different from the quick responses we would have made in life-threatening situations. If the fight or flight response is triggered chronically and over the long term, repair and important processes in the body, such as bolstering immunity, are depressed for long periods of time. Over time, this activation of the stress response makes us sick. This is why we get ulcers whereas zebras do not.

The effects of too much stress

If the stress process happens too often, side effects build up: nutrients are used up too quickly and become depleted; digestion is slow and disrupted; resistance to infection declines; and minor problems occur, such as headaches, stiffness, insomnia or moodiness. Many of the disorders that arise from stress are the result of nutritional deficiencies, especially deficiencies of B-complex vitamins. If nothing is done, major problems can occur, such as heart disease, diabetes, arthritis, and even cancer.

Stress can also lead to inflammation in the body, as confirmed by a study in 2002,[80] which showed that 25 stressed parents, whose children were being treated for cancer, were less likely to respond to cortisol (they had reached the exhaustion stage); their cells continued to produce cytokines (inflammatory chemicals); and the process of inflammation was not properly shut down in their bodies.

Why we need stimulants to keep going

It is not only the adrenal glands that can become exhausted from overstimulation. The thyroid, which works closely with the adrenals, can also be affected. A vicious circle is then created whereby more and more stimulation is needed to get them working, leading to cravings for harmful stimulants like sugar and coffee. As the systems become worn down, there may be weight gain, higher blood cholesterol, slower thinking and reduced energy (more about this in Chapter 16).

In a healthy person, adrenal hormones (such as cortisol) are actually released in a cycle with the highest value in the morning and the lowest value at night. This 24-hour cycle is called the circadian rhythm. People who find getting up in the morning particularly difficult, or who suffer with a low energy level during the day, often have abnormal adrenal rhythms and poor blood sugar regulation. Maintaining stable blood sugar levels depends on food choice, lifestyle, how well your adrenals are functioning and insulin activity (see Chapter 16 for more information about how to balance blood sugar levels).

Immune health

The body conditions and nourishes the immune cells (white blood cells) within the spleen and bone marrow during the cortisol cycle. So, if the cycle is disrupted, the immune system will be adversely affected.

How do you sleep?

Stress, as we have seen, raises cortisol. High cortisol levels at night and in the morning will interrupt your ability to enter REM (rapid eye movement) sleep cycles, which are the regenerative phases of sleep. Chronic lack of REM sleep can reduce a person's mental vitality and vigour as well as inducing depression and reducing immune function.

A lack of sleep can also be caused by depressed melatonin levels. Melatonin is a naturally occurring hormone that is involved in regulating our circadian rhythm. You can supplement this if you are having sleeping problems; however, although it is available over the counter in the US, in the UK you will need a prescription from your doctor. Ask for a dosage of 3mg.

Interestingly, a lack of melatonin is also thought to increase a person's cancer risk. In patients with breast cancer, melatonin levels were found to have been halved compared to those with non-malignant breast disease, and in patients with prostate cancer they were reduced by two-thirds compared to those who had benign prostate disease. Similar results have been found in patients with colorectal cancer.[81] Melatonin has also been found to complement the actions of anti-oestrogen drugs such as tamoxifen, leading to the suggestion that melatonin is a natural anti-oestrogen. In a review of ten studies published between 1992 and 2003, including 643 patients, melatonin reduced the risk of death from cancer at one year by a third.[82] All of this suggests great potential for melatonin as a future cancer treatment.

A measure of stress

Stress overload can be measured by determining a person's levels of cortisol and another key stress hormone called DHEA (the anti-ageing adrenal hormone and a precursor for stress hormones). A standard stress test involves analysing four saliva samples at different intervals over a 24-hour period. These tests, available through nutritional therapists (see Resources), can determine whether a person needs to pursue a nutritional or a hormonal strategy, or perhaps other therapies such as meditation, to restore a proper stress response. A number of studies have reported an increase in DHEA or a decrease in cortisol in people who meditated, as well as quality of life improvements.[83]

As always, however, prevention is better than cure, and your goal should be to reduce your stress, or at least how you respond to it. I'll give you some tips on how to do this in Chapter 23.

Emotional health

It is becoming increasingly clear that no thought occurs without an emotion, and that emotions, either positive or negative, have a massive effect on our health and the whole way our bodies operate. Through recent developments in neuroscience, we can now measure emotion to an extent, and its effects on both our mental and physical health. A 2003 study, published in the journal *Proceedings of the National Academy of Sciences*, linked 'negative' brain activity with a weakened immune system. Dr Richard Davidson, who led the research, said: 'Emotions play an important role in modulating bodily systems that influence our health.'[84]

The past affects our present

Our experiences through life mean that we inevitably accumulate emotional tension and unresolved memories. The more disturbing of these become deep-rooted negative emotional patterns that unconsciously determine how we react to the stresses of life.

The word 'emotion' comes from the Latin *e* for exit and *motio* for movement. So emotion is a natural energy, a dynamic experience that needs to move through and out of the body. As children, however, we are often taught not to express our emotions; for example, we might have been told, 'boys don't cry', or 'don't be a baby'. Or when we are angry we are taught that it's not appropriate to express it: 'Don't you dare raise your voice to me!' At some level most of us are taught that emotions are not OK.

As healthy adults, we need to let go of the emotional patterns from the past that mess up our lives and no longer serve us. As Fritz Perls, the founder of Gestalt Therapy, often said, 'The only way out is through.' It's not easy, and the vast majority of people deny the symptoms or anaesthetise themselves through work, TV, food, alcohol or some kind of drug. By discharging negative emotions attached to past memories we become more able to respond spontaneously in any given moment, allowing us to be more present in our relationships and to the gifts of the world around us.

The body expresses what the mind represses

These emotions literally store in our cellular memory through our lives. They can manifest as physical tension, causing a variety of health problems, including headaches, ulcers, irritable bowel syndrome (IBS) and more serious illnesses, such as cancer. Extreme emotions affect your heart function, depress the immune system and inhibit digestion. I remember one client who suffered from terrible IBS. Every nutritional treatment I tried failed to make any difference. Then, one day she confessed, for the first time, an act of infidelity. From that day on her IBS disappeared.

Grief is another example. It depresses immunity and may be one explanation as to why many people who are unable to come to terms with the death of their partner often die shortly after.[85]

The benefits of good emotional health

Emotional health is just as important as physical health, and emotional ill health causes us just as much, if not more, suffering. The World Health Organization says that mental health problems are the number-one challenge for the 21st century. Having a positive outlook on life makes a big difference. In one study by researchers at the University of Pittsburgh, which followed 100,000 women over eight years, optimists were 30 per cent less likely to die from heart disease, and 23 per cent less likely to die from cancer than those women who had a general distrust of people.[86]

Recognising the problem and dealing with it

So, what do you do when you become aware that stress and negative emotional patterns are messing up your life and your health? In the same way that we need to learn about optimum nutrition and how to choose the right foods and drinks to be healthy, we also need to learn how to cope with the stress that everyday life throws at us and how to discharge and let go of negative emotions and emotional patterns. As vital as these skills are, they unfortunately aren't taught in school and it isn't part of our culture to learn these things. I'll give you my top ten tips in Chapter 23.

CHAPTER 10

Communication Breakdown

Rather than thinking of cancer as something 'out there' that must be destroyed, we should perhaps see it as the inevitable consequence of a major breakdown in communication.

Genes 'talk' to the chemicals that enter our bodies, telling them how to become incorporated into this highly complex and intelligent structure. The chemicals, in turn, 'talk' to the genes, adapting and altering their expression. If this conversation is harmonious, the body's cells continue to work for the good of the whole. On the other hand, if the conversation goes haywire, certain cells stop talking to their co-workers and stop respecting their boundaries and their duties. They then start to multiply, then spread and disrupt the integrity of our bodies – that is, our health.

In most cases this scenario – cancer – is caused by a number of factors, which can be summarised as follows:

- Excessive exposure to carcinogens, including hormone-disrupting chemicals and oxidants

- Insufficient intake of antioxidants

- A weakened immune system

- Decreased ability to detoxify

The relative importance of each of these factors is different for each of us and is certainly different in different kinds of cancer.

However, from this perspective you can see more clearly how to prevent cancer.

Cancer prevention

There are six key measures you need to take:

1   Reduce your exposure to carcinogens

2   Increase your intake of anti-carcinogens (such as antioxidants)

3   Boost your immune system

4   Improve your liver's ability to detoxify carcinogens

5   Test and, if necessary, correct your homocysteine level

6   Make sure stress and/or negative emotions are not affecting your health and leaving you vulnerable

Creating a good environment for healthy cells

When it comes to reversing the cancer process once it has started, all the above measures are equally important. All of these are about creating an environment that supports cells staying healthy. However, there are also ways of targeting cancer cells to destroy them. The latest cancer therapies attempt to find more intelligent ways of giving the cancer mass a hard time than conventional surgery, chemotherapy and radiation. These treatments take the form of drugs that target only the cancer cells, or they involve different methods of cutting off a tumour's blood supply; for example, a number of drugs that can inhibit a tumour's ability to build its own blood supply (angiogenesis) now exist. These are known as anti-angiogenic. There are also anti-angiogenic factors in foods, such as curcumin in turmeric and resveratrol in red grapes (discussed in detail in Part 4), which are proving to be quite potent anti-cancer agents.

Changing the pattern

It is a rare cancer specialist who applies these anti-cancer strategies with the six key prevention measures. I have often spoken to cancer patients who have had one treatment or another but have never been given any advice about changing their diet or lifestyle. Yet it makes no sense to keep doing the same things and expecting different results. Even when a cancer has apparently been successfully treated, if you do not understand and change the circumstances that led to its development in the first place, why should the disease not reoccur?

By all accounts, cancer is the symptom of a disease process that usually begins at least a decade or more before symptoms develop. True cancer prevention should therefore start with making changes to your diet and lifestyle now (instead of when the first signs of a problem appear or at the final hour).

How you can change your lifestyle

This book draws together the available evidence, and aims to define what you need to eat and how you need to live to minimise your chances of ever developing the crisis of communication in the body known as cancer.

Part 2 looks at what you need to eat and drink, and what you should avoid; Part 3 looks at lifestyle factors and the art of chemical self-defence; and Part 4 examines the benefits of increasing your intake of anti-cancer nutrients and natural remedies. Part 5 puts it all together into a Daily Action Plan that will help you to say no to cancer. Parts 6 and 7 are for those who have cancer, or who have had cancer in the past.

PART 2

GOOD AND BAD CANCER FOODS

CHAPTER 11

Why Too Much Meat is Bad News

What you eat provides you with your greatest risk of, or protection from, cancer – even greater than stopping smoking. Thanks to the work of the World Cancer Research Fund (WCRF), there are now some very clear indications of how important diet is in cancer prevention. In their 1997 report, they concluded that by making a few simple changes to your diet you can reduce your risk by 30 to 40 per cent. Since then, the WCRF has painstakingly reviewed thousands of studies investigating the link between diet and cancer risk, and they have published the findings in their latest report (2007) entitled *Food, Nutrition, Physical Activity, and the Prevention of Cancer: A Global Perspective.*[1]

One of their latest recommendations is to limit the intake of red meat and avoid processed meat ('red meat' includes beef, pork, lamb and goat; 'processed meat' refers to meat preserved by smoking, curing or salting, or with chemical preservatives added to it). Their main advice is that, if you do eat red meat, you should eat less than 500g (1lb 2oz) a week and very little, if any, should be processed. What's interesting is that their 'public health goal' for meat is even lower: 300g (11oz) a week. This equates to a 150g (5½oz) serving (roughly the size of your palm) twice a week. So, if you enjoy eating red meat, you don't have to give it up completely, although it is preferable to choose fish, organic poultry or meat from non-domesticated animals in place of red meat.

The WCRF even go so far as to say that that 'many foods of animal origin are nourishing and healthy if consumed in moderate amounts'. The main issue with that, as always, is what does 'moderate' mean? To put this into perspective, when you go to a restaurant and choose a 175g (6oz) steak (or larger) from the menu, you will have used up at least one of your two servings of red meat for the week!

Why processed meat and cancer?

Processed meats have been implicated in stomach cancer. Compounds found in these meats (N-nitroso) damage DNA, and the high cooking temperatures may also produce additional carcinogens.

According to researchers at the University of Hawaii, in a study involving almost 200,000 people followed over seven years, eating too many hot dogs, sausages and other processed meats can also increase the risk of developing pancreatic cancer. Those who ate the least pro-cessed meat cut their risk of developing pancreatic cancer by almost half compared to those with the highest intake. People who ate a lot of pork and red meat also increased their pancreatic cancer risk by around 50 per cent, compared to those who ate less meat. There was no increased risk linked to eating poultry, fish or dairy products.[2]

Dr Ute Nothlings of the Cancer Research Center at the University of Hawaii, who led the research, suggests that the link could be due to the chemical reactions that occur during the preparation of pro-cessed meats, rather than its fat or cholesterol levels. He said such reactions could produce carcinogenic chemicals. Since vegetarians avoid these foods, this could explain the difference in cancer rates between vegetarians and meat-eaters.

Red meat – bad news for breast cancer

A team at the University of Leeds monitored 35,000 women over a period of seven years. Older women who ate one 57g (2oz) portion of red meat a day had a 56 per cent increased risk compared with those who ate none. And those who ate the most processed meat, such as bacon, sausages, ham or pies, had a 64 per cent greater risk of breast cancer than those who refrained.[3] This increased risk was strongest in post-menopausal women.

Another study in the US involving 90,000 pre-menopausal women found that eating one and a half servings of red meat per day almost doubled the risk of hormone receptor-positive breast cancer, compared to three or fewer per week.[4]

However, not all studies have confirmed the link between meat and cancer, which, says the WCRF, is strongest for colorectal cancer; for example, one smaller study that followed 3,660 adults in Britain over a seven-year period found no associations between increased meat consumption and a higher risk of cancer.[5]

What's wrong with meat?

It may not be meat, per se, that increases the risk of cancer but what's added to it and what we do with it. Generally, studies on Americans show the strongest association between meat consumption and cancer risk. One possible reason for this could be that animals in the EU are not given growth hormones, which are widely used for animals in the US.

Another suggestion is that different cooking methods, combined with a low fruit and vegetable intake in the US, partly explain why findings in the UK and the US are different. Also, eating a lot of meat means having a high-protein diet. Protein intakes consistent with a 'meat and two veg' diet have been shown to increase the incidence of all types of cancer in animals, according to cancer experts Dr Linda Youngman of Oxford University and Dr Campbell from Cornell University in the US.

A Swedish study also suggests that it's what we do to meat. They found that meat consumption in itself didn't increase kidney cancer risk except in those eating lots of fried or sautéed meat.[6] The fat in meat, if burned, generates oxidants and carcinogens. Grilling (broiling), barbecuing and frying meat all increase the risk, particularly of stomach and colorectal cancer. The high saturated fat content of most meats is also a factor (this is discussed more fully in Chapter 15).

It is not surprising to find that a diet of cooked meat, high in protein and fat, and low in fibre, together with carcinogens created from burning, creates havoc with the digestive tract. All this explains the link with cancer of the stomach, colon, rectum, pancreas (the organ responsible for digesting protein) and kidneys (the organ that has to eliminate the breakdown products of protein and other toxins). Why, though, the link with breast and prostate cancer?

The hormone connection

The higher incidence of these hormone-related cancers among meat-eaters suggests that such a diet introduces a different kind of cancer promoter. One candidate, of course, is simply the naturally occurring hormones and growth factors in meat. Such hormones are also present in milk products, excessive consumption of which has been linked to an increased risk of both prostate and breast cancer (see Chapter 12).

On top of the naturally occurring hormones and growth factors in meat, most non-organic meat, particularly in the US, whether from chicken, beef, pork or lamb, also receives hormone treatment of one kind or another. Cows, for example, are given hormone pellets to increase their growth or milk yield. This practice has been officially banned in the EU since 2006, but some unscrupulous farmers still give growth-enhancing hormones to increase profit. Of course, it isn't easy to find out what long-term effects these artificially introduced hormones are having, and have had, on us prior to their being banned.

Dr Malcolm Carruthers, a specialist in male hormone-related disease, investigated over seven years 1,000 patients complaining of symptoms of the 'male menopause'. The most common symptoms are fatigue, depression, loss of libido, testicular atrophy, impotence and breast enlargement, plus an increased risk of prostate cancer. Of those 1,000 cases, the highest occupational risk group was farmers (the 'front-line' troops in the agrochemical arms race). According to Carruthers:

> For some the causative agent appeared obvious. They had worked on farms caponizing chickens or turkeys with oestrogen pellet implants, to make the birds plumper and more tender. Unfortunately, though it might be considered poetic justice, they must have taken in large amounts of oestrogen which caused them to become partly caponized themselves.

Although we might be incensed to find that our food has been tampered with in this way, in some respects the UK is tame in comparison to the US, where many hormones banned in Europe are still widely used. One of these is bovine somatotrophin (BST), given to increase milk yield. With world trade legislation increasingly moving towards the removal of trade barriers, the US are putting pressure on EU countries to lift their ban on BST residues, which can be found in US milk and other dairy products.

Is it healthier to have a meat-free diet?

You may have seen in the newspapers in July 2009 that the risk of certain cancers was 45 per cent lower in vegetarians than in meat-eaters. Those who followed a vegetarian diet developed fewer cancers of the blood, bladder, ovary and stomach. In the case of multiple myeloma, a relatively rare cancer of the bone marrow, vegetarians were 75 per cent less likely to develop the disease than meat-eaters. Taking all cancer types together (including the more common types, such as breast and prostate), vegetarians were reported as having a 12 per cent lower risk than meat-eaters. However, what was interesting is that this study, published in the *British Journal of Cancer*, also included a group of non-meat-eaters who ate fish, and these were 18 per cent less likely to get most cancers. And yet this was not reported in any of the press articles at the time!

Led by Professor Tim Key, a Cancer Research UK epidemiologist at the University of Oxford, researchers from universities in the UK and New Zealand followed 61,566 British men and women. Overall, their results suggested that while in the general population about 33 people in 100 will develop cancer during their lifetime, for those who do not eat meat that risk is reduced to about 29 in 100.[7] Another large study involving 63,550 people in Britain, known as the EPIC study (European Prospective Investigation into Cancer and Nutrition), also concluded that the incidence of all cancers combined was lower among vegetarians than among meat-eaters.[8]

Vegetarian diets tend be lower in fat and higher in fibre, but they can require careful planning to ensure adequate levels of protein and vitamins – particularly vitamin D and B_{12}, which are mainly derived from animal products, as well as omega-3 fats from fish.

Summary

The weight of evidence is in favour of decreasing meat intake to reduce cancer risk. Those wishing to maintain optimal health and minimal risk of cancer should follow these guidelines:

- Preferably avoid or, at least, limit your intake of red meat to a maximum of 300g (11oz) a week, which equates to two small servings of 150g (5½oz) twice a week (roughly the amount that would fit into the palm of your hand).
- Choose lean meat, especially game, in preference to red meat or meat from domesticated animals.
- Avoid, or rarely eat, burned meat, whether grilled, fried or barbecued.
- Avoid processed meats including most burgers, sausages and pies, unless you are sure they are made from lean meat.
- Choose organic meat or free-range chicken.

CHAPTER 12

Why Milk is a Four-letter Word

It may come as a surprise that drinking milk isn't necessary when you're pregnant, breastfeeding or at any other time of your life, apart from when you are a baby. The only requirement for us humans is *breast* milk, ideally for the first year of life, and certainly the first six months. To be consuming dairy products – milk, cheese, yoghurt and butter – as an adult is a bit like breastfeeding from another animal. It's certainly not part of our evolutionary design.

Let's look at a few facts. Half the people of the world don't drink milk (and still have healthy babies and bones). Seven out of ten people don't have the enzyme to digest it and get digestive problems when they eat it as a result. It's Britain's number-one allergy-provoking food, linked to asthma, ear, sinus and throat infections. The largest ever UK health and diet survey, the 100% Health Survey (published in 2010, involving over 55,000 people), found that the more milk a person drinks the worse their overall health, their digestion, immune and hormonal health. That's the 'big picture', which certainly suggests that many of us are not well suited to drinking milk – and perhaps that includes you.

Links with cancer

But there's a much more serious reason for me to discourage you from making dairy products a staple part of your diet – and that's cancer. There is now consistent and substantial evidence that the higher the milk consumption of a country the greater their breast and prostate cancer risk. The highest risk of cancer death is found in Switzerland, Norway, Iceland and Sweden, countries with the biggest consumers of milk. In stark contrast, in most Asian countries the risk is minimal.[9] In such countries, where the diet consists mainly of wholegrains, vegetables, fruits, tofu, soya milk and other soya products, and where milk is not a normal part of the diet, people are generally healthier, and breast and prostate cancers are much rarer than in the US and Europe.

The problem with milk

The connection between milk an increased risk of cancer has been known for some time. Back in 1937 a group of 4,999 children in the UK took part in a long-term study recording their dietary habits year on year. Sixty-five years later a study has found that those with a high dairy intake during childhood had tripled their odds of having colorectal cancer.[10] There was a weaker association with prostate cancer risk and no association, in this study, with increased breast cancer risk.

According to the National Cancer Institute (NCI), 19 out of 23 studies have shown a positive association between dairy intake and prostate cancer: 'This is one of the most consistent dietary predictors for prostate cancer in the published literature ... In these studies, men with the highest dairy intakes had approximately double the risk of total prostate cancer, and up to a fourfold increase in risk of metastatic or fatal prostate cancer relative to low consumers.'[11]

Further analyses of the EPIC study, which I mentioned in relation to meat and cancer, found no clear association between milk consumption and breast cancer, but it did find a trend towards a higher risk for premenopausal women partial to butter, and also in those with high intakes of processed meats.[12]

To date it appears that countries that are virtually milk-free have the lowest risk, and that, among Western countries, low milk intake means a low risk of colorectal cancer and prostate cancer in particular.

What's in milk?

Why would milk increase risk? Milk contains 38 different hormones and growth promoters. After all, that's its job: to make cells grow. But one in particular is attracting a lot of attention. It's called insulin-like growth factor, or IGF-1. It's a naturally occurring hormone, found both in cow's milk, breast milk and your blood. The more milk you drink the higher your level. What this hormone does is stimulate growth. Blood levels of IGF-1 peak during adolescence, stimulating development of breasts in girls or the prostate in boys, then levels rapidly drop off as you get older. Not so if you keep guzzling milk and cheese. Milk not only contains IGF-1, a small part of which is absorbed into your blood, but it also stimulates the body to produce more of its own. It simply does what it's meant to do – stimulate growth. It also stops overgrowing cells from committing suicide, a process called apoptosis. While you are a rapidly growing baby this is good news. But when the only overgrowing cells are cancer cells, this is especially bad news, because IGF-1 has also been found to directly stimulate the growth of cancer cells, with high levels being linked to an increased risk of breast, prostate, colon and lung cancer.[13] Having a high IGF-1 level as a pre-menopausal woman just about doubles your risk of cancer overall.[14]

Studies on high IGF-1 levels

A Harvard University study showed that men who had the highest levels of IGF-1 had more than four times the risk of prostate cancer compared with those who had the lowest levels.[15] Two other major Harvard studies have shown that milk-drinking men have a 30 to

60 per cent greater prostate cancer risk than men who generally avoid dairy products.[16] In one of these, involving more than 20,000 male doctors (known as the Physicians' Health Study), those who consumed more than two dairy servings daily had a 34 per cent higher risk of developing prostate cancer than men who consumed little or no dairy products.[17]

According to Professor Jeff Holly, from Bristol University's Faculty of Medicine, one of the world's leading experts in IGF, 'those in the top quarter for blood IGF-1 levels have approximately a three- to fourfold increase in risk of breast, prostate or colorectal cancer. This level of increased risk is in the same order as the risk of having cardiovascular disease from a high level of cholesterol.' His research, and that of others at Harvard and Montreal, show that a non-milk-drinking 30-year-old might have an IGF level of 130ng/ml, while a high dairy consumer might have a level of 200ng/ml, and that's more than enough to dramatically increase your risk. The evidence is compelling and any scientist who denies this is simply not up to speed. Holly doesn't drink milk and actively discourages anyone with a diagnosis of these cancers to have any dairy produce. Although we do not know whether a high milk intake could initiate cancer we can be pretty confident that a high milk intake, by increasing IGF-1 and possibly other growth promoters, speeds up the growth of pre-existing cancer cells.

Dairy and ovarian cancer

A high dairy intake is also linked to increased ovarian cancer risk. This link, however, is thought to be more due to the way that the milk sugar, lactose, breaks down in the body. Lactose breaks down into another sugar called galactose, which appears to be able to damage the ovary. A review in 2006 found that for every 10g of lactose consumed (the amount in one glass of milk), ovarian cancer risk increased by 13 per cent.[18]

I don't mean to scare you unnecessarily, unless it might save your life, and I don't mean to put you off ever touching the white stuff. But I do recommend two things. Firstly, give yourself a dairy-free week. You may find relief from some niggling symptoms you have suffered from in the past. If you find your indigestion or bloating stops, the headaches you have suffered from have stopped, your energy increases or your sniffs and snuffles clear up, get yourself tested for dairy intolerance. There's a simple food intolerance test you can do at home for this (see Resources). Secondly, add up all the milk you have in teas, coffees and cereals, plus servings of yoghurt and cheese, and if it's over half a pint a day, cut back. Try rice milk, oat milk or soya milk instead. Milk is a food designed for baby cows, but not for you.

How to get your calcium without the cow

Many people believe that you have to have milk for calcium, vitamin D and protein. You do need these nutrients, but you don't need milk. You can easily achieve all the protein, calcium and vitamin D you need from nuts, seeds, beans and fish – and getting enough sun exposure in the case of vitamin D. If you don't, vitamin D can be supplemented (more on this in Chapter 27). Milk isn't even that good for minerals. Sure, it's high in calcium, but it's low in magnesium, the other key bone-building mineral. Also, the common belief that drinking milk reduces bone mass loss is highly contentious. Although some studies support this, others show the exact opposite: that high milk consumers have low bone-mass density.

A moderate amount of calcium from a variety of plant sources seems to be best. There's plenty of easily absorbed calcium in all kinds of greens – kale being one of the best, as well as broccoli, beans, seeds (especially sesame), nuts (especially almonds), calcium-fortified juices, soya milk and other non-dairy milks. Plus, these foods contain other cancer-fighting nutrients that aren't present in dairy products, as you'll see in the next chapter.

The best no-dairy foods for calcium are included in the chart overleaf.

cont ▶

Common sources of calcium: how they compare

Milk – 250 ml = 315 mg calcium

Firm cheese – 50g = 350mg calcium

Yoghurt – 175ml = 275mg calcium

Food	Serving (mg)	Calcium	Rating
Almonds	125mg (½ cup)	(200)	**
Baked beans	250mg (1 cup)	(163)	**
Beet greens, cooked	125mg (½ cup)	(87)	*
Brazil nuts	125mg (½ cup)	130	*
Bread, wholewheat or white	1 slice	25	
Broccoli, cooked	125mg (½ cup)	38	
Cauliflower, cooked	125mg (½ cup)	18	
Chickpeas, cooked	250mg (1 cup)	84	*
Dates	60mg (¼ cup)	12	
Figs, dried	4 medium	61	*
Kale, cooked	125mg (½ cup)	103	*
Lentils, cooked	250mg (1 cup)	40	
Nuts, mixed	125mg (½ cup)	48	
Orange	1 medium	52	*
Pak choi, cooked	125mg (½ cup)	84	*
Prunes, dried, uncooked	60mg (¼ cup)	18	
Raisins	60mg (¼ cup)	21	
Red kidney beans, cooked	250mg (1 cup)	(52)	*
Rhubarb, cooked	125mg (½ cup)	(184)	**
Rice, white or brown	125mg (½ cup)	12	
Rice drink (fortified)	250mg (1 cup)	300	***
Salmon, canned with bones	½ 213g can	225	**
Sardines, canned with bones	½ 213g can	210	**
Sesame seeds	125mg (½ cup)	(104)	*
Sesame paste (tahini)	30mg (2 tbsp)	(40)	
Shrimps, cooked/canned	70g (12 large)	41	
Soya beans, cooked	125 (½ cup)	(93)	*
Soya drink	250mg (1 cup)	28	
Soya drink (fortified)	250mg (1 cup)	300	***
Spinach, cooked	125mg (½ cup)	(129)	*
Tofu, regular processed[†]	100g (⅓ cup)	(150)	*
White beans, cooked	250mg (1 cup)	(170)	**

cont ▶

( ) – Calcium from these foods is known to be absorbed less efficiently by the body.

† The calcium content shown for tofu is an approximation based on products available on the market. Calcium content varies greatly from one brand to the other and can be quite low. Tofu processed with magnesium chloride also contains less calcium.

Rating as established according to Canadian Food and Drugs Regulations
* Source of calcium
** Good source of calcium
*** Excellent source of calcium
Source: Health Canada, Canadian Nutrient File, 1993

Summary

- If you have cancer, especially any hormone-related cancer such as breast or prostate cancer, or colorectal cancer, I recommend the complete avoidance of dairy products.

- If you don't have cancer, keep your intake of dairy products low; that is, below half a pint a day and ideally less than 1.2 litres (2 pints) a week. If your aim is to minimise your chances of prostate or colorectal cancer, it would make sense to be largely dairy-free.

CHAPTER 13

The Best Anti-cancer Fruits and Vegetables

Most people are aware that they should be eating at least five portions of fruits and vegetables daily. The World Health Organization takes this one step further and recommends eight to ten servings daily, particularly in relation to cancer prevention. Our 100% Health Survey of over 55,000 people finds that the healthiest eat eight servings of fruit and vegetables a day. This might sound like a lot but it only means fruit with your breakfast, two servings of vegetables with each main meal, and two additional servings of fruit or vegetables as snacks (such as a carrot with some hummus). The more you can eat the better.

The average adult eats fewer than three portions daily, as shown in a 2003 survey of 1,724 adults in the UK, aged 19–64. Consumption was highest in the older age group (50–64), while in the younger age group (19–24 year olds) only 4 per cent of females but no males achieved the five-a-day target.[19] In our 100% Health Survey the average intake was two pieces of fruit and two veg daily.

Top protection

Of all the dietary factors, increasing your intake of fruit and vegetables provides the greatest protection from cancer – and there's no cut-off point. In other words, the more of these foods you eat, the lower your risk.

The evidence is equally strong for eating fruits as well as vegetables, and this is one reason why the government encourages us all to eat at least five servings of these foods per day. One study compared people on a Mediterranean diet – high in fruits, vegetables and cereals – with others on a control diet (similar to the American Heart Association's 'prudent' diet for heart disease). After four years, those on the Mediterranean diet showed a 61 per cent reduction in cancer risk and half the risk of death.[20] Over the last ten years more and more evidence confirms the health benefits of consuming a traditional Mediterranean diet. According to a study of almost 400,000 people with an age range of 50 to 71, eating a Mediterranean-style diet, rich in fruit, vegetables, legumes (peas, beans and lentils), olive oil and fish reduced the risk of dying from cancer by 17 per cent for men and 12 per cent for women. The people who stuck most closely to a Mediterranean diet were significantly less likely to die during the first five years after the surveys were taken.[21]

Which cancers are we most protected from?

The link between increasing intake of fruit and vegetables and decreasing risk is most convincing for cancers of the digestive tract (mouth, pharynx, stomach, colon and rectum). It is also quite strong for lung cancer.

It was this strong link that led to investigations into what the protective factors in these foods were. Certain foods appear to be especially protective. Among these are carrots – some studies have indicated that eating probably the equivalent of a carrot a day meant cutting cancer risk by a third.[22] Tomatoes are also great. Men consuming at least ten servings of tomato-based foods a week are almost 50 per cent less likely to develop prostate cancer, whereas those consuming four to seven servings a week are only 20 per cent less likely to develop the disease.[23]

Antioxidant power

According to Dr Richard Cutler, Director of the US Government Anti-Aging Research Department, 'the amount of antioxidants that you maintain in your body is directly proportional to how long you will live'. Living in a polluted area, smoking or regularly eating barbecued or deep-fried foods can all create an increased need for antioxidants.

Both carrots and tomatoes are high in antioxidant nutrients, which are known to protect against cancer-causing oxidant damage. Although fruits and vegetables are rich in a wide variety of antioxidants, the most research has been carried out on the amount of vitamins A, C and E in foods. While these are important in preventing cancer, along with other antioxidants explained in Chapter 25, it is becoming clear that there is much more to fruit and vegetables than their vitamin content. There are literally hundreds of active compounds in plants, collectively known as phytonutrients (phyto = plant). Many of these active compounds are cancer-protective antioxidants. Others, like salvestrols, harness the power of nature's defence mechanisms (see the next chapter).

The benefits of A, C and E

The higher a person's intake of vitamin A (or more particularly beta-carotene, the fruit and vegetable source of vitamin A), the lower their risk of lung cancer. A study in Japan, of 265,000 people, found that those with a low beta-carotene intake had a much higher risk of lung cancer.[24] This was confirmed by a study published in the *Lancet*, which showed that a heavy smoker with a high beta-carotene status had the same risk of developing lung cancer as a non-smoker with a low beta-carotene status.[25] This study illustrates just how important both sides of the cancer equation are: exposure to carcinogens (in this case oxidants from smoke) versus protection factors (in this case the antioxidant beta-carotene).

Carrots, broccoli, sweet potatoes, cantaloupe melons and apricots are particularly high in beta-carotene. Fresh vegetables and fruit are high in vitamin C. Eating these foods appears to prevent DNA damage (stopping the initiation of cancer)[26] and also to stop the cancer developing.[27]

The effects of vitamin E

Vitamin E may protect against the development of cancers by enhancing immune function[28] and it is also thought to block the formation of nitrosamines: carcinogens formed in the stomach from nitrites consumed in the diet (from processed meat, for example). Vitamin E is principally found in nuts, seeds and, especially, oily fish.

A large study, the Nurses Health Study, which involved over 80,000 women, showed that pre-menopausal women with a family history of breast cancer who consumed the highest quantity of vitamin E had a 43 per cent reduction in breast cancer incidence compared to only a 16 per cent risk reduction for women without a family history of breast cancer.[29]

A comprehensive review of the evidence in 2002, published in the *Journal of Nutritional Biochemistry*, showed that certain vitamin E compounds found in food confer a significant protective effect in breast cancer.[30] There is also some evidence that associates a higher intake of vitamin E with a decreased incidence of prostate and oesophageal cancer.[31]

Measuring the strength of antioxidants

Rather than focusing on individual antioxidants in foods, such as vitamin A, C and E, the total antioxidant power of a food can be measured by a test developed at Tufts University in Boston, which determines a food's 'oxygen radical absorbance capacity', known as ORAC for short. Each food can now be assigned a certain number of ORAC units. Foods that score high in these units are especially helpful in countering oxidant, or free radical, damage in the body.

Increase your antioxidant power

Your goal is to obtain 3,500 ORAC units a day, although 5,000 to 6,000 will give you even more protection against ageing and many diseases, including cancer. How do you achieve this?

The list below shows the ORACs of 20 different foods that are easy to incorporate into your daily diet. Each serving contains approximately 2,000 ORACs. Just pick at least three of these daily to hit your optimal score of 6,000. The complete list is available on my website at www.patrickholford.com/ORAC.

1 ⅓ tsp cinnamon, ground
2 ½ tsp oregano, dried
3 ½ tsp turmeric, ground
4 1 heaped tsp mustard
5 ⅕ cup blueberries
6 ½ pear or grapefruit or 1 plum
7 ½ cup blackcurrants or berries, raspberries, strawberries
8 ½ cup cherries or a shot of Cherry Active concentrate (see page 387)
9 An orange or apple
10 4 pieces of dark chocolate (70% cocoa solids)
11 7 walnut halves
12 8 pecan halves
13 ¼ cup pistachio nuts
14 ½ cup cooked lentils
15 1 cup cooked kidney beans
16 ⅓ medium avocado
17 ½ cup red cabbage
18 2 cups broccoli
19 1 medium artichoke or 8 asparagus spears
20 medium glass (150ml/5fl oz/ ¼ pint) red wine

Oxygen Radical Absorbance Capacity of Selected Foods – 2007, US Department of Agriculture

Go for colour

Generally speaking, where you find the most colour and flavour you will also find the highest antioxidant levels. The reds, yellows and oranges of tomatoes and carrots, for example, are due to the presence of beta-carotene. Artichoke has the highest ORAC rating of vegetables whereas other vegetables, such as carrots, peas and spinach, although great for you, are lower in ORACs, so aim for five to ten servings daily of a range of fruits and vegetables including the highest ORAC scorers, to keep your antioxidant intake high. Too much fruit and fruit juices can mean too much sugar, however, so aim for two to three fruit and three to seven vegetable portions daily.

Fruits that have the highest levels are those with the deepest colour such as blueberries, raspberries and strawberries. These are particularly rich in powerful antioxidants called proanthocyanadins. One cup of blueberries will provide 9,697 ORACs. You would need to eat 11 bananas to get the same benefit as a cupful of blueberries! But bananas have a greater effect on your blood sugar, so they can cause weight gain; as I explain in Chapter 16, the GL (glycemic load, or the effect on our blood sugar) of a banana is 12 whereas a whole 120g (4¼oz) punnet of blueberries is only 5 so, if you are watching your weight, the punnet of blueberries is a far better option.

How many daily portions do you need?

The number of portions needed per day really does depend on your choices, as you can see in the two daily 'menus' below. Both days have five portions selected, but the Day 1 selection is 8,000 ORACs less than for Day 2! That's a massive difference. So you need to learn which foods are putting money in your antioxidant bank.

Our daily choices *do* make a difference!

DAY 1		DAY 2	
Fruit/vegetable portion	**ORAC**	**Fruit/vegetable portion**	**ORAC**
⅛ large cantaloupe melon	315	½ pear	2,617
1 kiwi fruit	802	½ cup strawberries	2,683
1 medium carrot, raw	406	½ avocado	2,899
½ cup green peas, frozen	432	1 cup broccoli, raw	1,226
1 cup spinach, raw	455	4 asparagus spears, boiled	986
Total score	2,410	Total score	10,411

Top Tips

1 Aim to eat 6,000 ORACS a day.
2 Have seven or more servings of fruits and vegetables a day, plus nuts, herbs and spices.
3 Have a multi-coloured diet with each meal, containing three or more colours.
4 When preparing meals, aim to fill at least half your plate with vegetables.
5 Heating destroys antioxidants, so aim to eat most of your fruits and vegetables raw or lightly cooked or steamed.
6 Stock up on frozen berries when fresh berries aren't in season.
7 Keep a bowl of fruit on your desk at work and at home. When you are hungry have some fruit.
8 Snack on fruit and raw nuts rather than crisps and other processed foods. A handful of nuts with fruit will also help to keep your blood sugar balanced.

Antioxidant overload?

In case you are wondering, you cannot have too many antioxidants in your diet – your body will use what it needs and excrete the rest. However, antioxidants work synergistically, so if taking in supplement form, it is better to supplement a combination, rather than just one antioxidant in isolation, especially in large amounts (more on this in Chapter 25).

There are also many other antioxidant nutrients, which can be found in nutritional supplements, such as quercetin (from cranberry); rutin (from buckwheat); catechin (from grapes); pycnogenol (from pine bark); silymarin (from milk thistle); bilberry and anthocyanidins (from berries). Their role as supplements is discussed in more detail in Part 4. Many of these phytonutrients determine the colour of food. The carotenoids, including beta-carotene, are responsible for the orange colour of carrots, while anthocyanidins give berries their red/blue hue. In general terms there is good reason to recommend not only eating plenty of fruits and vegetables but also choosing those that give a good variety of colour, including oranges, blues and reds.

Cruciferous vegetables – are you eating enough?

Another protective factor in plants is a family of phytonutrients called glucosinolates. These help the body detoxify potential carcinogens. They are found particularly in cruciferous vegetables, a family of vegetables whose leaves grow as a cross: broccoli, cabbage, cauliflower, Brussels sprouts, cress, horseradish, kale, kohlrabi, mustard, radish and turnip. Eating cruciferous vegetables three times a week may halve your risk of colon cancer[32] among others.

In one study, the volunteers first ate glucosinolate-containing Brussels sprouts for seven days and then glucosinolate-free sprouts for the same period. After the week of glucosinolate-rich Brussels sprouts the level of detoxification enzymes in the colon was 30 per cent higher, compared to the glucosinolate-free period.[33] More recent studies have shown that a high intake of cruciferous vegetables, including broccoli and cauliflower, is associated with a reduced risk of aggressive prostate cancer,[34] and bladder cancer.[35] Raw or lightly steamed foods are better for you.

Glucosinolate-rich foods also contain a substance called indole-3-carbinol (I3C), which helps to detoxify harmful oxidants and breaks down excess oestrogens in the body.[36] As we have seen, high oestrogen levels are strongly linked with breast and uterine cancer. Animal studies using I3C have shown a reduced incidence of cancer.

Soya and cancer prevention

Glucosinolates aren't the only factor in plant food that may protect against hormone-related cancers. Asian people who swap their traditional diets of bean curd and soya milk for burgers and fries are increasing their risk of cancer as well as heart disease. Collaborative research between Hong Kong's Chinese University and Manchester University indicates that soya beans may protect people from developing prostate and breast cancer.

Soya beans contain large amounts of phytoestrogens, which probably explains their protective effect. The traditional oriental diet is particularly high in isoflavonoids, one type of phytoestrogen. Levels of isoflavonoids in the blood have been found to be up to a hundred times higher in Japanese men with a low incidence of prostate cancer, compared to Finnish men, who have a high incidence.[37] However, we still don't understand exactly how phytoestrogens help. Professor Sir Norman Blacklock from Manchester University believes they may exert a 'weak oestrogen effect', and it is thought that phytoestrogens may block oestrogen receptor sites, thereby lowering the body's levels of active oestrogen. If this proves to be so, it is consistent with accumulating evidence that many modern diseases, including breast and prostate cancer, are the result of too much oestrogen and other growth-promoting hormones.

There is also reason to believe that a protease inhibitor in soya, Bowman-Birk inhibitor (BBI), may be another key anti-cancer compound. In a study at the University of Pennsylvania School of Medicine, BBI was added to the diet of rats that had previously been fed a substance known to induce colon cancer. None of the rats developed tumours. In another animal study, BBI suppressed the formation of tumours by 71 per cent.[38] Human trials are now under way.[39]

The importance of phytoestrogens

Whatever the mechanism, phytoestrogens have consistently been associated with reduced cancer risk. Women whose diets are abundant in soya beans have a lower risk of getting breast cancer, whereas men with a high soya intake have a substantially lower risk of prostate cancer. Research has focused mainly on two isoflavones – genistein and daidzein. Japanese women, who generally have a lower risk of breast cancer than women in other industrialised societies, have been found to have higher levels of these in their bodies. They may protect against the harmful effects of unopposed oestrogen. One study suggested that long-term regular soya intake, which exposes tissues to these two isoflavonoids, enhances their protective effects.[40] And further studies have illustrated the role of other phytonutrients in soya – the isoflavone equol and the lignan enterolactone – in lowering the risk of breast cancer.[41] Researchers also believe that soya beans may offer protection partly by inhibiting the development of new blood vessels, thus starving the tumour of nourishment. Soya may therefore both protect against the initiation of hormone-related cancers and inhibit the development of cancer.

Endometrial cancer

Regular intake of soya foods has been shown to reduce the risk of endometrial cancer. A study involving 1,678 women in Shanghai, China, found that regular consumption of soya foods, measured as an amount of either soya protein or soya isoflavones, significantly reduced the risk of endometrial cancer. The risk reduction was most pronounced among overweight women.[42]

Getting enough in your diet

Tofu, a curd made from the soya bean, is the richest source of isoflavonoids, whereas highly processed soya products are the poorest source,[43] which is why I would advise eating soya foods and other foods containing phytoestrogens in their natural form.

To help people understand how to boost levels of phytoestrogens in their diet, Dr Margaret Ritchie, an expert in phytoestrogens at the University of St Andrews, has spent over a decade measuring levels of the isoflavone family of phytoestrogens in commonly eaten foods. She's created a database that's a world first, as it assesses levels based not only on the actual food content but is also corroborated with what's absorbed and excreted after eating. 'Put simply, we're pin-pointing foods which you can introduce to your diet – or that of your teenage son or daughter – so they can build up cancer protection in later life,' Dr Ritchie told me.

For the best results, she recommends having some phytoestrogen-rich foods at least once a day, as blood levels of the beneficial compounds they contain start to decline six hours after eating. 'Asians eat small quantities of soya and other plant-based foods regularly throughout the day and this seems to be the most beneficial,' she says.

Based on her research, I recommend you aim for around 15,000mcg (15mg) of phytoestrogens a day. This is easily achieved by having a small portion of tofu – a 100g (3½oz) serving provides 78,000mcg, or a 100ml (3½fl oz) glass of soya milk or soya yoghurt (11,000mcg) and a portion of chickpeas, perhaps as hummus (2,000mcg). Eating rye bread, beansprouts, beans, lentils, nuts and seeds also helps to boost your levels – these are the very foods that are staples in the East and unheard of by many in the West, although hummus is a staple food in the Mediterranean diet.

The phytoestrogen content of commonly eaten foods

Food	mcg per 100g	Food	mcg per 100g
Soya flour, full fat	166,700	Soy sauce	1,800
Soya beans	142,100	Multigrain crispbread	1,187
Miso	126,500	Wholemeal bread	830
Soya mince	121,100	Beansprouts	758
Tofu	78,700	Rye bread	757
Soya cheese	33,000	Premium sausages	620
Vegetarian sausages	26,300	Currant bread	547
Vegeburger	26,200	Granary bread	370
Tofu burger	24,200	Pitta bread	321
Soya milk, plain	11,815	Malt loaf	293
Soya yoghurt, plain	11,815	Currants	250
Chickpea channa dahl	1,960	Runner beans	222

cont ▶

Food	mcg per 100g	Food	mcg per 100g
Mung beans	212	Passion fruit	17
Nut and seed roast	162	Prunes, ready-to-eat	13
Brown rice	133	Apples	12
Chickpeas	124	Brown rice and red kidney beans	12
Mixed nuts and raisins	100	Hummus	11
Fruit cake, wholemeal	96	New potatoes	8
Fruit loaf	94	Waldorf salad	8
Ice cream, dairy	91	Mangoes	7
Sage and onion stuffing	90	Dates, dried	7
Sausage and bean hotpot	85	Okra	7
Nut cutlets	62	Mixed bean salad	5
Muesli, Swiss-style	52	Sesame seeds	5
Red kidney beans	40	Strawberries	5
Turkey burgers, breaded	40	Mixed nuts	5
Green beans/French beans	38	Sun-dried tomatoes	5
Blackeyed beans	32	Apricots, dried	4
Hazelnuts	24	Tomatoes, stuffed with rice	4
Haricot beans	24	Cranberries	4
Peanuts, plain	24	Tomatoes	3
Noodles, wheat	23	Sweetcorn	3
Lentils, green and brown	22	Tuna pasta	2
Mung bean dahl	21	Curly kale	2
Aubergine, stuffed with		Lentil soup	2
lentils and vegetables	19	Peppers, stuffed with rice	2

Adapted from the Phytooestrogen Database 2004, compiled by Dr Margaret Ritchie, Bute Medical School at the University of St Andrews

Other important sources of phytoestrogens

Although Dr Ritchie's database contains sources of isoflavone-rich foods, there are other classes of phytoestrogens that also contain cancer-protecting properties. These include the following foods overleaf:

- Lignans – rich in linseeds, black/green tea, coffee, fruits and vegetables, split peas, lentils and beans

- Flavones – rich in fruits, nuts, green vegetables

- Coumarins – in cabbage, peas and liquorice

- Acyclics – in hops (Belgium beer is the richest source of acyclics)

- Triterpenoids – in liquorice and hops

- Coumestans – in alfalfa, beans, split peas and lentils

Garlic

Adding garlic to your vegetable dishes will add flavour and simultaneously reduce your risk of cancer. Garlic contains around 200 biologically active compounds, many of which protect against cancer. Other 'allium' compounds – the active component in garlic, onions, leeks, chives and shallots – have been shown to inhibit cancer in the test tube and in animals. Garlic is especially rich in the sulphur-containing amino acids, glutathione and cysteine, which are powerful antioxidants. Not only does it help protect against the formation of tumours, including metastases, it also inhibits the growth of established tumours, strengthening the immune system and detoxifying the liver. A National Cancer Institute study carried out in China in 1989 found that provinces that used garlic liberally had the lowest rate of stomach cancer.[44] The results of a large study involving 41,837 women aged between 55 and 69 from Iowa, USA, indicated that garlic was the most protective type of vegetable against colon cancer. Women who said they ate garlic at least once a week were half as likely to contract colon cancer as those who said they never ate it.[45]

A review of all research up to 2000, at the University of North Carolina at Chapel Hill, reported that people who consume raw or cooked garlic regularly run half the risk of stomach cancer and two-thirds the risk of colorectal cancer of people who eat little or none.[46] Garlic's sulphur compounds, from which the body can make the most powerful antioxidant of all, glutathione, may offer particular protection against cancers of the breast, oesophagus, prostate, skin and stomach.

Detoxing with garlic

Garlic also appears to stimulate the body's production of an enzyme called glutathione-S-transferase, which helps detoxify potential carcinogens. It's also associated with general detoxification, and, as we have learned, when glutathione levels increase, homocysteine levels are lowered (see Chapter 8). Whether or not this alone is the reason, there's no doubt that garlic is an excellent food for lowering your homocysteine level, according to the results of a trial with some very smelly rats!

Dr Yu-Yan Yeh and his team of researchers at the Pennsylvania State University put young rats on a diet low in folate. Not surprisingly, they developed high homocysteine. They were then given aged garlic (which is more potent). Those that had the highest homocysteine scores had up to a 30 per cent reduction! Those with lower homocysteine scores still had a reduction, proving that garlic does lower your homocysteine – which may be yet another reason why it's good for the heart.[47]

That's why I say 'a clove of garlic a day keeps the doctor away'. It's essential. One to three cloves a day, or the equivalent in capsules, provides good support for the immune system and may help protect against cancer. This means that when you are making dinner, you need to add a clove of garlic per person to the main dish. Garlic is another staple food of the Mediterranean diet. But cooking decreases the potency of the garlic, so it's even better to crush and stir it in just before serving. If you really don't like the taste or smell, you can take a garlic capsule instead. Some are deodorised.

Eat organic

While there is good reason to be concerned about the use of herbicides and pesticides, the strong worldwide association between eating lots of fruit and vegetables and reduced cancer risk suggests that the positive factors in these foods outweigh any such negative effects. Having said that, eating organic fruit and vegetables (which are cultivated without the use of pesticides and herbicides) may confer extra protection by minimising your exposure to toxins. They have also been found to contain more minerals.

If you want to know what the worst foods are for pesticides residue, take a look at the Pesticide Action Network (PAN) UK website (or contact them, see Resources). PAN is an independent, non-profit organisation which works nationally and internationally with like-minded groups and individuals concerned with health and the environment. They have used data from the UK government's Pesticide Residue Committee to determine pesticide levels in various foods. They looked at how often pesticides at any level were detected, how frequently legal levels were exceeded and how often more than one pesticide was found on a sample. The list was then sorted for the best and worst foods.

Top ten worst foods for pesticide residues

According to PAN in the UK, the worst foods are flour, potatoes, bread, apples, pears, grapes, strawberries, green beans, tomatoes and cucumber.

Which came up tops?

The worst offender in terms of exceeding legal limits was green beans. What was astonishing was that almost half the samples tested had pesticide residues above legal limits! The list of offending pesticides is too numerous to list, but what is more worrying is that five of the pesticides listed – namely dicofol, dimethoate, cypermethrin, chlorothalonil and carbendazim – are classified as possible human carcinogens (cancer-causing) by some international experts. Not only that, but three of these are also possible endocrine-disruptors (see Chapter 3). Unfortunately, what happens with these and many other chemicals we are exposed to is that regulators cannot even agree on what is, and what is not, a cancer-causing or an endocrine-disrupting chemical. PAN uses classifications from the International Agency for Research on Cancer (IARC), the US Environmental Protection Agency (EPA) and the European Union (EU), and their classifications of individual chemicals are often different.

What is particularly worrying is the evidence that children consume more pesticide residues than adults – exposure during the 'developing years' significantly increases risk. This is probably because they eat more fruit and food in general in relation to their body size. (The link between pesticide exposure and cancer is discussed further in Chapter 20).

There is good reason, both from the point of view of cancer risk and general health, to eat organic and feed your children organic fruit and vegetables whenever possible. If your budget does not stretch to buying everything organic, then research from the US Department of Agriculture (USDA) and the Food and Drug Administration (FDA) may help you choose. According to the Environmental Working Group (EWG), consumers can reduce their pesticide exposure by almost 80 per cent by avoiding the top 12 most contaminated fruits and vegetables and eating the least contaminated instead (see table below).[48]

The 'Dirty Dozen':

Top 12 foods to eat organic	15 foods you don't have to buy organic
Fruits	
Peaches	Avocados
Apples	Pineapples
Nectarines	Mangoes
Strawberries	Kiwi
Cherries	Papayas
Grapes	Watermelon
Pears	Grapefruit
Vegetables	
Sweet bell peppers	Onions
Celery	Sweetcorn
Kale (and leafy greens in general)	Asparagus
Lettuce	Peas
Carrots	Cabbage

cont ▶

Top 12 foods to eat organic

Potatoes*

15 foods you don't have to buy organic

Aubergine

Broccoli

Tomatoes **

Sweet potatoes

*EWG analyst Chris Campbell points out that potatoes are now 'just off the list', so you should still try to buy organic when possible. Potatoes also get the double whammy of fungicides that are added to the soil for growing.[49]

** In a change that surprises some, tomatoes have moved from the previous Dirty Dozen list to the EWG's most recent 'clean' list of safest conventional produce. According to Chris Campbell, the researchers aren't sure exactly why this is the case. 'It could be any number of reasons. It could be increasing awareness, better washing, substitution with better pesticides, changes in weather patterns or something else.' It's still true that the thin skin of tomatoes can allow pesticides to enter the fruit, so it's always a good idea to buy organic when possible, even if the popular food is no longer among the worst offenders.[50]

Summary

To maximise your protection against cancer:

- Eat as much fruit and vegetables as possible – at least seven servings a day. Pick those that have a high ORAC rating.
- Have a variety of 'colours' of fruits and vegetables, including something orange/red every day (such as carrots, sweet potato, tomatoes, watermelon, peaches) and something red/purple (such as berries, grapes or beetroot).
- Use herbs in your cooking, especially oregano, and have lots of turmeric, ginger and other spices.
- Include at least one serving of cruciferous vegetables every day. These include broccoli, Brussels sprouts, cabbage, cauliflower and kale.
- Eat organic whenever possible.
- Have a clove of garlic a day.
- Eat more phytoestrogen-rich foods, aiming for 15,000mcg of phytoestrogens a day, by having some beans, lentils, nuts or seeds, or miso, tempeh, soya milk or tofu every day.

CHAPTER 14

The Secret of Salvestrols

In terms of cancer treatment, most current anti-cancer chemo-therapy is beset by serious side effects: fatigue, hair loss, nausea and vomiting, mouth sores, appetite loss ... the list goes on. It isn't difficult to kill cancer cells – many chemotherapy drugs are already doing this effectively. However, they cannot discriminate between healthy and cancerous cells, and this is why they cause such horrible toxic side effects. The holy grail of cancer treatment is to find a treatment that targets only cancer cells and leaves healthy cells alone.

Thanks to a dedicated team of research scientists, led by Professor Dan Burke, a pharmacologist, and Professor Gerry Potter, Professor of Medicinal Chemistry and Director of the Cancer Drug Discovery Group at Leicester's De Montfort University, this goal could be closer than you think. They believe that a group of naturally occurring compounds in certain plants, called salvestrols, could be a major breakthrough in both cancer prevention and treat-ment.[51] Because salvestrols are activated only within cancer cells, they offer the possibility of anti-cancer treatment without the awful side effects.[52]

Professor Burke describes salvestrols as 'the most significant breakthrough in nutrition since the discovery of vitamins'; similar comments were made by Dr John Briffa in the *Observer* in 2005.[53] But how can salvestrols be so selective?

Salvestrols: nature's defence against attack

Since plants cannot run away from predators and pathogens, how do they defend themselves? The answer is by chemical warfare. Plants produce chemicals that act as repellents. The repellents are synthesised in response to microbial attack and fight off microbial pathogens such as fungi (mould) or bacteria.

When ripe fruits and vegetables are attacked by fungus, which happens all the time, they develop a group of chemicals (salvestrols) as a natural defence. When we eat these fruits and vegetables as part of our diet, the salvestrols they contain are activated by a particular enzyme found only in pre-cancerous or cancerous cells, and chemicals are produced that attack the cancer cells in the same way as they attacked the fungus. So, instead of using a synthetic drug to fight cancer, it may be possible to plug into one of nature's existing natural defence mechanisms.

Professor Potter believes that salvestrols have evolved as 'a rescue mechanism' that causes a cascade of events that can kill cancerous cells before they have a chance to develop into tumours, possibly explaining the protective effects of a diet high in fruits and vegetables.

How salvestrols target only cancer cells – the CYP1B1 story

It all started with the discovery of an enzyme in 1995, called CYP1B1 (pronounced 'sip one bee one'), by Professor Burke and his team at Aberdeen University Medical School.

It is now well established that CYP1B1 is present in the tumour cells of a wide variety of human cancers but is virtually undetectable in the normal cells of the corresponding healthy tissues.[54] This has been described as 'one of the most important revelations in cancer research for the past 25 years'[55] and has since been confirmed by at least 12 different studies by a number of eminent laboratories around the world, including the Dana-Farber Cancer Institute[56] and the Gray Cancer Institute in London.[57] According to the Dana-Farber

Cancer Institute, 'Chemotherapeutic agents generally do not differentiate between cancer and normal cells, resulting in considerable toxicity. Since CYP1B1 expression is limited in normal tissue, and highly expressed in human cancers, immunotherapy directed against CYP1B1-expressing cells is far more specific'. CYP1B1 is found inside cancerous cells of tumours within the bladder, brain, breast, colon, kidney, liver, lung, oesophagus, ovary, skin, small intestine, stomach and uterus[58] and is considered to be a tumour-marker enzyme, since it is virtually exclusive to cancer cells.

What's interesting to note is that where the CYP1B1 enzyme is artificially inhibited, the salvestrols will not succeed in destroying the cancer cell. So, CYP1B1 can be thought of as a Trojan horse inside cancer cells, which merely has to be provided with salvestrols in the diet in order to unleash a stream of chemical agents that are deadly to cancer cells. In other words, the presence of CYP1B1 in cancer cells seems to have provided cancer cells with the seeds of their own destruction – if you happen to eat foods high in salvestrols.

What are salvestrols?

The salvestrol molecules themselves are not new discoveries, since their chemical structures and the plants in which they occur have been known about for many years. But never before have these chemicals been grouped together on the basis of this particular set of anti-cancer actions.[59]

Salvestrols were discovered in 2002/3 as a result of the combined research of Professors Burke and Potter. Because Professor Burke is an expert on CYP enzymes, he knew that the discovery of CYP1B1, being unique to cancer cells, opened up the possibility of designing a better and safer type of anti-cancer drug; that is, one that is initially inactive and innocuous but which is then converted to a potent anti-cancer molecule by the CYP1B1 in the cancer cells (this is known as a prodrug). Normal cells would remain unharmed, because they lack the CYP1B1 enzyme and therefore lack the ability to activate this prodrug. Professor Burke teamed up with Professor Potter, who had spent almost 20 years designing synthetic cancer drugs, in 1996, in order to design and make the drug.

Professor Burke said:

> Gerry is a brilliant medicinal chemist, and already had stunning anti-cancer drug design achievements to his name by the time we teamed up. We produced the novel anti-cancer prodrugs in partnership, and then Gerry had the brilliant realisation that equivalent molecules are likely to be found in fruit and vegetables. Of course, he was right – and we found them and he called them salvestrols.

How salvestrols were discovered

Having developed a synthetic prodrug which could be activated by CYP1B1 to kill cancer cells and which is currently going through clinical trials, the science behind salvestrols really began when Potter realised that the molecule he had synthesised was very similar in structure to resveratrol (a chemical found in grape skins and red wine), which is widely credited with cancer-preventative properties. Potter found that resveratrol is changed by the CYP1B1 enzyme to produce a toxic substance, which brings about 'cell death' (apoptosis) and therefore destroys the cancer cells. This substance is called piceatannol (pronounced 'piss-see-at-inol'), known to be highly toxic to cancer cells.[60] This defines resveratrol as a salvestrol. Since salvestrols are highly selective and only active in cancer cells, they are non-toxic to non-cancerous cells.

However, Potter discovered that although resveratrol could work in the predicted way, the level of desired activity was quite low and so he started to look for other plants that have similar chemicals,[61] which might provide new natural anti-cancer remedies.

Potter and his team have been busy analysing many kinds of foods and have discovered that there are dozens of natural molecules similar to resveratrol, found in common foods and plants, some that have an even stronger anti-cancer activity than resveratrol. Salvestrol is the name used to describe this group of natural compounds (from the Latin word *salve*, meaning 'to save'). The formal definition of a salvestrol is 'a natural dietary anti-cancer prodrug'.

Potter's team searched for plants that had the highest level of salvestrols. Their definition of a salvestrol is that it is not an actual compound, like vitamin C, but an actual effect. So, any plant that could activate the production of an anti-cancer agent only within cancer cells, but not normal cells, is deemed to have a salvestrol effect. As I'll illustrate shortly, Potter's team identified the potency of each plant in salvestrol 'points'.

Professor Potter then started testing to see if the compound would fight an active cancer if taken in a concentrated form as a supplement. Results were impressive. I've seen a film of this actual process occurring within cancer cells and found it very convincing. If they can really do to cancer cells in the body what they can do in the laboratory, this is a really big breakthrough!

As explained in Chapter 1, single cancer cells are continually forming in our bodies to some extent, but most are destroyed before they develop into malignant tumours. Salvestrols in the diet may be a main mechanism by which this ongoing prevention of cancer can occur. What is now becoming clear is that there is more than one single mechanism whereby plants are able to help prevent and reverse the cancer process.

The key feature of salvestrols is that they are initially inert. They are activated only inside the cancer cells, which they arrest or kill. The anti-cancer effects are due, not to the plant chemicals themselves, but what they turn into within the cancer cells triggered by the presence of the CYP1B1 enzyme.

Where do we get salvestrols from?

Resveratrol, the first – but limited – salvestrol to be discovered, has been the subject of much research and has been shown to have many health benefits, including anti-cancer properties, especially for breast cancer.[62] Resveratrol is found most abundantly in red and green fruits and vegetables, mainly in organic produce (explained in more detail later on).

Importantly, some varieties contain salvestrols whereas others do not. So, it's no use saying 'eat an orange', for example, because many varieties have little if any intrinsic levels of salvestrols. Investigations have revealed that the salvestrol concentration of foods varies enormously and depends very much on where and how the plant is grown and the particular variety of fruit or vegetable.

Since salvestrols have a bitter taste, the problem is not only that we don't eat enough of these foods, but that salvestrols are depleted in the diet because of commercial food processing, often selecting and developing particular hybrids of plants to satisfy the demands for ever sweeter-tasting fruits and vegetables. Higher levels of salvestrols have been found in older, more bitter varieties of fruits and vegetables. In many cases salvestrols are extracted and filtered out – for example, in cranberry juice and olive oil. Unfortunately, these practices are removing the life-protecting salvestrols from our diet. Salvestrols are highest in stone-ground, unfiltered olive oil (if you can find it!) and in organic fruits and vegetables.

Nature's sources

There are thought to be around 50 salvestrols present in nature, found in a variety of different plants. The table opposite shows the main ones tested to date. As explained, it is not possible to rank foods in order of potency; for example, two Golden Delicious apples bought from different parts of the UK may vary, depending on where and how they were grown, regardless of the fact that they may both be organic. And a Gala apple will vary from Golden Delicious apples, and so on. Salvestrol activity ('points') can only be consistent ('standardised'), in supplement form. However, to give you an idea of how these points relate to the foods you eat, you can download a FREE recipe book – 'Salvestrol Richest Recipes' from http://www.naturesdefence.com.sg/dietrecipe.html.

Fruits	**Vegetables**	**Herbs**
Apples	Artichokes (globe)	Basil
Blackberries	Aubergines	Chamomile
Blackcurrants	Avocado	Dandelion
Blueberries	Beansprouts	Milk thistle
Cranberries	Broccoli	Mint
Grapes (and wine)	Brussels sprouts	Parsley
Oranges and tangerines	Cabbage	Rosemary
Pears	Cauliflower	Sage
Strawberries	Celery	Thyme
Redcurrants	Chinese leaf	
	Olives	
	Red/yellow peppers	
	Rocket	
	Watercress	

Diet and supplements

Salvestrols are good for all of us and need to be part of your daily diet. How many points you need on a daily basis will depend on what you are trying to achieve (see the table overleaf). Realistically, a non-organic diet will probably deliver 20 points a day if you eat lots (for example, at least five or more portions) of fruit and vegetables, and an organic diet probably 60–70, but it all depends on what specific foods you select. We are far removed in the practical sense from the Palaeolithic hunter-gatherer diet of our ancestors, estimated to provide around 100 points a day. And yet genetically, we are not that different.

To get the higher amounts means concentrated salvestrol food supplements. These were made available as a result of the demand from cancer patients when the original 'proof of principle' work was made public. A salvestrol supplement generally provides between 100 and 2,000 points per capsule. The lower dose being a preventative dose for a healthy individual while 4,000 points is for therapeutic purposes. However, please bear in mind that it is important to ensure that you get the right guidance from a nutritional therapist to ensure that you are taking the right supplements for your particular type of cancer.

Salvestrol points per day

Healthy (Palaeolithic) diet	100
Extra protection	350
Rescue recovery (2 × 2000 doses)	4,000

Why you don't get enough from food

Although some salvestrols can be obtained by eating lots of organic fruit and vegetables, extra virgin olive oils and unfiltered juices, for some of the reasons explained, it is difficult to get enough from diet alone. Generally, organic produce has a much higher salvestrol content compared to more intensively grown fruit – up to 30 times if grown without fungicides.

In modern agriculture, chemical fungicides are used extensively to prevent rot and fungal infections in fruits and vegetables. These dramatically reduce the natural salvestrol content of the food – if there is no fungi threatening the plant, there will be no stimulus for the plant to synthesise salvestrols. Also, many fungicide agents used in modern-day farming can interfere with the CYP1B1 mechanism and therefore block salvestrols' anti-cancer action within the body. In the context of the changes in farming methods, these findings could help explain rising cancer rates since we stopped eating organic and started eating foods sprayed with fungicides.

Decreasing salvestrol levels in wine

Even today's wine-making methods can deplete salvestrol levels. Traditionally, grape pulp is fermented with the skins still on, which results in resveratrol in wine. A bottle of wine made this way can contain 20mg of resveratrol, a significant salvestrol effect. Today, many red wines provide around 2mg of resveratrol – a tenth of traditional wine. This is because the grapes for the wine are fermented without the skins on. White wines, including champagne, are also produced this way, so there is no extraction of resveratrol and therefore no resveratrol in the wine.

Also, since some salvestrols can be extracted in hot water, it is best to use cooking liquids for sauces and gravy and generally to eat vegetables raw or steamed.

Should you supplement salvestrols?

Although there are now many thousands of people, mainly cancer patients, using salvestrols, and some extraordinary stories of recovery confirmed by their doctors, the hard evidence to date is specifically on human cancer cells tested in the laboratory in what's called 'in vitro' research. We do not yet have any published trials in cancer patients and will no doubt have to wait a few years for this level of evidence. As a review concluded,[63] the main issue is that randomised clinical trials (the so called 'gold standard' for medical evidence) are very costly and time-consuming, and are generally only carried out for patentable compounds. Since salvestrols are natural compounds, they cannot be patented and there is therefore not the funding available to perform such trials. It may be possible to carry out clinical trials, which are smaller and over a shorter period. However, for ethical reasons, such trials could initially only involve either those who fail to respond to standard conventional treatments, or individuals who reject conventional cancer treatment. However, five case reports were published in 2007 in the *Journal of Orthomolecular Medicine*. These included patients with various stage cancers of the lung, melanoma, prostate, breast and bladder.[64] In all cases the response was positive and, for some, apparently curative. (See www.patrickholford.com/salvestrolcasestudies.) If you want to take salvestrols in a concentrated amount, you may wish to explore the possible benefits of a salvestrol supplement. As TV doctor Chris Steele, who has been impressed with the results using salvestrols in some of his cancer patients, points out, 'it is extremely difficult to obtain all these phytonutrients from the diet, even if you have access to everything organic'. In fact, it is estimated that we now have only 10–20 per cent of the salvestrol component in our diet that we had 100 years ago. It seems that even an organic 'five-a-day' diet is unlikely to contain sufficient salvestrols and certainly not enough if you're fighting cancer.

So, should we all be supplementing salvestrols?

There's certainly a good case for supplementing. I take an antioxidant formula every day that contains salvestrols, and also a vitamin C supplement containing black elderberry and bilberry extracts. Time will tell if that's enough. If I had specific cancer concerns, I would certainly take an additional supplement of salvestrols from food concentrates.

Since salvestrols are natural extracts from organic foods, there is little danger or risk of harmful side effects, although some people may develop loose bowels from the high fruit concentrate used in some supplements.

Summary

The pedigree of the researchers is first class and the science is robust. The clinical evaluation of salvestrols is ongoing and will hopefully reveal their true importance to the maintenance of well-being in due course.

In the meantime, salvestrol supplements are available, generally providing between 100 and 2,000 points per capsule. As explained above, the lower dose is generally for those without cancer wanting to prevent it, whereas the higher doses are more for therapeutic purposes. However, if you have cancer, please bear in mind that it is important to ensure you get the right guidance from a practitioner who is knowledgeable in the use of salvestrols (see Resources).

CHAPTER 15

Good Fats and Bad Fats

O ur modern diet is too high in fat, which accounts for around 40 per cent of our total calorie intake. The ideal figure is around 20 per cent, with most government targets set at reducing fat intake to 30 per cent. Even more important than the quantity, however, is the kind of fat we eat and how we eat it.

Too much hard or saturated fat (the type found mainly in meat and dairy products) means a higher risk of cardiovascular disease and is tentatively linked to an increased risk of cancers of the lung and breast, according to the latest report from the World Cancer Research Fund (WCRF).[65] The World Health Organization's International Agency for Research on Cancer has also reported an association between increased risk of breast cancer in people who ate high-fat diets as children.

Interpreting the conflicting messages

A 2003 Harvard University study that included more than 90,000 premenopausal women showed that the women who had eaten the most animal fat had a significantly higher rate of breast cancer compared with women who ate the least.[66] However, a large study of American nurses showed that those who limited fat to 27 per cent of their calories were not any better off in preventing cancer than those consuming more fat.[67] It seems that while some studies have established a link between dietary fat intake and breast cancer risk, others, most of them involving postmenopausal women, have not supported this association.

There are many possible interpretations of the data. Since the associated cancers are primarily hormone-related, and since most saturated fat comes from intensively reared animals it may well be that eating a high-fat diet happens to increase a person's exposure to hormone-disrupting chemicals and hormones, and other growth promoters. Also, the higher the percentage of body fat, the more the hormone oestrogen is likely to be stored rather than removed.

A deficiency in essential fats

Perhaps even more significant is the fact that modern people are grossly deficient in essential or polyunsaturated fats, especially omega-3 fats – found in seeds, nuts, fish and their oils. Essential fats (which come in two families, known as omega-3 and omega-6 fats) are vital constituents of a healthy diet; they are unquestionably essential for the immune system and cell health.

Although polyunsaturated fats from fish, seeds and nuts are essential for health, they are also much more prone to damage – to becoming oxidised – than saturated fat. High temperatures or processing can make these good fats bad (hydrogenated fats and trans fats). Instead of getting our essential fats from raw seeds, nuts and their cold-pressed oils or fish, most of the polyunsaturated fats we take in are already damaged through heating or processing in the form of processed foods, margarine and refined oils used for frying. When coupled with a poor intake of antioxidants, this is a recipe for disaster.

Consequently, studies that have examined the association between polyunsaturated fats and cancer without determining what kind of polyunsaturates were being eaten, or how they were being processed, have produced mixed findings.

Fats that heal

There is, however, growing evidence that an increased intake of omega-3 fats (found in flaxseeds and fish, such as salmon, herring, mackerel and tuna) may reduce the risk of cancer. It is well documented that these fats help reduce inflammation and it is thought they prevent the expression of genes that promote cancer. Also, when the body is in a state of inflammation there is an increased chance of a cancer progressing into the metastatic phase with secondaries developing. Minimising inflammation through the use of omega-3 fats reduces the likelihood of this progression.[68] Studies have shown that lowering total dietary fats, limiting saturated fats and improving the ratio of omega-3 to omega-6 oils is likely to reduce the risk of breast cancer.[69] Omega-3 fats derived from fish oils appear to be the most protective.[70] A study involving more than 6,000 Swedish men aged 55 for a period of up to 30 years concluded that those eating fatty fish such as salmon, sardines, herring and mackerel cut their risk of prostate cancer by a third.[71] Another study from Korea found that a higher intake of fatty fish and omega-3 fats correlates with a lower risk of breast cancer.[72]

Fish oils seem to be protective in many ways. Animal studies have found that omega-3 fish oils encourage apoptosis, the process by which cancer cells commit suicide.[73] They can also boost immunity, as shown by a group of Greek scientists. They gave fish oil supplements (18mg fish oil, 115mg DHA and 200mg vitamin E) to malnourished cancer patients for 40 days and found significantly higher T-cell levels and an improved ratio of T-helper to T-suppressor cells, indicating improved immune strength.[74]

But if you eat more of all types of fish does it help prevent cancer?

A study undertaken by the Division of Human Nutrition, Wageningen University in the Netherlands, on people with colorectal polyps, the precursor of colorectal cancer, investigated this by giving either a serving of salmon or cod twice a week compared to basic dietary advice for six months. Both those eating salmon and cod showed no further progression of their pre-cancerous status. Since cod is not an oily fish and therefore not a good source of omega-3 fats this suggests there's more to fish than just the benefit of omega-3. Fish is also a rich source of many nutrients including B_{12}, selenium, zinc and vitamin D, all of which have anti-cancer properties.

Avoiding contamination in fish

For those dealing with hormone-related cancers it is also worth considering that many fish are polluted with PCBs and possibly mercury. PCBs tend to accumulate up the food chain, and store in fat, and are more likely to be concentrated in oily fish. Mercury is also higher in larger oily fish, generally in higher concentrations in fish bigger than salmon, such as tuna, swordfish and marlin. For purists, you can opt for a purified omega-3 fish oil supplement, free from PCBs and mercury. Arctic cod and halibut are among the least polluted fish.

Healthy choices

Both for cancer prevention and overall health, it is best to reduce your intake of saturated fats (principally from meat and dairy products) and processed or damaged fat (from fried and pro-cessed foods), and increase your intake of seeds, nuts and their cold-pressed oils or fish. The best seeds are those high in omega-3 fats, namely flax, followed by pumpkin seeds. Walnuts are good too. They are high in antioxidants and are anti-inflammatory.[75] An animal study in the US showed that the omega-3 fatty acids in walnuts may play a key role in reducing the risk of breast can-cer. Mice fed the human equivalent of 56.7g (2oz) of walnuts per day developed fewer and smaller tumours. Researcher Dr Elaine

Hardman, of Marshall University School of Medicine, said that although the study was carried out in mice, the beneficial effect of walnuts was likely to apply to humans too. These need to be eaten raw (not roasted or salted) and the fats are protected by vitamin E, which is naturally present in seeds. Taking a multivitamin that contains vitamin E further protects these important essential fats from oxidation.

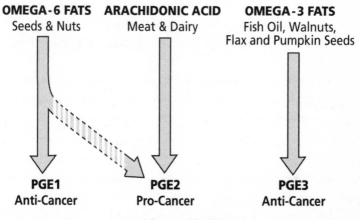

Good fats and bad fats

Fats that we eat are converted in the body into a number of hormone-like substances, called prostaglandins (or PGEs), which participate in a wide range of functions in the body, including modulation of inflammation. PGE 1 and 3 are predominantly anti-inflammatory (and therefore anti-cancer), whereas PGE2 is pro-inflammatory (and therefore more likely to be cancer promoting).

Cold-pressed is best

It's important to use only cold-pressed oils for salad dressings. Cold-pressed olive oil, rich in monounsaturated, not polyunsaturated fats, is associated with a reduced cancer incidence, as is a Mediterranean diet, with more fish, less meat and lots of fruit and vegetables.[76] Eating fried food, whatever the oil, has been linked to an increased risk of a number of cancers.

Summary

To maximise your protection from cancer:

- Eat oily fish two to three times a week – herring, mackerel, sardines and salmon – but also eat non-oily fish.
- Minimise your intake of saturated fat from meat and dairy products.
- If you are a vegetarian, make sure you have flaxseeds or flaxseed oil every day. If you are not a 100 per cent strict vegetarian I would recommend taking an omega-3 fish oil supplement.
- Minimise your intake of fried food. Boil, steam, poach or bake food instead.
- Add flaxseeds and pumpkin seeds to your breakfast, snack on walnuts or pumpkin seeds and use flaxseed oil in salad dressings. Generally avoid refined vegetable oils, using only cold-pressed oils.

CHAPTER 16

The GL Factor – Why Sweet Foods are Bad News

One of the most consistent recent findings is the link between sugar, weight gain and the increasing risk of cancer; for example, children whose diets are high in calories are at greater risk of developing cancer in later life. A report in the *British Medical Journal* examined a 1937 study of the diets of nearly 4,000 youngsters who were then traced in later life. The researchers found that the children who had had the highest-calorie diets had a 20 per cent higher risk of dying from cancer.[77] An analysis of the diets of colon cancer patients and a control group showed that a high calorie intake was associated with a higher risk of getting the disease.[78]

Take it slowly

Restricting calories doesn't mean you have to starve yourself; for example, the Japanese have a saying *hara hachi bu*, which means 'eat until you are 80 per cent full'. Stopping at 80 per cent capacity works because the stomach's stretch receptors take about 20 minutes to tell the body (via the brain) that it is full. So, the worst thing you can do is to eat 'fast' food that allows you to stuff yourself in ten minutes. Eating more slowly gives your body time to tell you that you are full.

Apart from the obvious benefit of maintaining an ideal body weight, which you will see is an important factor in protection against cancer and improving the prognosis of cancer patients, fewer calories also mean lower insulin levels. As you'll see later, high insulin levels are associated with many types of cancer.

Obesity and cancer

To put this into context, being obese puts you at almost as great a risk of cancer as smoking. According to Dr Walter Willett of the Harvard School of Public Health, being obese accounts for 14 per cent of cancer deaths in men and 20 per cent in women, compared with about 30 per cent each for smoking.[79] However, one of the most significant new risk factors for breast cancer are indicators of blood sugar problems.

Out-of-control blood sugar is bad for you

As I explain in detail in *The Low-GL Diet Bible* (Piatkus) one of the main drivers of weight gain, apart from excess calorie consumption, is what's called a high glycemic-load (GL) diet, meaning a diet that raises blood sugar levels.

The glycemic load (GL) is the measure of what a food does to your blood sugar. Neither protein nor fat (for example, meat, fish, cheese or eggs) has any substantial effect on your blood sugar balance, so I am talking here about sugary or carbohydrate-rich foods.

The sugars and starches in foods with a high GL (these are refined carbohydrates, such as white bread, sweets and biscuits) are broken down and absorbed quickly into the bloodstream making your blood glucose levels soar. You are likely to experience an increase in energy followed by an energy crash when your blood sugar drops, and you will probably reach for something sweet in order to relieve the symptoms of low blood sugar. Meanwhile, the sugars and starches in foods with a low GL (these are complex carbohydrates such as wholegrains, vegetables, beans or lentils, or simpler carbohydrates such as fruit) take longer to digest than refined carbohydrates. As a result, the glucose released from these foods trickles slowly into the bloodstream. This means that it's used for energy rather than being stored, leaving blood glucose levels on an even keel, and preventing dramatic changes in your mood, behaviour and energy.

When fast-releasing carbs become fat

When you eat a diet high in fast-releasing carbohydrates the body tries to compensate by releasing lots of insulin, whose job is to take excess sugar out of the blood and dump it into storage as fat. Then you feel hungry again, triggered by low blood sugar levels. The more this happens, the more insulin you make, but the more resistant your body becomes to its effects. This is called insulin resistance, which is a hallmark of what's called metabolic syndrome. Now your blood sugar level is going up and down like a yo-yo.

What happens when blood sugar fluctuates?

When blood sugar is too high, the excess sugar damages both your blood and arteries. This is called glycosylation, which is quite similar to oxidation; for example, red blood cells, called haemoglobin, become glycosylated. By measuring your level of glycosylated haemoglobin (also called HbA1c) you get one of the best measures as to whether you are losing your ability to control blood sugar. The other measure is your insulin levels.

Blood sugar lows also promote the release of the stress hormone cortisol, effectively getting you ready to hunt for food. Out-of-control blood sugar, if it continues long term, results in adrenal exhaustion (as explained in Chapter 9), while increasing blood sugar problems also tend to raise insulin-like growth factor (IGF-1), which as we saw in Chapter 12 promotes the growth of cancer cells.

The reason I tell you all this is that every single one of these factors is associated with quite a dramatic increase in cancer, especially of the breast. A high calorie intake, a high sugar intake, a high glycosylated haemoglobin level, a high insulin level, and high IGF-1 all correlate with increased risk of cancer. These are also all signs of a shift in your metabolism, the equivalent of your own internal 'global warming', called metabolic syndrome, again a major promoter of certain cancers.

Let's look at some of the evidence

Eating foods with a high glycemic index (GI) and/or glycemic load (GL) have been linked to a higher risk of many cancers, including breast,[80] colorectal,[81] pancreatic,[82] ovarian,[83] thyroid,[84] endometrial (womb),[85] and gastric.[86] Conversely, low-GI and/or low-GL diets are associated with a reduced risk of breast, colorectal, ovarian and endometrial (womb) cancers.[87]

GI and GL

It is worth explaining here the difference between GI and GL (glycemic index and glycemic load). The 'index' is a measure of the effects of carbohydrates on blood sugar levels, based on a fixed quantity of the food being measured, usually 50g (2oz). High-GI foods break down quickly during digestion and release glucose rapidly into the bloodstream, whereas low-GI foods break down more slowly, releasing glucose more gradually into the bloodstream. The 'load' is calculated by taking into account the GI of the food in question and the portion size, which is more useful since a high-GI food consumed in *small* quantities would give the same effect on blood sugar as *larger* quantities of a low-GI food.

For example, researchers in Italy in 2005 found that regularly eating sweet foods, including biscuits, brioches, cakes, ice cream, honey and chocolate, increased the risk of breast cancer. As the authors point out, these foods also contain other nutrients that are potentially involved in causing breast cancer, including saturated fats.[88] It is believed that a high-GL diet increases levels of insulin-related growth factors, primarily IGF-1, which are promoters of breast cancer. Insulin also stimulates hormones, including oestrogens, which have been related to excess breast cancer risk. Postmenopausal women with high insulin levels have been shown to have twice the risk of developing breast cancer.[89]

Women who gain weight throughout adulthood rather than maintaining a stable weight may have an increased risk of breast cancer, according to a report in the *Archives of Internal Medicine*. Women who were not obese or overweight at age 18 but were at ages 35 and 50 were 40 per cent more likely to develop breast cancer than women who maintained a normal weight.[90] Obesity is known to be a risk factor for developing breast cancer after menopause. Oestrogens can accumulate in fat tissue, potentially initiating or promoting the growth of cancerous cells in the breast.

Cancer risk has been found to be elevated in those with diabetes. A 2005 review of studies ranging from 1966 to 2005 found an 82 per cent increase in risk of pancreatic cancer.[91] Two other reviews by Swedish researchers reported a 30 per cent increase in risk of colorectal cancer and a 20 per cent increase in risk of breast cancer.[92]

The ups and downs of glucose

The level of glucose in your blood largely determines your appetite. When the level drops you feel hungry. The glucose in your bloodstream is available to body cells to make energy. When the levels are too high the body converts the excess to glycogen (short-term fuel mainly stored in the liver and muscle cells) or fat, our long-term energy reserve. When the levels are too low we experience a whole host of symptoms, including fatigue, poor concentration, irritability, nervousness, depression, excessive thirst, sweating, headaches and digestive problems. An estimated three in every ten people have glucose intolerance (an inability to keep an even blood sugar level). Their blood sugar level may go up too high and then drop too low. The result, over the years, is that they become increasingly fat and lethargic. On the other hand, if you can control your blood sugar levels, the result is even weight and constant energy.

Glucose tolerance check

If you answer 'yes' to eight or more of the questions below there's a strong possibility that your body is having difficulty keeping your blood sugar level even.

- Are you rarely wide awake within 20 minutes of rising?
- Do you need tea, coffee, a cigarette or something sweet to get you going in the morning?
- Do you really like sweet foods?
- Do you crave bread, cereal, popcorn or pasta?
- Do you feel like you 'need' an alcoholic drink on most days?
- Are you overweight and unable to shift the extra pounds?
- Do you often have energy slumps throughout the day or after meals?
- Do you have mood swings or difficulty concentrating?
- Do you get dizzy or irritable if you go six hours without food?
- Do you often find you overreact to stress?
- Do you often get irritable, angry or aggressive unexpectedly?
- Is your energy level now lower than it used to be?
- Do you ever lie about how much sweet food you have eaten?
- Do you ever keep a supply of sweet food close to hand?
- Do you feel you could never give up bread?

Fast-release and slow-release foods

So what makes your blood sugar level unbalanced? Obviously eating too much sugar and sweet foods. However, the kinds of food that have the greatest effect are not always the ones you might expect.

Alcohol, a chemical cousin of sugar, also upsets blood sugar levels. So do stimulants, such as tea, coffee, cola drinks and cigarettes. These substances, like stress itself, stimulate the release of adrenalin and other hormones that initiate the 'fight or flight' response. This prepares the body for action, by releasing sugar stores and raising blood sugar levels to give our muscles and brains a boost of energy. Unlike

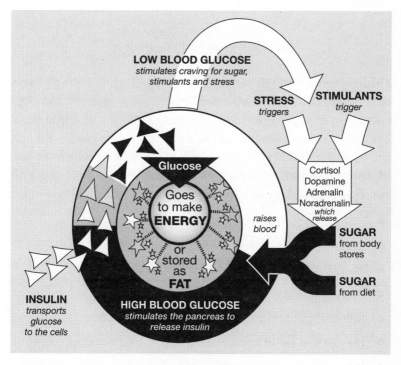

The sugar cycle

Eating sugar increases blood glucose levels. The body releases insulin into the blood to help escort glucose out and into body cells, to make energy or convert into fat. The result is low blood glucose. Either stress, causing more adrenalin, or induced stress, caused by consuming a stimulant such as caffeine, which raises adrenal hormones, causes breakdown of stores of sugar in the liver and muscles, called glycogen, which raises blood sugar levels. Low blood glucose causes stress or cravings for either something sweet or a stimulant.

our ancestors, whose main stresses required a physical response (like climbing up a tree to avoid being eaten for dinner), 20th-century stress is mainly mental or emotional. It still provokes the same response though, so the body has to cope with the excess of blood sugar by releasing yet more hormones to take the glucose out of circulation. The combination of too much sugar, stimulants and prolonged stress taxes the body and results in an inability to control blood sugar levels, which, if severe enough, can develop into diabetes.

Getting the balance right

The only way out of this vicious circle is to reduce or avoid all forms of concentrated sweetness as well as tea, coffee, alcohol and cigarettes, and to start eating foods that help to keep your blood sugar level even. The best foods are all kinds of beans, peas and lentils, oats and wholegrains. These foods are high in complex carbohydrates and contain special factors that help to release their sugar content gradually. They are also high in fibre, which helps to normalise blood sugar levels.

The golden rules for blood sugar balance

1   Eat low-GL foods
2   Eat protein with carbohydrate
3   Graze, don't gorge – eat little and often

The carbs that keep blood sugar even

The chart on pages 147–9 gives the GL score of an average serving of a range of common foods. Foods with a GL of less than 10 (shown in bold) are good and should be the staple foods of your diet. A GL of 11–14 (shown in regular type) can be eaten in moderation. A GL that is higher than 15 (shown in italics) should be avoided.

Glycemic load of common foods

Food	Serving size in grams	Serving	GLs per serving
Bakery products			
low-carb muffin	**60**	**1 muffin**	**5**
muffin – apple, made without sugar	**60**	**1 muffin**	**9**
muffin – apple, made with sugar	60	1 muffin	13
crumpet	50	1 crumpet	13
croissant	*57*	*1 croissant*	*17*
doughnut, plain	*47*	*1 doughnut*	*17*
sponge cake, plain	*63*	*1 slice*	*17*
Breads			
wholemeal rye or pumpernickel-style rye bread	**20**	**1 thin slice**	**5**
wheat tortilla (Mexican)	**30**	**1 tortilla**	**5**
wholemeal wheat-flour bread	**30**	**1 thick slice**	**9**
pitta bread, white	**30**	**1 pitta bread**	**10**
baguette, white, plain	*30*	*⅓ baton*	*15*
bagel, white	*70*	*1 bagel*	*25*
Crispbreads and crackers			
rough oatcakes (Nairn's)	**10**	**1 oatcake**	**2**
fine oatcakes (Nairn's)	**9**	**1 oatcake**	**3**
cream cracker	25	2 biscuits	11
rye crispbread	25	2 biscuits	11
water cracker	*25*	*3 biscuits*	*17*
puffed rice cakes	*25*	*3 biscuits*	*17*
Dairy products and alternatives			
yoghurt (plain, no sugar)	**200**	**1 small pot**	**3**
non-fat yoghurt (plain, no sugar)	**200**	**1 small pot**	**3**
soya yoghurt (Provamel)	**200**	**1 large bowl**	**7**
soya milk (no sugar)	**250ml**	**1 glass**	**7**
low-fat yoghurt, fruit, sugar (Ski)	**150**	**1 small pot**	**7.5**

cont ▶

Food	Serving size in grams	Serving	GLs per serving
Fruit and fruit products			
blackberries, raw	120	1 medium bowl	1
blueberries, raw	120	1 medium bowl	1
raspberries, raw	120	1 medium bowl	1
strawberries, raw	120	1 medium bowl	1
cherries, raw	120	1 medium bowl	3
grapefruit, raw	120	½ medium	3
pear, raw	120	1 medium	4
melon/cantaloupe, raw	120	½ small	4
watermelon, raw	120	1 medium slice	4
apricots, raw	120	4	5
oranges, raw	120	1 large	5
plum, raw	120	4	5
apple, raw	120	1 small	6
kiwi fruit, raw	120	1	6
pineapple, raw	120	1 medium slice	7
grapes, raw	120	16	8
mango, raw	120	1½ slices	8
apricots, dried	60	6	9
fruit cocktail, canned (Del Monte)	120	small can	9
papaya, raw	120	½ small papaya	10
prunes, pitted	60	6	10
apple, dried	60	6 rings	10
banana, raw	120	1 small	12
apricots, canned in light syrup	120	1 small can	12
lychees, canned in syrup and drained	120	*1 small can*	16
figs, dried, tenderised (Dessert Maid)	60	*3*	16
sultanas	60	*30*	25
raisins	60	*30*	28
dates, dried	60	*8*	42

cont ▶

Food	Serving size in grams	Serving	GLs per serving
Jams/spreads			
pumpkin seed butter	16	1 tbsp	1
peanut butter (no sugar)	16	1 tbsp	1
blueberry spread (no sugar)	10	2 tsp	1
orange marmalade	10	2 tsp	3
strawberry jam	10	2 tsp	3
Snack foods (savoury)			
eggs (boiled)	–	2 medium	0
cottage cheese	120	½ medium tub	2
hummus	200	1 small tub	6
olives, in brine	50	7	1
peanuts	50	2 medium handfuls	1
cashew nuts, salted	50	2 medium handfuls	3
potato crisps, plain, salted	30	1 small packet	7
popcorn, salted	25	1 small packet	10
pretzels, oven-baked, traditional wheat flavour	*30*	*15*	*16*
corn chips, plain, salted	*50*	*18*	*17*
Snack foods (sweet)			
Fruitus apple cereal bar	**35**	**1**	**5**
Euroviva Rebar fruit and veg bar	**50**	**1**	**8**
muesli bar with dried fruit	30	1	13
chocolate bar, milk, plain (Mars/Cadbury/Nestlé)	50	1	14
Twix biscuit and caramel bar (Mars)	*60*	*1 bar (2 fingers)*	*17*
Snickers bar (Mars)	*60*	*1*	*19*
Polos, peppermint sweets (Nestlé)	*30*	*16*	*21*
Jelly beans, assorted colours	*30*	*9*	*22*
Kellogg's Pop-Tarts, double choc	*50*	*1*	*24*
Mars bar	*60*	*1*	*26*

A comprehensive list of the GL values of foods is also available online at www.holforddiet.com. This allows you to 'build a menu' and also work out your total GL intake for the day.

Healthy snack options

Try these alternatives:

- **Instead of crisps**, have oatcakes with some nut butter or hummus, pumpkin seeds, roasted snack mix or plain popcorn.
- **Instead of biscuits**, have a sweet oatcake biscuits (such as Nairn's) or fruit or nut bars (such as Fruitus bar by Lyme Regis Foods).
- **Instead of sweets and chocolate**, have fresh fruit (apple, pear, peach, plum, berries) or dried fruits such as apricots (these are a concentrated source of natural sugars, so eat in moderation).
- **Instead of sugar** (in drinks and home baking), have xylitol (it tastes just like sugar but doesn't upset blood sugar balance or cause tooth decay).
- **Instead of sweetened drinks**, drink water, fruity/herbal teas, diluted fruit juice (gradually increase the amount of water to let your taste buds adjust), diluted apple and blackcurrant concentrate, such as Meridian or cherry concentrate such as CherryActive.

Important: stay off the caffeine

Sugar isn't the only factor in blood sugar problems. Stimulants are, too. And as caffeine is a powerful one, it can be highly disruptive to your blood sugar balance. The biggest culprits are cola and energy drinks, chocolate bars and chocolate drinks, tea and coffee. Instead, have herbal teas or rooibos (redbush) tea or green tea in moderation (a maximum of three cups a day). You can also have decaf tea or coffee, but these still contain some stimulants. A stimulant-free alternative, such as a grain or dandelion coffee substitute, is better. My favourite coffee substitutes are Teeccino and Caro Extra. These are available in health-food stores. You may experience 'withdrawal' symptoms, such as headaches, when you give up caffeine, but these will disappear within a couple of days – unless you have a serious addiction to caffeine. In that case, as the first symptoms subside you may begin to experience some of the ongoing abstinence symptoms. Stabilising your blood sugar is an important part of decreasing their severity.

Eat protein with carbohydrate

The more fibre and protein you include with any meal or snack, the slower the release of the carbohydrates, which is good for blood-glucose balance. So, combining protein-rich foods with high-fibre carbohydrates at *every* meal (and even with snacks) is an excellent rule of thumb. Here are some ways to combine carbohydrates and protein:

- Eat unsalted seeds or nuts with a whole fruit snack.

- Add seeds or nuts to carbohydrate-based breakfast cereals.

- Top wholemeal toast with eggs, baked beans or nut butter.

- Serve salmon or chicken with brown basmati rice.

- Add kidney beans to pasta sauce served over wholemeal pasta.

- Put cottage cheese on oatcakes, or hummus on pumpernickel-style wholegrain rye bread.

- Make sandwiches with sugar-free peanut butter and wholemeal bread.

What about high-protein diets?

Very high-protein diets have proved effective in managing blood sugar, but they are not great for your health in the long term. This is because too much protein, especially from meat and dairy products, can have negative effects on the kidneys and bones, as well as being associated with a higher incidence of breast, prostate and colorectal cancer.

A better way

You can get the best of both worlds, however: you can have good health as well as a rich supply of amino acids – by eating protein-rich foods together with low-GL carbohydrates.

> ## Remember
>
> You need some protein with every meal, because protein provides
> essential amino acids, and you need low-GL carbs to give you energy.

For breakfast, you can achieve the correct balance and amount
of protein and low-GL carbohydrate by, for example, eating some
seeds, yoghurt or either skimmed milk or soya milk, with your cereal
and fruit. If you have an egg on toast, or kippers and oatcakes you've
done it already.

The fibre factor

Most people think of fibre as roughage – the indigestible part of plant
foods that helps to clean out our insides. What fibre actually does is
absorb water in the digestive tract, thereby bulking out faecal matter,
which then passes more easily through the body. This means that our
exposure to carcinogen-containing foods is shorter. It also minimises
the formation of carcinogens, which can occur if the food passes
through slowly, and, in effect, rots inside us.

Fibre offers protection

Not surprisingly, having enough fibre in your diet correlates with a
lower risk of colorectal cancer, and possibly oesophageal cancer too.[93]
Diets high in complex carbohydrates and low in fat are also high in
fibre, and a high-fibre diet is associated with protection against colon
cancer.[94] There is little doubt that the modern diet – high in alcohol,
sugar and fat, and low in fibre – wreaks havoc on the digestive tract.
Such a diet disrupts the sensitive balance of beneficial bacteria there
(see Chapter 30), inflames the digestive tract wall and disturbs the
gut-associated immune system.

All this is known as 'dysbiosis' and can easily be tested by stool
analysis, which measure the presence of certain markers of digestive

disease. These include butyric acid and beta-glucoronidase. Butyric acid is a kind of fat that actually feeds and nourishes the digestive tract. A certain proportion of fibre is fermented into butyric acid. Without this source of fuel, the digestive tract is more likely to become inflamed, paving the way for colon cancer.[95] Having too much beta-glucoronidase is another useful marker for cancer risk, both of the digestive tract and of the breast. Beta-glucoronidase is a carcinogen made within a digestive tract in a state of dysbiosis. It interferes with the liver's ability to break down oestrogen, which results in its continued circulation, thereby contributing to oestrogen dominance, a known risk factor for breast cancer.

This may explain why a study in China concluded that consumption of foods rich in fibre (as well as vitamin C and carotene) helped protect against breast cancer.[96] In another study from Uruguay an examination of the diets of over 700 women found a strong link between dietary fibre intake and a reduction in the risk of breast cancer in both pre- and post-menopausal women.[97] In a more recent study, pre-menopausal women with the greatest intake of fibre cut their risk of breast cancer in half.[98]

Fibre favourites

The best way to increase your fibre intake is to eat wholefoods, such as wholegrains, lentils, beans, nuts, seeds and vegetables, all of which contain fibre. Some of the fibre in vegetables is destroyed by cooking, so you should also eat something raw every day.

The correct balance

The simplest way to plan your meals, as far as lunch and dinner are concerned, is to think of them divided into quarters. Visualise a protein-rich food portion (roughly the size of the palm of your hand), filling one-quarter of your dinner plate, and an equivalent-sized serving of any carbohydrate-rich food filling the other quarter, then a large salad or two servings of vegetables filling the remainder of the plate. So, half of what's on your plate is vegetables, one-quarter is a protein-rich food and one-quarter is a carbohydrate-rich food.

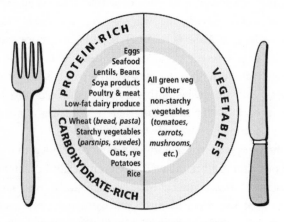

The perfectly balanced dinner plate

Summary

- Eat low-GL foods.
- Eat protein with carbohydrate to help balance blood sugar.
- Eat little and often.
- Eat wholefoods, such as wholegrains, lentils, beans, nuts, seeds and vegetables every day – all of which contain fibre.
- Balance your meals by filling half your plate with vegetables, one-quarter with a protein-rich food and one-quarter with a carbohydrate-rich food.
- Avoid alcohol and cut back on caffeine, sugar and fat.
- Maintain a healthy weight and engage in regular physical exercise to help reduce insulin levels.

The most practical way to learn how to eat a low-GL diet is to follow *The Low-GL Diet Bible*. This book, and *The Low-GL Diet Cookbook*, provides many excellent recipes. There are even more in *Food Glorious Food*, all published by Piatkus.

CHAPTER 17

Alcohol, Coffee and Tea – the Whole Truth

There is no question that alcohol is a powerful carcinogen. It damages intestinal bacteria, converting them into secondary metabolites that increase proliferation of cells in the colon, hence initiating cancer. It can also be absorbed directly into the mucosal cells that line the digestive tract, and is converted into aldehyde, which interferes with DNA repair and promotes tumour development. In addition, alcohol consumption may lead to nutritional deficiencies, affecting the absorption of cancer-fighting nutrients.

When a number of studies were 'pooled together' to evaluate a total of 322,647 women, researchers found a greater risk of breast cancer among those who drank alcohol and concluded that, in women who consume alcohol regularly, reducing alcohol consumption is a potential means to reduce breast cancer risk.[99] Another study reported a suppression of the immune system during acute alcohol intoxication as well as an increased risk of cancers 'metastasising' or spreading, due to decreased activity of the natural killer immune cells (which protect against both cancer cells and infections).

A 2006 review of more than 20 research studies, published in the medical journal *Lancet Oncology*, came to the conclusion that there is an especially strong relationship between alcohol consumption and cancers of the breast, colorectum, liver, oral cavity, pharynx, larynx and oesophagus. There is also a suspected link for cancers of the pancreas and lung.[100] According to the 2007 report from the World Cancer Research Fund, the evidence that all types of alcoholic drink are a cause of a number of cancers is now stronger than it was in the 1990s and they cite hundreds of studies associating alcohol with increased cancer incidence.[101] The question is, how much is too much?

Alcohol: how much can you drink?

The World Cancer Research Fund advises that even small amounts of alcoholic drinks should be avoided and, if consumed at all, should be limited to no more than two drinks a day for men and one drink a day for women. For breast cancer, the risk increases at even one drink a day, and less if your homocysteine level is high and/or you have low levels of folate, in which case the risk increases above three drinks a week. Another study in Finland, which followed over 27,000 men for up to eight years, found that the risk of colorectal cancer increased with the amount of alcohol consumed.[102]

Are any alcoholic drinks less harmful?

If you are going to drink, red wine is probably your best choice. It has been well publicised that substances in red wine have shown a protective effect against heart disease. As with many foods, it is likely that this is due to its antioxidant properties. One study, which involved feeding mice a diet including red wine, found that those given the wine were free of tumours for 40 per cent longer than those not given wine.[103] You could, of course, eat grapes or drink red grape juice instead and obtain the antioxidants from grapes without the alcohol! Juice made from 'concord' grapes is the best in this regard, but don't have more than half a glass a day due to the high sugar content.

Bad partners

Drinking alcohol and smoking is a lethal combination. Both can initiate cancer. Alcohol's suppressive effect on the immune system means it increases the risk of any cancer spreading; hence it is considered a 'co-carcinogen' for many cancers.

The dangers of caffeine

Although some studies have shown an increased incidence of pancreatic cancer with coffee consumption,[104] further studies have not shown such an association. Over the last decade considerable research has been undertaken on the cancer–coffee link. Most of these studies have come to the conclusion that coffee is unlikely to increase the risk of any cancer, except possibly for that of the bladder.

However, caffeine may increase symptoms of fibrocystic breast disease, a common but benign breast condition – a significant association was found in those drinking four or more cups a day.[105]

Caffeine also raises levels of the stress hormones adrenalin and cortisol (see Chapter 9) and also substances that reliably indicate inflammation, such as interleukin-6, TNF, C-reactive protein and homocysteine[106] (see Chapter 8). A Greek study from 2004 that involved over 3,000 participants found that those consuming 200ml of coffee – two cups – had between 28 and 50 per cent higher levels of three kinds of inflammatory markers compared to non-coffee consumers.[107] It is highly unlikely that the consumption of fewer than two cups of coffee a day adds any cancer risk.

Tea – is it good for you?

On the other hand, tea is good or bad depending on which kind you drink and how you drink it. Green tea is associated with decreasing risk of colorectal cancer.[108] Scientists have been researching green tea for decades[109] and some clinical trials investigating green tea consumption by cancer patients have found potential benefits.[110] The health benefits of green tea stem from the antioxidant properties of catechins, or polyphenolic compounds that are especially high in green tea due to its unique preparation. It is known that antioxidant levels increase in the blood after green tea consumption, which could prevent free radicals from damaging the body (see Chapter 2). However, drinking a lot of tea or coffee is not recommended from an overall health point of view. Both contain addictive stimulants, and too many stimulants have negative effects on mental performance, stress and energy levels.

One tea, maté, drunk in large quantities in South America, appears to increase the risk of mouth and oesophageal cancer. This is most likely due to the high temperature and the fact that it is drunk through a metal straw. However, so too does drinking very hot drinks, as this can damage the membrane that lines the throat and oesophagus.

Summary

Overall, the general advice is:

- Don't drink alcohol and, if you do, limit your intake to two drinks a day (if you are male) and one drink a day (if you are female).
- Drink green tea and 'red' herb teas, such as rooibos, rosehip, hibiscus and berry teas, which are rich in antioxidants, or regular tea in preference to coffee. However, for general health, don't drink excessive amounts of either.

PART 3

ANTI-CANCER LIFESTYLE FACTORS

CHAPTER 18

Protecting Yourself from Radiation

There is no question that radiation initiates cancer and that we are all exposed to substantial levels of it. The questions are: what kind and how much radiation significantly affects your risk of developing cancer and what can you do to reduce your exposure?

We are all exposed to radiation from the atmosphere, and not just from man-made sources – in fact, two-thirds of our radiation exposure is from nature. There are naturally occurring radio-active materials in air, food and water. We receive the majority of our radiation from natural sources, and the minority from X-rays, nuclear incidents or leaks, and possibly from other factors such as mobile phones. Air travel also increases exposure.

'Radiation' is a broad term, which includes such things as light waves, radio waves and microwaves. However, it is most often used to mean ionising radiation – that is, radiation that produces free oxidising radicals, which, in turn, can initiate cancer (see Chapter 2). The long-term consequences of excessive exposure can include leukaemia and other kinds of cancer (breast and thyroid, for example), as well as infertility, eye cataracts and skin damage.

How radiation works

Not all radiation, however, is ionising radiation. To understand what does and doesn't put you at risk, it's helpful to understand how radiation works. Atoms, when 'excited', give off energy. This energy travels as a wave that radiates out from the source – hence the term 'radiation'. If the wave has a high frequency, it has a lot of energy – it can pass through things and can trigger changes (that is, it can generate those harmful 'free radicals' in the body). The radiation that comes off uranium, for example, fits into this category. The sun also emits high-frequency radiation. UV radiation from sunlight or sunlamps causes both malignant melanoma and non-melanoma skin cancer. Although UVB rays are the most damaging to our DNA, UVA rays damage DNA through the generation of free radicals (see Chapter 2).

However, it isn't just the frequency that determines how potentially harmful the radiation is. It's also the intensity – the power of the signal. So, although the sun emits high-frequency radiation, by the time it gets to us across millions of miles of space, especially if passing through layers of clouds, it's relatively harmless. Not so, however, if you spend an hour in the scorching heat at the equator. So, the higher the frequency, the stronger the signal, and the closer you are to the source, the more high-energy particles you are exposed to, with an accompanying increase in the generation of harmful free radicals. On the other hand, a low-frequency signal, like a radio wave, may produce a bit of heat but doesn't contain anything like enough energy to generate free radicals and harm you.

The dangers of computers and TV

The radiation that comes off your radio, TV and computer screens is not likely to present any health risk, because it is low energy, although it's a good idea to have some ventilation, as many appliances dry the air and generate heat. Watching TV a foot away from the screen 24 hours a day might, however, pose a health hazard. Some people choose to fit filters on their computer screens to cut down the radiation. Generally, it is a good idea to sit as far away from the screen as you realistically can so that the energy in the particles dissipates before it gets to you.

Microwave ovens

Although microwave ovens are high energy, the waves are relatively contained within a metal box, so you are not exposed – at least providing you have a more modern and better-quality unit. However, the intense heat generated by microwaving fatty foods generates free radicals, much like frying, so this is not a recommended cooking technique.

Mobile phones – are they a health hazard?

The frequency of the signal from a mobile phone is quite low. However, the strength of the signal and, most importantly, the fact that the source (the phone) is right next to your brain, has raised concerns about whether the energy is strong enough to generate free radicals and hence increase cancer risk.

In the late 1990s, Australian research found a doubling of tumours in mice exposed to radiation at mobile phone frequencies. In research led by Dr Michael Repacholi (who headed the WHO programme studying the possible hazards of electromagnetic fields until his retirement in June 2006), the mice were exposed to pulsed radiation for one hour a day for nine to 18 months. At the end of the trial, the mice showed twice as many B-cell lymphomas.[1] (B-cell effects are implicated in roughly 85 per cent of all cancers.) Additional research by Lester Packer and colleagues also linked electromagnetic fields to increases in cancer.[2] Although mice are not human beings, these findings are worrying, because there is evidence of an increase in the incidence of brain cancer in correlation with the widespread use of mobile phones. Dr Andrew Davidson, at the Fremantle Hospital in Australia, analysed the incidence of brain cancer in Australia from 1982 to 1992. His survey showed double the number of cases.[3] Brain cancer is also on the increase in Britain and the US for no apparent reason.

Safety levels around the world

Over four billion people around the world now use mobile phones. Many scientific experts believe that safety standards in the UK are inadequate, and that we must protect ourselves from exposure to radiation from sources such as mobile phones. A detailed summary of the science behind these concerns was compiled by 27 experts in the field and published, in 2007, in a report called the Bioinitiative Report.[4] Among its many recommendations was one that the safe level of exposure to the kind of microwaves used in mobile phones should be 1,000 microwatts per square metre. In the UK the level, set a decade ago, is 10,000,000 microwatts. The safety level in Russia, China, Switzerland and Luxemburg is 100 times lower at 100,000.

Has there been any recent research about risk?

In September 2009, the Radiation Research Trust held a major conference in London where academics from both the safe and not-safe camps sat side by side for the first time.

The most striking report came from a Swedish researcher, Dr Lennart Hardell, an oncologist at University Hospital in Orebro in Sweden, who had already found a connection with long-term mobile phone use and brain cancer in adults. He has found that the brain cancer risk for children who regularly use a mobile phone before the age of 20 goes up five times.[5] 'Our study showed that children under 20 who regularly use a mobile phone have a four or five times greater risk of brain cancer than adults,' he told the conference. He went on to say that the effect of mobile phone radiation is different in children's brains from adult ones, as more of their brain is exposed to it and the cancer risk rises the earlier they start using it. What's more, the risk showed up as the same whether they were using mobile phones or cordless ones that transmit a signal back to the base station. This view was supported by a senior Russian academic, Professor Yuri Grigorie of the Russian Federal Medical Biophysical Centre.

What is shocking about this increasing evidence of a risk to children is that it was first flagged up officially eight years ago in the UK, in what is known as the Stewart report. It made precisely the same point about children's skulls being more vulnerable and advised taking a 'precautionary approach' that is still the basis of the official policy today. So you might imagine that since then government agencies such as the Health Protection Agency (HPA) would have made a serious effort to both warn parents of the possible dangers and to set up research projects to prove or disprove them. In fact, very little has been done on either count.

So what exactly is a 'precautionary approach'? It is explained in a Department of Health leaflet, put out after the Stewart report, which recommended that children under 16 should only make mobile phone calls for essential purposes and that they should be kept short. But have you ever seen such a leaflet? If you blinked you could well have missed it, and since then there has certainly been no attempt to reinforce it. And there are no warnings on mobile phone packaging or talks about the dangers in schools.

When asked about the new brain cancer research at the London conference, an official with the HPA commented that the study only involved a small number of subjects and if people were concerned 'they could take protective action if they want to'.

Mobile phone warnings

Many health authorities around the world, rather than relying on individuals taking precautions, are now warning about mobile phones in a more direct way:

● Toronto Public Health in Canada asked parents to think twice before giving their children a mobile phone. It advised teens to limit their time on a phone and recommended that prepubescent children should only use landlines.

- The French Health Ministry, at the beginning of 2008, gave even more specific advice, saying that children should avoid calling when reception is poor (which means the emitting signal has to be stronger) and should keep phones away from sensitive areas of their bodies with a hands-free kit. At the same time, a group of 19 French scientists concerned about mobile phone dangers stated that parents should forbid all children under the age of 12 to use mobiles! This is supported by Dr Lennart Hardell, who advises that children under 12 should not use mobiles except in cases of emergency and that teenagers should use hands-free devices or headsets and use texting instead of calls.

- The University of Pittsburgh Cancer Institute, a leading cancer centre in the States, has advised all employees to keep mobile use to a minimum because of the possible cancer risk. The director, Dr Ronald B. Herberman, said he was basing his alarm on early unpublished data, saying, 'It takes too long to get answers from science and I believe people should take action now, especially when it comes to children.'

Until we know for sure, it would seem prudent to use your mobile phone infrequently or use them with earphones.

Mobile phone safety guidelines

The current measure used to classify a mobile phone as 'safe' is called the specific absorption rating (SAR). The SAR level relates to the intensity of the signal, which is measured as watts per kilogram (W/kg). Although the current control on mobile phones is 2W/kg, the best phones on the market have an SAR of less than 0.5. To discover the SAR of your personal phone, visit the Mobile Operators Association website www.mobilemastinfo.com or call your mobile phone company.

X-rays

Another definite source of high-energy radiation is X-rays. For this reason it is not advisable to have them frequently. This, of course, raises a dilemma when it comes to mammograms, introduced as an early warning system for identifying breast cancer. Some argue that if these were used as a regular screening programme, the cumulative effects of the X-rays might counteract the small benefit achieved in early diagnosis.

While the general recommendation in the UK is to have three-yearly screens, Dr Karol Sikora, honorary Consultant Oncologist at Hammersmith Hospital, believes that, under the age of 47, there is no benefit from screening and he doesn't recommend it. Since the first issue of this book, the age has been reduced by the Department of Health to 47 rather than 50, based on new data, and the new digital machines have more than halved the radiation dose. Having a mammogram is certainly not something a pregnant woman would be advised to do. The late Dr John Lee said that mammograms often pick up microcalcifications (small calcium deposits) in the breast. Whether or not these warrant treatment is a matter of debate, since microcalcifications may not be cancer as we know it. Both Sikora and Lee favour regular breast examination to identify any suspect changes.

Ironically, another major source of radiation exposure is radio-therapy, used to treat cancer. This is only recommended when there is an advanced malignant tumour that can be pinpointed in order to minimise surrounding damage. The radiation damages the DNA of the cancer cells and there is obviously the risk of damaging some healthy cells too. Radiation treatment is carcinogenic in itself, and, as such, requires serious consideration for cancer treatment (I discuss this more in Chapters 36 and 37).

Nuclear power – is it safe?

Despite denials by the nuclear industry, there is some evidence to show an increased incidence of childhood leukaemia in certain regions adjacent to nuclear power generators; for example, research published in the *British Medical Journal* in October 1987 looked at two groups of children: 1,068 born near Sellafield in Cumbria and 1,564 born outside the area but attending nearby schools.[6] The leukaemia and cancer cases occurred only in those children born near the Sellafield nuclear reprocessing plant. And there are other areas of 'leukaemia clusters' adjacent to nuclear installations. However, it is also true that major improvements have been made in safety standards and it is quite possible that such risk is confined to old reactors and errors, such as leaks. However, there are good grounds for society to remain extra vigilant about the safety measures surrounding the handling of nuclear fuel.

Natural radiation

Apart from the effects of sunlight (discussed in the next chapter), the largest 'natural' source of radiation is radon. Radon is a naturally occurring gas that is present in some areas due to the underlying geology. As uranium in rocks decays, it produces radon, which escapes – colourless and odourless – into the air. Uranium and its decay product radium are found naturally in rocks and soil and also in building materials such as wood, bricks and concrete. When the decay by-products are inhaled (contained in small dust particles), the radioactive molecules settle in the lungs and irradiate intensely at close range for many years.

In the open air any radon is mixed and diluted with air and quickly dispersed. Inside buildings, however, it is released from construction materials and from the ground, and is then inhaled by the occupants.

Where you live will make a difference

Recent surveys carried out in the UK suggest that residents in some parts of the country are at greater risk than others. The south-west seems to be the most affected area, but there are also other local 'hot spots'. Areas with high levels of granite are the most affected. In some cases the radiation dose from radon accounts for over 50 per cent of the total natural radiation. At this level, it could be responsible for several hundred deaths from cancer per year. A study by the Imperial Cancer Research Fund shows that people exposed to radon have a 20 per cent higher chance of contracting lung cancer; indeed it attributes 1,800 lung cancer deaths a year to radon exposure.[7]

If you live in an area that is largely granite, most common in the south-west of England, contact your local environmental health officer to find out what your radon exposure is likely to be. When radon levels are high, it is better to use certain building materials than others. Adequate ventilation under floorboards is also important to remove the radioactive compounds before they can build up to significant levels.

Protecting yourself from radiation

Radioactive elements can be taken up by the body and incorporated into your tissues where they continue to emit radiation. An example is radioactive iodine, which is taken up by the thyroid gland. By ensuring a more than adequate intake of minerals (in this case iodine), tissues are saturated with non-radioactive elements and are therefore protected.

However, the more forms of radiation we are exposed to (for example, from the sun or mobile phones), the more free radicals (oxidants) are likely to be generated that can harm body cells. So, in addition to minimising exposure, the most important protection factor is to ensure an optimal intake of antioxidant nutrients, such as vitamins A, C and E, and the minerals zinc and selenium. These help protect against the damage caused by ionising radiation.

If you are concerned about your exposure to electromagnetic radiation (EMR) fields, you can buy a device called an electrosmog detector, which turns EMR into sound. The louder and dirtier the sound, the more aggressive the EMR signal. Turning this invisible energy into sound could be a real eye-opener; for example, I turned on my microwave oven and the electrosmog detector howled, and only stopped howling 4½m (15ft) away, even if I stood behind a solid brick wall. It is important to keep at least 3m (10ft) away from a microwave oven while it is on.

Summary

- Get an electrosmog detector and check out your appliances and hot spots in your home and office (available from Totally Nourish, see Resources). Don't buy a new house without checking it out.
- Place your bed and desk in a low signal area.
- Make sure your cordless phone base station is neither in your bedroom nor close to where you often sit. Ideally, don't have one.
- Make sure you are at least 3m (10ft) away from your microwave oven when it is on.
- Only have an X-ray if it is absolutely essential.
- If you use a mobile phone, buy one with a low SAR rating, use it infrequently and use an earphone attachment. To use an earpiece safely, it should be at least three feet away from your mobile phone – an easy way to do this is to put it on a table or chair next to you, or on the passenger seat if you are in your car. Ideally, install a hands-free unit in your car.
- Don't use it when the signal is bad, or have long conversations in the car.
- Don't keep a clock radio right by your bed.
- If you spend a lot of time in front of a computer, place the monitor about two feet or more away from you. Try increasing the print size on the screen so that you can read it from further away.
- If you suspect you live in a high radon area, check with your local environmental health office and make sure your house is well ventilated.
- Take antioxidant supplements daily (see Chapter 34).

CHAPTER 19

The Two Sides of Sunbathing

The link between skin cancer incidence and sun exposure is far more tenuous than we have been led to believe. Did you know, for example, that the closer you get to the equator, the lower the incidence of cancer? Sunlight, it appears, is both good for us and bad for us. On the one hand, there is evidence that light-skinned people exposed to strong sunlight have more skin cancer. On the other hand, there is some evidence that people deprived of natural sunlight, spending hours in artificial lighting, may actually have a higher cancer incidence.

Natural sunlight does generally boost immunity and improve health. One major reason for this could be that exposure to sunlight stimulates vitamin D synthesis in the skin. Although the mechanism by which this may happen is not yet clearly understood, vitamin D has been shown to slow down the proliferation of some cancer cells.[8] (The connection between vitamin D and cancer is explored more fully in Chapter 27.) This is consistent with evidence that patients with advanced breast cancer who have high vitamin D levels have a better chance of survival. It may also explain why breast cancer rates are lower in sunnier parts of the world. Interestingly, natural sunlight actually stimulates cell growth but not during exposure or the first hour thereafter.[9] So, we have an hour's grace to mop up oxidants and repair any DNA damage in readiness for the burst of increased cellular activity following exposure to sunlight.

Fair-skinned people need to take care

There is a limit to the benefits of sunshine, especially if you are fair-skinned. People with fair skin (low in melanin), who burn easily and rarely tan when they sunbathe, do have a higher risk of skin cancer when exposed to the high-energy UV radiation of the sun. As research proceeds, it is becoming more and more evident that it is the combination of a certain skin type with excessive sun exposure that increases the risk of cancer. Other research has, however, shown that genetic factors (such as the number of moles a person has, or their natural skin colour) can be more important in determining cancer risk than the amount of time they spend exposed to the sun.

Not all skin cancers are equal

Most skin cancer, although quite common, is easily treated and rarely fatal. However, about 2 per cent of all skin cancers are of a more insidious nature and are likely to metastasise quickly, spreading to other parts of the body. These are melanomas. Some experts think that one big, blistery burn as a child can also increase risk as an adult, perhaps by damaging the skin's immune cells. Since 1935 the risk of developing melanoma has increased twenty-fold. Dr Marianne Berwick, of the Sloan-Kettering Cancer Center in New York, found that those with a large number of moles, or with red or blond hair and lighter-coloured eyes or with pale skin, had a six times higher risk. However, the rapid increase in melanoma does suggest that factors other than inherited characteristics are involved – greater UV exposure due to changes in holiday habits and ozone layer depletion are two possible candidates. Over the past decade there has been a 7 per cent increase in UV exposure in Europe.

Alcohol and smoking can make matters worse

The combination of fair skin, excessive exposure to strong sun-light and alcohol or smoking is definitely bad news. During strong sunlight exposure, the risk of oxidant damage to the skin (burning) is at its highest. Smoking introduces oxidants into the lungs and bloodstream. Alcohol, meanwhile, suppresses the immune system, weakening the body's natural defences. This is also not a good time to be eating a lot of fried food.

Use sunscreens

If you are lying on a sunny beach, it is therefore best to use a sunscreen that also contains antioxidants. I am particularly impressed with the Environ products, rich in vitamin A and C and their sunscreen RAD (see Resources). These are the nutrients that protect your skin from damage. So, by increasing the level in your skin you protect it from damage, and from increased oxidative stress to an extent greater than the SPF would suggest. Also, eat plenty of antioxidant-rich foods, such as fresh fruit and vegetables. These high antioxidant foods are exactly those found in parts of the world where the sun shines long and strong.

Sunscreens do their job by absorbing UV energy before it gets through to our skin. There are two kinds of UV rays: UVA, an excess of which depresses the immune system and is more associated with ageing and less with cancer; and UVB which causes sunburn and damage to skin cells and can initiate cancer. Ideally, you want to limit exposure to both, since UVA can weaken immune responses vital for dealing with damaged cells.

But not all sunscreens are equally effective. Research has shown that chemicals found in some sun creams may actually pass on excess energy from the sun's rays into the skin, where it damages DNA. These chemicals are Padimate-O, PABA-O or Escalol 507, says Dr John Knowland of Oxford University. The research was done in test tubes, so it has yet to be discovered whether the same effect takes place in humans.[10]

Octyl methoxycinnamate, octyl salicylate, tea salicylate and homosalate all effectively absorb the dangerous portions of UVB light. Titanium dioxide and zinc oxide also absorb part of the UVA spectrum and scatter or reflect the sun's rays. These two are often employed in higher SPF (sun protection factor) blocks. The SPF number indicates how long you can stay in the sun without burning, so SPF2 means twice as long, because these blocks absorb 50 per cent of the energy hitting the skin. Better sunscreens, such as Environ's RAD, also contain antioxidants, which protect the skin by mopping up oxidants as well as improving immune defences.

The Australian motto is 'slip, slap, slop': slip on a shirt, slap on a hat, and slop on some sunscreen, especially if you're fair-skinned. Melanomas start from moles, so it's a good idea to check for any changes in moles, especially on the feet, genital folds, breasts, armpits and scalp. If detected early, the success rate is good. However, if melanomas go undetected for six months this type of cancer is often fatal.

Summary

- Minimise the amount of time you spend in strong sunlight, especially if you have fair skin, light-coloured eyes and lots of moles.
- Use a good sunscreen that contains antioxidants, not lower than SPF7.
- Eat plenty of antioxidant-rich foods – especially fruits and vegetables.
- Take a supplement containing antioxidants.

CHAPTER 20

Pesticides and Plastics

Possibly one of the most underestimated contributors to the epidemic of cancer is the combined effect of humanity's exposure to manufactured chemicals. However, this statement must be qualified for two reasons. Firstly, we know remarkably little about most of the thousands of chemicals to which we are all unwittingly exposed, and virtually nothing about their effects in combination. Secondly, some of the cancer research organisations are very closely linked to, and funded by, the medical/industrial chemical industry who can influence the direction of their research; consequently, little research is being done into the effects of such chemicals. However, the investigations that have been done raise some serious questions about certain pesticides and chemicals, particularly those used in the plastics industry.

Problem pesticides

Currently, the three areas of most concern in relation to pesticides are their links with breast cancer, childhood cancers and increased cancer incidence among farmers.

Each year in the UK 12,000 women die of breast cancer. A study by Greenpeace and several women's groups looked at the possible links between various environmental pollutants and breast cancer.[11]

They found that women have up to ten times the normal risk of getting cancer when they are shown to have high levels of pesticides and other toxic chemicals in their body. The groups specifically looked at dioxin, PCB and DDT. These chlorine-based chemicals – organochlorines – are commonly found in fish and waterfowl and can end up in many women's diets. The researchers say that when similar chemicals were banned in Israel, breast cancer rates dropped sharply.

It may surprise you to know that almost half of all food eaten throughout Europe is contaminated by pesticides. Currently licensed pesticides include known and suspected carcinogens and hormone-disrupting chemicals. Infants, children, pregnant women and the developing foetus are particularly vulnerable to pesticides.

Let's consider some of the facts:[12]

- The annual application of synthetic pesticides to food crops in the European Union (EU) exceeds 140,000 tonnes. This amount corresponds to 280g (10oz) per EU citizen per year.

- More than 300 different pesticides are known to contaminate food products in the EU.

- In 1993, Pesticides News (a PAN publication, see Resources) listed 70 possible carcinogens – now the list has grown to over 240.[13]

- One out of 20 food items exceeds the current EU limit for an individual pesticide.

- Over 25 per cent of fruits, vegetables and cereals are known to contain detectable residues of at least two pesticides.

- Processed food and non-organic baby foods are also commonly contaminated.

- Several approved pesticides are considered carcinogenic and may contribute to the development of malignant diseases, such as breast cancer, colon cancer, leukaemia and lymphomas.

If that list doesn't convince you to eat organic, nothing will!

Positive developments in Europe

The European Parliament has long been pressing for radical controls, despite opposition from some governments, especially Britain. Those opposing the controls fear that such bans could make crop production impossible and result in a dramatic drop in yields. However, in 2009, the European Parliament, following long negotiations with individual governments, voted to tighten rules on hazardous pesticides in the EU by listing pesticides to be eliminated from use in food production. Despite determined resistance to the safety measures from the British government, Britain has to comply.[14]

Scores of pesticides suspected of causing cancer, DNA damage and 'gender-bender' effects are to be phased out under new EU rules, which are being hailed as a revolution in the way the public is protected against poisonous chemicals.

The new rules will eliminate – or severely restrict – pesticide use near schools, parks and hospitals, and other public places, with aerial spraying banned anywhere in the country unless given exceptional approval by safety authorities.

A total of 22 particularly hazardous chemicals used in scores of herbicides, fungicides and insecticides will gradually be phased out over the next decade to avoid abrupt withdrawal from the market. Some exemptions will be made, as the National Farmers' Union believes that the ban could make vegetable production impossible and result in a dramatic drop in wheat yields. They said that growing carrots, parsnips and onions would be more difficult because the herbicides that MEPs voted to phase out killed weeds that affect these crops.[15] The exemptions will last for five years.

Hiltrud Breyer, the German Green MEP who steered the proposals through the parliament, called them a 'milestone for the environment, health and consumer protection', although PAN and other critics believe the ban doesn't go far enough. 'Banning 22 harmful substances out of over 400 is barely a start,' said Manfred Krautter of Greenpeace. 'Food in Europe will continue to be contaminated by many dangerous chemicals for years to come.'

The effects of banned chemicals live on

Krautter's concerns are illustrated by a study published in the *Journal of the National Cancer Institute*, showing that a chemical that comes from the pesticide DDT (banned more than 30 years ago but still present in all of us) may raise a man's risk of developing testicular cancer. Researchers found a clear link between testicular cancer and DDE, which is created when the body or the environment breaks down the pesticide DDT. Men with the highest levels of DDE were 70 per cent more likely to have developed testicular cancer than those with the lowest levels.[16]

The researchers also found a somewhat lower increased risk of testicular cancer in men with higher levels of chemicals related to chlordane, which was used to kill termites and was banned in the US in 1988.

Testicular cancer has been increasing in recent decades in many countries. Lead researcher, Katherine McGlynn of the US National Cancer Institute, said the findings suggested that about 15 per cent of the testicular cancer cases in the men in the study could be attributed to DDE. She says that 'DDE remains ubiquitous in the environment even decades after DDT was being banned in the United States – and is present in about 90 per cent of Americans.' It is possible some of the men who later developed cancer of the testicles were exposed to DDE at very young ages – in the womb or through breastfeeding. 'The trouble with these chemicals is they hang around a long time. It's in the food chain now,' McGlynn added. For example, people who eat fish from areas contaminated with DDT can absorb it.

Pesticides, children and cancer

Research from New Zealand has clearly shown that pesticide levels are highest in children, especially young children.[17] This is probably because they consume more food in relation to their body mass than adults and generally consume more fruit, which is heavily sprayed. The New Zealand survey found that intake of organophosphate pesticides was twice as high in young children, aged one to three, than in male adults. This finding is particularly worrying, because the introduction of either carcinogens or hormone-disrupting chemicals while a child is still developing has greater implications for their future health. Animal studies have certainly shown that young animals are much more susceptible to the effects of a wide range of pesticides in use today.

Studies looking at the association between lifestyle factors and childhood cancer have frequently identified chemical exposure as an associated risk factor. A study of 84 children in Maryland, USA, who had developed brain cancer, versus those who hadn't, found that those with brain cancer were more likely to have been exposed to insecticides in the home.[18] The US Children's Cancer Study Group found an increased risk of leukaemia in 204 children whose parents used pesticides in their home and garden,[19] a finding reported by other researchers.[20]

Dangerous chemicals can still be used in pharmaceuticals

One source of organophosphates to which some children are exposed is anti-head-lice lotions, which can contain a chemical called lindane. Although lindane has been targeted for global elimination since May 2009, it can still be used for pharmaceutical purposes (see box). With some manufacturers suggesting that children leave these products in the hair overnight, it seems that there is a reasonable cause for concern. Natural alternatives include suffocating the lice by soaking the hair with olive oil and covering it with a shower cap; the lice can then be combed out. Another method is to add tea tree oil to the children's shampoo and leave it on for 10 minutes. If you don't want the hassle of having to wash out olive oil and tea tree oil, then another tried-and-tested method is to wash and rinse the hair, apply lots of conditioner (cheap is fine), and then use a nit comb to comb through the hair from root to end, rinsing the comb out regularly. Then rinse thoroughly.

Lindane banned by international convention

In May 2009, the international community added lindane to the Stockholm Convention list of persistent organic pollutants (POPS) targeted for global elimination. The US withdrew agricultural uses, but pharmaceutical use will still continue in some countries including the US and Canada (this exemption is set to expire in 2014). Lindane is banned in at least 52 countries and severely restricted in more than 33 others. According to PAN, lindane is long overdue to be phased out in every country of the world.

Eight other toxic chemicals were added to the list of poisonous substances that are to be eliminated under the Stockholm Convention.

The UN Under-Secretary General Achim Steiner said, 'The tremendous impact of these substances on human health and the environment has been acknowledged today by adding nine new chemicals to the Convention. This shift reflects international concern on the need to reduce and eventually eliminate such substances throughout the global community.'

The nine chemicals that member states have committed to eliminate are:

1   Lindane – used in the treatment of head lice and scabies, and in insecticides.
2   Alpha hexachlorocyclohexane – a by-product of lindane.
3   Beta hexachlorocyclohexane – a by-product of lindane.
4   Hexabromodiphenyl ether and heptabromodiphenyl ether – used in flame retardants.
5   Tetrabromodiphenyl ether and pentabromodiphenyl ether – used in flame retardants.
6   Chlordecone – used in agricultural pesticides.
7   Hexabromobiphenyl – used in flame retardants.
8   Pentachlorobenzene – used in fungicides and flame retardants.
9   Perfluorooctane sulfonic acid, its salts and perfluorooctane sulfonyl fluoride – used in electric and electronic parts, photo-imaging and textiles.

Farmers suffer the effects of using chemicals

Another indication that exposure to agrochemicals is of real concern comes from statistics on the incidence of cancer among farmers. Generally speaking, farmers are healthier than the average person. Yet there is a disproportionate increase in the incidence of several cancers, including leukaemia, non-Hodgkin's lymphoma and cancers of the brain and prostate. In the US the amount of pesticides sprayed annually has gone from 50 million pounds in the 1940s to one billion pounds in the 1980s. This means that the average person now has up to a gallon of pesticides and herbicides sprayed on the fruit and vegetables they eat each year. When I first made this statement back in the 1980s I received a stern letter from the Ministry of Agriculture who had received complaints from the agrochemical lobby questioning the figures and the implications, which I substantiated.

Why are pesticides and herbicides so dangerous?

The bottom line is that agrochemicals are designed to kill, often by acting as nerve poisons, and there is no doubt that human exposure is undesirable. It's just a question of how much we can tolerate and for how long. Although a number of pesticides, herbicides and fungicides are known to act as carcinogens, it is very hard to prove which ones are a problem and at which doses, and what their combined effects are. Broadly speaking, there is plenty of evidence that eating fruit and vegetables reduces risk, but perhaps the benefit would be even greater if the fruits and vegetables were organic.

There is certainly a logical case for choosing organically grown foods on the basis that these chemicals are 'guilty until proven innocent'.

Plastic dangers

Perhaps even more worrying is the discovery that a number of chemicals used in plastics are also potentially carcinogenic. These include

alkylphenols, such as nonylphenol and octylphenol, biphenolic compounds such as bisphenol A, and phthalates. These chemicals are
used in domestic detergents and toiletries, so the chances are that
you have some of them in your bathroom. If they had to be listed
on food packaging, you'd probably find them in your kitchen too.
They are often used to coat metal containers such as food cans, and
they can also be in soft plastic liners in juice cartons, film wrapping
and other plastic wrappers. The trouble is that they don't have to be
declared. So, until they are banned or legislation is passed requiring
declaration of such chemicals, there's really no way of knowing.

Why are these plastics potentially dangerous?

The problem with this group of chemicals is that they can disrupt hormone signals – they generally have an oestrogenic effect (see Chapter
3). It is this effect that is associated with the increasing risk of hormone-
related cancers. Fuelled by concerns about rising cancer incidence and
falling sperm counts, many environmental groups are campaigning
for the disclosure, if not the banning, of such hormone-disrupting
chemicals. Included in this list are chlorine compounds such as organochlorines, polychlorinated biphenyls (PCBs) and dioxins. These
are used in farming, in paper production, and in industrial processes.
Even though PCBs and DDT (an organochlorine) have been banned,
they are non-biodegradable, which means that significant levels can
still be detected in each of us. Also on the suspect list is the food addi-
tive butylated hydroxyanisole (BHA), or E320, which is used as an
antioxidant/preservative, particularly in fat-containing foods, confec-
tionary and some medicines. The International Agency for Research
on Cancer (IARC) says that BHA is possibly carcinogenic to humans.
It is not permitted for food use in Japan. So, check food labels!

The quantity of chemicals is staggering

According to Dr Theo Colborn, co-author of the book *Our Stolen
Future* (see Recommended Reading), there are now 100,000 synthetic

chemicals on the world market, including 15,000 synthetic chlorinated compounds – a category of chemicals that has come under attack because of their persistence in the environment and record of causing health problems. The US exports 40 million pounds of compounds known to be endocrine-disrupters each year, and anyone willing to spend the money on tests will find at least 250 contaminants in his or her body fat.

Plastic linings

In Spain, an analysis of 20 brands of food in cans which are now lined with plastic (as are many drinks cartons) showed that most contained significant levels of bisphenol-A, some at a level 27 times higher than that known to cause the proliferation of breast cancer cells. This is just one of the disturbing statements in Dr Colborn's book, which links such chemicals to endocrine-related diseases including breast cancer, endometriosis, prostate problems – and the decline in male fertility.

Reduce your risk

Once again, until more research is carried out, it is impossible to quantify the real dangers of exposure to these chemicals. While it is impossible to avoid them all, there are many changes you can make to your diet and lifestyle that are likely to substantially decrease your exposure to such hormone-disrupting and potentially carcinogenic chemicals. These are as follows:

- **Eat organic** This instantly minimises your exposure to pesticides and herbicides. When you are eating non-organic produce, wash it in an acidic medium, made by adding 1 tablespoon vinegar to a bowl of water. This will reduce some, but not all pesticides.

- **Filter all drinking water** I recommend getting a water filter that you install under the sink, made from stainless steel (not plastic or aluminium), employing some kind of carbon-filtration system (see Resources). Although not proven to remove all hormone-disrupting chemicals, this should decrease your load. The alternative is spring water, bottled in glass.

- **Reduce your intake of fatty foods** Non-biodegradable chemicals accumulate in the food chain in animal fat. Minimising your intake of animal fat – meat and dairy produce – lessens your exposure. There is no need to limit essential fats in nuts and seeds.

- **Never heat food in plastic*** This means saying goodbye to micro-waved TV dinners. If you have to have them, transfer the food into a glass container before heating.

- **Minimise fatty foods exposed to flexible plastics*** Some chemicals that keep plastics flexible easily pass out of the plastic into fatty food such as crisps, cheese, butter, chocolate, pies, and so on.

- **Minimise liquid foods exposed to flexible plastics*** This not only includes fruit juices in cardboard packs, which have a plastic inner lining, but also some fruits and vegetables in cans, which may again have a plastic inner lining.

- **Minimise exposure of food to flexible plastics*** This means using paper bags whenever possible as opposed to buying everything in plastic trays, covered with clingfilm.

- **Switch to natural detergents** Use only ecological detergent products for washing up, washing clothes and body washing, made by companies who declare all their ingredients. And check that the ingredients exclude the suspect chemicals listed on pages 192–3 [agricultural chemicals]. Also, rinse dishes and cutlery after washing up.

- **Don't use pesticides in your garden** Some pesticides are hormone-disrupters. Unless you're sure yours isn't, it is better not to spray. The incidence of childhood cancer is higher in homes where the gardens are sprayed with pesticides.

- **Read the summary** in Chapter 18 for further advice on protecting yourself from radiation.

*It is currently impossible for you to know whether the plastics you use contain hormone-disrupting chemicals or not.

CHAPTER 21

Active and Passive Smoking

The association between smoking and cancer is, without question, the major reason why lung cancer is now the most common cause of cancer deaths in the world for men and the second for women (after breast cancer). Incidence from country to country correlates very closely with the number of cigarettes smoked, except in certain parts of the world; for example, in Japan and in rural China there is a weaker correlation between the number of cigarettes and the incidence of lung cancer. There is therefore a very real possibility that at least two other factors need to be taken into account: diet and exposure to exhaust fumes or industrial pollution.

Antioxidants from the diet protect

Few people realise how important our intake of antioxidant nutrients is in protecting us against the harmful effects of smoking. Cigarette smoke is a powerful carcinogen – containing at least 80 known mutagenic carcinogens, including arsenic, cadmium, ammonia, formaldehyde and benzopyrene – and also a source of oxidative stress (see Chapter 2). Compared with non-smokers, smokers have lower levels of several antioxidants, including alpha-carotene, beta-carotene, and vitamin C.[21]

Back in the 1980s a study of 265,000 people in Japan found that those with a low intake of beta-carotene (the form of vitamin A found in fruits and vegetables) had a higher risk of lung cancer.[22] Furthermore, a study of employees of Western Electric, published in the *Lancet* medical journal, found that beta-carotene status was as significant as smoking in determining risk of lung cancer.[23] In this study they found that 6.5 per cent of heavy smokers with a low beta-carotene status developed cancer. This percentage dropped to 0.8 per cent for heavy smokers with a high beta-carotene status. Conversely, non-smokers with a low beta-carotene status also had a 0.8 per cent risk, while non-smokers with a high beta-carotene status had no risk at all.

These studies demonstrated that smoking and diet each play important roles in the lung cancer process. Smoking also increases the risk of other kinds of cancer, including other parts of the airways (mouth, pharynx and larynx), oesophagus, cervix (smoking makes a woman twice as likely to develop cervical cancer) and bladder,[24] although diet offers protection against these forms of cancer too.

Early smokers are more at risk

Although it is known that the number of years a person smokes, the number of cigarettes they smoke, and the tar content, all increase risk, research shows that another highly critical factor is the age at which a person starts smoking. The risk of death from lung cancer is almost double for those who start smoking before the age of 15, compared to those who start in their twenties.[25] This underlines the importance of campaigns dissuading teenagers from taking up the habit.

Other causes of lung cancer

However, there are undoubtedly other risk factors involved in lung cancer that have been downplayed in the rush to point the finger at smoking alone. The importance of considering such factors is evident when you look at some surprising facts: the incidence of lung cancer in non-smokers has doubled over recent decades; the incidence of adenocarcinoma of the lung (which is less clearly related to smoking) has also continued to increase; and in the US, the incidence is much higher in black men than in white. Professor Samuel Epstein believes that occupational exposure to carcinogens used in a wide variety of industries, and exposure to industrial pollutants and exhaust fumes, particularly from diesel, play an important part in non-smoking-related lung cancer.[26]

Passive smoking

For non-smokers, the key issue is to what extent other people's smoke contributes to their cancer risk. A number of studies have been conducted over the past decade, many of which have shown a slightly higher risk of lung cancer, and, in women, for breast cancer, when exposed to other people's smoke. One such study looked at deaths from lung cancer in women living in Pennsylvania.[27] Women who neither smoked nor were exposed to smoke had a quarter of the incidence of death from lung cancer of women exposed to other people's smoke. The incidence of death from lung cancer among smokers was approximately ten times that of passive smokers. Other studies confirm this trend, although more research is needed. One analysis of studies to date concludes that 'the relative risk [of a passive smoker contracting lung cancer] is about two-fold higher [than a non-exposed, non-smoker]'.[28] There is also some evidence that women who are exposed to other people's cigarette smoke have an increased risk of breast cancer.[29]

Despite the general decline in smoking in the Western world a staggering number of people do smoke. In the US, it is estimated to be more than 43 million adults. In the UK the figure is about 10 million. There is a long way to go before this major contributor to cancer risk is eliminated.

CHAPTER 22

The Art of Chemical Self-defence

Many common substances to which we are exposed are known carcinogens. Some of these, but by no means all, have been discussed in earlier chapters. Although the levels that trigger cancer may be a lot higher than most people are normally exposed to, a cursory look through the lists below will show that, like most people, you are probably exposed to a large number of potential carcinogens. You may wonder what the cumulative effect is of such exposure, albeit at low doses. In truth, no one knows, but the results from the laboratory of Professor Ana Soto and Professor Carlos Sonnenschein at Boston's Tufts University are alarming. They were investigating the levels at which known hormone-disrupting chemicals would cause proliferation of breast cancer cells. They then exposed these cells to combinations of five or ten chemicals, each at a tenth of the dose that would produce proliferation. Sure enough, there was a cocktail effect such that, in combination, these chemicals were ten times as powerful, producing rapid proliferation of breast cancer cells.[30]

How to decrease your exposure to known carcinogens

The following factors are carcinogenic only at certain concentrations. Although it is ideal to minimise your overall exposure or intake, the presence of these in small amounts may not constitute a risk. After all, it is now impossible to avoid all carcinogens, no matter where or how you live. Below you will find chemicals divided into groups and our suggestions of ways to cut down your exposure to them.

Household, and daily living and working

- Tobacco smoke, whether or not you are a smoker.

- Coal tar and petrochemical derivatives used in some hair oils, lipsticks and cosmetics, perfumes, soaps, deodorants and antiperspirants.

- Plastics containing vinyl chloride, polystyrene and certain plasticisers (such as phthalates), used in food containers, kitchen utensils, clothes, furniture, curtains, bedding, and so on.

- Fluoride in water supplies and in toothpaste.

- Epoxy resins, glues, and so on.

- Carbon tetrachloride (used in cleaning fluids).

- Industrial detergents containing alkylphenols.

- Many factory emissions; for example, iron and steel founding, the rubber industry and especially those containing sulphuric acid.

- Car, lorry, bus and boat exhausts, and fumes from central heating boilers (oil, coal or gas-fired).

- Working daily in boot and shoe manufacture and repair, furniture manufacture, painting, and so on.

- Dioxins produced by incineration of chlorine-containing chemicals and some processes, such as the production of chlorinated hydrocarbons and paper.

- PCBs (polychlorinated biphenyls), although now banned in Europe, are very persistent; they used to be added to ink, paint, plasticisers, capacitators and electricity transformers.

- Brominated flame retardants (BFRs): chemicals added to many products (such as carpets and computers) to reduce fire risk.

- Fluorocarbons, used in many products, from refrigerants and anaesthetics to pesticides and industrial surfactants.

What you can do:

- Don't smoke, and avoid spending much time around people who do.

- Choose your cosmetics carefully. Most health-food shops stock less chemical-laden alternatives.

- Use glass, paper and wooden containers, and utensils, as much as possible in the kitchen.

- Minimise the amount of food you eat that is covered in plastic, especially fatty food such as cheese.

- Use 'environmentally friendlier' detergents.

- If your job involves particularly high exposure to chemicals, wear a mask and gloves and make sure your workplace is well ventilated.

Food and drink

- Chlorine in tap water.

- Pesticides and their residues (see Agricultural Chemicals, below).

- Smoked meats and fish (such food often contains creosote and formaldehyde).

- Food preservatives, especially nitrates in bacon, processed meats, non-organic fruit and vegetables, and water (from overuse of nitrogen fertilisers in agriculture).

- Coffee is suspect, because roasting produces matrol.

- Decaffeinated coffee contains matrol and other solvents.

- Saccharin and cyclamates (chemical sweeteners).

- Fats heated to high temperatures (above 200°C/392°F) in preparing food.

- Alcohol – risk is significant above one drink a day for women and two drinks a day for men.

- Parsley, celery and parsnips – these and other members of the Umbelliferae family contain carcinogenic psoralens.

- Burned (charred or dark brown) food (such as toast, cakes, bread) produces heterocyclic amines (HCAs) and acrylamides.

- Barbecued, charred meat and fish – which produce heterocyclic aromatic amines.

- Bleaches (for white bread, and so on).

- Moulds on foodstuffs (such as *Aspergillus flavus*, the toxin aflatoxin and other mycotoxins found in certain moulds); for example, on nuts, cheese, milk, jam, bread.

- Some antioxidant preservatives such as butylated hydroxyanisole (BHA).

What you can do:

- Get a good water filter or drink spring water from glass bottles.

- Eat and drink organic produce whenever possible.

- Wash non-organic produce in acidic water – add 1 tablespoon of vinegar to a bowl of water.

- Minimise your consumption of saturated fats (meat and dairy products), processed meats and smoked foods – choose fish and soya products instead.

- Avoid fried food.

- Eat grilled or barbecued meat and fish infrequently – poach, bake or boil it instead.

- Have no more than one alcoholic drink a day – have an alcohol-free week every now and then.

- Avoid all processed, refined food, especially foods that are high in preservatives and other additives.

- If you drink coffee, go for the organic varieties. Choose water-processed decaffeinated coffee.

- Don't eat food that's starting to go mouldy.

Medical carcinogens

- Chloroform.

- Liquid paraffin.

- X-rays (including radioactive dyes and radio isotopes).

- Mineral oils.

- All coal-derivative products.

- Hormone therapy (contraceptive pills and HRT).

- Certain antibiotics and sulphonamide drugs are strongly suspect.

- Psoralens (used for treating skin complaints).

- Tamoxifen, the anti-cancer drug.

- Dental lacquers that contain bisphenol A.

- Analgesics containing phenacetin.

What you can do:

- Have X-rays only when you absolutely have to.

- Use natural alternatives to artificial hormone therapy.

- Use natural alternatives to drugs whenever possible.

Agricultural chemicals

- Atrazine, the most common pesticide found in UK drinking water.

- Captan, a fungicide.

- Chlorothalonil, a fungicide.

- Chlorpyrifos, an organophosphate.

- DDE, a very persistent breakdown product of DDT.

- Dichlorvos, an organophosphate.

- Dithiocarbamates or EBDCs, fungicides including mancozeb, metiram, thiram and zineb, which break down to form ethylene thiourea (ETU).

- Endosulfan, an organochlorine.

- Fenitrothion, an organophosphate.

- Iprodione, a fungicide.

- Malathion, an organophosphate, used in several head-lice lotions.

- Permethrin.

- Pirimiphos methyl, an organophosphate.

- Procymidone, a fungicide.

- Vinclozolin, a fungicide.

What you can do:

- Choose organic produce whenever possible.

- Don't use any products in your garden or pot plants that contain these chemicals.

- Choose natural alternatives.

Others

- Background nuclear radiation polluting atmosphere, crops, meat and water.

- Certain viruses.

- Radiation from TV sets, computers and mobile phones.

- Radiation from the sun.

What you can do:

- Avoid being out in strong sunlight for too long. If you are, cover up or use a good sunscreen, around factor 15.

- If you use a mobile telephone, use an earpiece.

Limit your exposure where you can

For many factors, such as smoking, the necessary action is clear-cut: don't smoke. The same can be said for pesticides: eat organic. However, with other factors, there is a limit to how much action we can reasonably take. Because we do not fully understand the effect of combinations of mild carcinogens and because it would take decades to find out, the only sensible way forward is to develop a diet and lifestyle that reduces exposure to as many as possible. Admittedly, all this is easier said than done. But, as long as you are doing all you can to minimise your exposure, it's not worth becoming completely obsessive. After all, stress and worry are not helpful either, as explained in Chapter 9. You will find out how to minimise the effects of stress on your health in the next chapter.

CHAPTER 23

Ten Ways to Reduce Stress and Emotional Baggage

As we explored in Chapter 9, stress and negative emotions play an important role in the cancer equation. It is not helpful to dwell on whether or not there is a so-called 'cancer personality', as that can lead to feelings of guilt and depression in some cancer patients, as if the illness is somehow their fault. However, those people who succumb to any kind of illness are often those who look after the needs of everybody else and put themselves last on the list. It is not selfish to look after your own needs and do whatever you have to do to keep yourself healthy and happy. Whether you are looking at cancer prevention or trying to avoid a recurrence, your mind and body have to be in balance. It's no good having treatment to rid your body of cancer cells if depression or the constant fear of a recurrence is wearing you down. As Deepak Chopra says, in his excellent book *Quantum Healing*, 'the vital issue is not how to win the war but how to keep peace in the first place'. He goes on to say:

> if you reacted to cancer as no great threat, the way you react to flu, you would have the best chance of recovering, yet a diagnosis of cancer makes every patient feel abnormal. The diagnosis itself sets up the vicious circle, like a snake biting its tail until there is no more snake.

So how do you cope with the daily challenges that life throws at you, particularly if you are also dealing with a diagnosis of cancer? And how do you give yourself the equivalent of a psychological detox, releasing stored-up patterns of negative emotions that keep you blocked, unhappy, over-reactive and generally low? Here are my top tips to help you to reduce stress, let go of emotional baggage and give your mind (and body) a chance to be the best that it can be.

Long-term stress control

What you really need is to counter stress at source. Try the following suggestions:

1 Work–life balance

The concept of a work–life balance is a bit of a myth. The reality is that many people are juggling too many balls in the air and have trouble 'switching off'. If you are 'switched on' all the time, you are still burning energy and activating your 'fight or flight' stress response. You need to be like a light bulb: switched on when you need to be and then be able to be switched off.

- At the very least, limit your working hours to, at most, ten hours a day, five days a week. And always have a proper lunch break – at least 30 minutes and preferably an hour.

- Keep at least one and a half days a week completely free of routine work. Use this free time to cultivate a relaxing hobby, do something creative or take exercise, preferably in the fresh air.

- Have a wind-down routine at bedtime so that you are ready for bed – don't watch the late-night news or horror movies.

2 Breathe!

A well-known effect of chronic stress is that it causes people to breathe too quickly and too shallowly. The result is a drop in the amount of carbon dioxide (CO_2) in the bloodstream. Although most people think of CO_2 as a waste gas, it is also vital for the proper functioning of nearly all body chemistry. A drop in CO_2 causes blood vessels and airways to narrow. The best thing to do in stressful situations is to stay calm and practise breathing slowly and deliberately.

The basic principle of all breathing exercises is to use your diaphragm (the dome-shaped muscle just below your lungs), rather than the top of your chest, as we tend to do when we are anxious or stressed. Learning how to breathe from the diaphragm is part of many health systems, such as yoga and the martial arts.

3 Exercise

In many stressful situations, the most we might do is drum our fingers or make a rude remark, or, even worse, keep our feelings bottled up inside, which can lead to hidden resentment. Such responses do not use up the hormones released into the blood, nor do they stimulate the physical mechanisms designed to burn them up.

This is one reason why exercise is important for people who are stressed in any way. Obviously, it is best taken at the time of stress – a brisk walk or vigorous exercise session is good first aid. If that is impossible, you will benefit overall from regular exercise anyway.

4 Relax

Adopt a relaxed manner – walk and talk more slowly. If you find this difficult, try acting 'as if' you were a relaxed person, almost as a game. Simple relaxation techniques also help the body and mind to get back to normal. Tense your muscles as hard as you can and then relax, starting with your feet and ending with your facial muscles. Or just clench your fists tightly and relax. Or take a deep breath, hold it for a count of ten, and then breathe it all out at once. Yoga breathing and meditation exercises are also excellent de-stressors.

5 Say no

Avoid obvious pressures, such as taking on too many commitments. Learn to say no, or 'not now'. Learn to see when a problem is somebody else's responsibility, and refuse to take it on.

6 Talk to a friend or join a support group

If you have an emotional problem you cannot solve alone, seek advice or join a support group. There are many charities and organisations that provide help and support to cancer patients and their families (see Resources). Breast Cancer Care, for example, offer emotional and practical support and bring people affected by breast cancer together. It is often the camaraderie and being with others in the same situation that aids the healing process. Perhaps the most powerful demonstration of the clinical power of emotional support was illustrated by a study conducted by Dr David Spiegel at Stanford University Medical School. Women with advanced metastatic breast cancer who went to weekly meetings with others survived twice as long as women with the same disease who faced it on their own.[31]

7 Live in the present

Concentrate on one task at a time, and focus all your attention on the present. The past is history, the future a mystery. Living life to the full is all about living in the moment, not rushing through life too busy to appreciate it and dreaming of the time when 'things will get easier'.

We have all said at some time or another, 'When this, that or the other happens … I will be happy', or 'If I can just … reach this deadline/finish this/and so on …' For many people, being happy is no longer immediate but something that will happen at some time in the future. A very good book to read to bring you into the present is the *Power of Now* by Eckhart Tolle.

8 Express yourself

Learn to say what is on your mind instead of suppressing it. You don't have to be aggressive – just state your point of view clearly and truthfully. More about this later.

9 Be self-aware

Listen to what other people say to you, and about you.

10 Take control of your life

Look long and hard at all the stresses in your life. Make a list of them. Try to take a positive attitude to things that can't be changed. If change is possible, take action. Don't let things wear you down.

There is more information on how to deal with stress in my book *Beat Stress and Fatigue* (see Recommended Reading).

Emotional baggage

You may think that stress and emotions are one and the same thing, and often they are. However, when emotions are as a result of a deep-seated pattern of behaviour that you recognise as being unhelpful or a hindrance to your health or recovery, then it is important to do something about it. Here are some suggestions to help you.

1 Learn to express your emotions

How you consciously experience your emotions makes all the difference. Here are two simple ways to do this:

Exercise: speaking about your feelings

1   When you feel an emotion and need to express it, take a breath and say clearly, 'I am feeling [*xyz (such as, angry, frustrated, sad)*] and that's OK.'

2   Take another breath and say this again two more times until you sense a different feeling.

In some circumstances it may be better to say this just to yourself, not aloud. Whichever way you do it, you are allowing the feeling, and yourself, to simply be, without judgement.

Exercise: breathe out your negative emotions

1   Bring to mind an emotionally charged situation that is still causing you some distress or unease.

2   Identify a place in your body where you feel the emotion this memory evokes. Put your hand there.

3   As you breathe in, imagine white light pouring into that area. As you breathe out, imagine the old pain of that memory leaving.

4   Breathe in warmth and light, and breathe out the negative emotions. With each breath you feel lighter and clearer until you feel a physical sense of relief in that place in your body.

It's OK to feel

The first step is simply to acknowledge how you feel in the moment. Sadness, anger and fear – and all the shades in between – are perfectly normal reactions when things happen in our lives that don't match our expectations. We all have the need for expressing, venting and releasing feelings in healthy, appropriate and conscious ways, thus avoiding getting stuck in negative emotional patterns. Some people decide to control their feelings rather than expressing them and letting them go.

Candice Pert, author of *Molecules of Emotion* (see Recommended Reading), points out that all emotions are healthy, and to repress them creates stress and blockages in the system that can lead to disease. She says,

> All honest emotions are positive emotions … health is not just a matter of thinking 'happy thoughts'. Sometimes the biggest impetus to healing can come from jump-starting the immune system with a burst of long-suppressed anger. How and where it's expressed is up to you – in a room by yourself, in a group therapy situation where the group dynamic can often facilitate the expression of long-buried feelings, or in a spontaneous exchange with a family member or friend. The key is to express it and then let it go, so that it doesn't fester, or build, or escalate out of control.

Our experiences from the past can affect the present

Often, what happens is that our rational mind is hijacked by a strong emotional reaction that has more charge because it plugs into some of our old history. Have you ever noticed how something that makes you react particularly strongly goes over the head of someone else? Perhaps your boss doesn't say 'Good morning' as he passes by, and you feel hurt. However, your colleague isn't concerned at all and says, 'Oh, never mind, he's probably just got his head in the clouds.' This is a good indicator that your reaction reflects just the tip of an emotional iceberg, a more deep-rooted negative emotional pattern, in this case one of feeling easily rejected.

Although you may not be able to recognise in that moment how you are feeling and what drives that feeling, and you may not be able to express it in a conscious and appropriate way, there may be a link with some deep-rooted emotional patterns from your childhood. You can explore this further if you wish to, by trying the options overleaf.

Learning from dreams

It's now also well established that dreaming sleep is vital for effective learning. Dreaming is how we process and help to release unexpressed emotions, so those emotions we didn't express and let go of during the day may surface in our dreams. It may be a way that our mind sorts out the emotional problems that we hadn't dealt with during the day, and if we don't do this, our brain would be permanently caught in a 'stress' mode. In fact, it appears that the period of sleep known as REM (rapid eye movement) sleep helps to release unexpressed emotions.[32]

Next time you wake up remembering a dream, become aware of the predominant feeling. Now, scan through yesterday and think of a time when you felt this feeling but didn't fully express it. You'll be amazed at how often these unexpressed emotions come out in our dreams. If you'd like to know more about this, I recommend you read *Dreaming Reality* by Joe Griffin and Ivan Tyrrell.

2 Describe your memories to a 'witness'

This technique was taught to me by Oscar Ichazo and is excellent if you have someone who is skilled in listening as your 'witness' to a charged memory.

Exercise: use a 'camera eye'

1 Think of an emotionally charged memory – perhaps the loss of someone close to you, the break-up of a relationship, or the loss of a job or an important opportunity.

2 Now describe this incident to your 'witness' factually in the present tense, as if you were watching the incident through a camera. Don't describe your feelings or thoughts about what happened. Just say what happens (what you see, hear, and so on); for example, 'I am sitting on the sofa in my living room. My husband comes in the room and says ... '

3   Be aware of the moment in the description where you feel an emotion. Initially you may find it hard to describe exactly what happened in the moment of charge. You may start to rationalise or say how you feel or get sleepy, or skip the actual moment of charge.

4   So, run through the incident more than once and you'll find the emotional charge starts to dissipate. It's important that the person listening doesn't interject, sympathise or pass judgement. Their role is simply to listen.

3 Let your troubled feelings out

This is a way to 'ventilate' troubled feelings.

Exercise: remembering an emotional event

1   Take a piece of paper and, without any censorship whatsoever, write down as quickly as you can one of the emotional scenes from your past that keeps having an impact upon your present. Put your real feelings in there: how you felt as a child, how you feel affected now. Make it emotional, specific and powerful.

2   When you are finished, take the piece of paper and burn it. Have in your mind the sense of the power of that negative pattern burned and destroyed – floating away with the smoke. (Burning the paper afterwards allows you to literally 'burn up' a stress that was previously confined to your body.)

James Pennebaker, a Southern Methodist University psychologist, uses this method with his patients. Those in the midst of emotional stresses are encouraged to write about their trauma for 15–20 minutes a day for about five days. This has resulted in enhanced immune function, significant drops in health-centre visits in the following six months, fewer days missed from work, and even improved liver function.[33]

This kind of writing exercise is good for discharging negative emotions you have in unresolved relationships, perhaps with an ex-partner or parent, and helps you to move on.

Exercise: remembering and forgiving

1   Make a list of people you still feel upset with or haven't forgiven. Choose one. Next, write a letter expressing all your negative feelings about their behaviour or attitude. Hold nothing back, but tell them that you won't accept their negative projections. Remember: *don't* send it!

2   Next, write a letter expressing everything you appreciate about them, all you have learned from them. Really open you heart to them and forgive them.

This simple exercise will make you clearer and more able to meet them, if you wish to, or move on, without always carrying the weight of the past with you.

4 Write a journal

Another writing method is journaling. The best time to do this is first thing in the morning, because this is the time when you will have the least noise from your own inbuilt critic (that's the voice in you that undermines you and stops you from doing certain things or trying something new).

Exercise: journaling

1   Get a couple of pieces of paper and write down whatever comes up. Don't worry about writing fine literature here, just write as you think.

2   You might find yourself repeating sentences, using colourful language or appreciating something beautiful around you; on the other hand you may find yourself pouring scorn on someone or something – it doesn't matter what emerges, just go with it.

3   Let your hand write faster than you can think, don't worry about spelling and grammar or even sticking to the margins.

4   If you are writing about a past situation and get stuck, start each sentence with the phrase, 'I remember...' and allow whatever comes to follow. It doesn't even matter if it feels made up – it's your emotional truth.

This method, called 'Morning Pages', was originally designed by Julia Cameron to help creative artists get past their blocks, but it is of value to each one of us. After all, we are all creative: we are creating our own lives, and we'll be more and more creative if we are freed from the chains of the past.

5 Use physical movement

A great way to discharge negative emotions is through movement itself. As you know, when you have a good walk or a run, you come back feeling refreshed. The effect will be doubled if you use that exercise to discharge negative emotions.

Exercise: moving it out of your body
If you are emotionally upset, go for a jog, swim or walk, and with each step or stroke imagine letting go of the emotion you are feeling.

One excellent and systematic way to do this is to join a Five Rhythms class (see Resources). Its founder, Gabrielle Roth, has pioneered a way of using music and movement to tap deeply into unexpressed emotions and release them. It incorporates five specific rhythms, from very quiet to very frenetic, that magically bring up the full spectrum of unexpressed feelings.

6 Read some helpful books

Gabrielle Roth's book *Maps to Ecstasy: Healing Power of Movement* is helpful in moving through and letting go of negative emotions. My favourite is Tim Laurence's *You Can Change Your Life*. Also excellent for understanding the effect of our family conditioning is Oliver James's *They F*** You Up*. If you are drawn to journaling a very good book to help you is *The Artist's Way* by Julia Cameron.

7 Try emotional therapy

Many therapies identify what's wrong, but don't find ways to help you let go of the past and develop new and healthier habits.

When we react emotionally, these reactions are automatic and physical, literally flooding your brain and body with neurotransmitters associated with the stress response. They take over the rational mind, stop you being able to listen and lead to irrational reactions and behaviour. Your heart rate can jump from 70 beats a minute to over 100 in a single heartbeat, muscles tense and your breathing changes. Daniel Goleman, author of *Emotional Intelligence*, calls this emotional hijacking.[34] The emotional reaction patterns that trigger emotional hijacking are learned in early life and can be changed into more functional responses by coming to an understanding of how our past has programmed us to respond automatically to current events.

Looking back

Cast your mind back to your early childhood. How did you see anger expressed? Did you ever see your mother or father shouting, or did they give you the silent treatment? Were you able to sense their anger underneath? What did you learn from this? If you had a raging, shouting parent, you've probably learned to shut down, as you had to do when you were a frightened and vulnerable child. Perhaps you said that you'd never be like that when you grew up, and swore that you would certainly never, ever treat your children in that way. Yet, in a moment of weakness or frustration, you might have reacted in just the same way your parents did, and felt really guilty afterwards. It can take a lot of energy to be different from how we were brought up, because we had years of 'emotional education', both positive and negative, from our parents as well as our schoolteachers.

A softer emotion than anger is sadness. Think back to how your parents dealt with sadness or grief. For example, if there was a death in the family how did your parents react? Sadness is an appropriate reaction, but if it is left unexpressed it leads to depression. Depression can also arise from suppressed anger; 'Don't get sad, get mad,' the saying goes. If you are depressed, is there something you are angry about but have been unable to express or do something about? Do you think that either of your parents was depressed, and, if so, how has this affected you?

Look at your own characteristics

Are you either always trying to be positive about everything or do you have an underlying sense of hopelessness – or perhaps you flip-flop between the two? Do you fear that any love relationships are doomed, a minefield that could explode at any time, or are they best avoided completely? What lessons did you learn about love and relationships when you were growing up? If you always fear being abandoned or not finding a loving relationship, that may very well stem from early memories of feeling abandoned or unwanted as a child.

Our emotional baggage

The real destructive power of the past can become manifest because we keep recreating history by subconsciously setting up situations that feel familiar, despite our best intentions. It's horrifying and strangely comforting at the same time; for example, if we had a critical parent we attract a critical partner or boss. Or if one of your parents was always blaming the other for his or her problems, perhaps you have inherited the victim role. It's never your fault, and you always have someone else to blame. That's the power these negative patterns have in our lives. Psychologists call this 'transference', whereby we bring our internalised parents into our present lives, along with their, and our, shared emotional baggage from the past.

Finding emotional therapy

A good psychotherapist can help you let go of negative emotional patterns and develop healthier ways of being. To find a psychotherapist or counsellor in your area contact the UKCP (the United Kingdom Council for Psychotherapy). Also, we have been particularly impressed by psychotherapists and counsellors trained at the Psychosynthesis and Education Trust. It also has an excellent two-weekend workshop called The Essentials, which enables you to look at your life, how you would like it to be and what needs to change (see Resources).

8 The Hoffman Process

By far the most powerful and effective course I have come across, which frequently receives excellent reviews, is a one-week residential course called the Hoffman Process. It thoroughly 'undoes' the negative patterns of behaviour we have inherited from childhood, resulting in a profound transformation in relating and relationships, and the sense of who we are. It crosses the fine line between psychology – healing the psyche – and spirituality: getting you back in touch with the higher 'self' or soul. Since 1967, more than 70,000 people worldwide have used the techniques of Hoffman to achieve personal strength, clarity and freedom from destructive emotional patterns. Participants have reported benefits such as much better relationships with family members and being able to communicate more effectively at home and at work. I often receive letters from people who want to express their gratitude for the introduction to this excellent course and the transformation they have received from doing it (see Resources for details).

9 Find your purpose

When asked how he managed to be so vibrant in his nineties, Bertrand Russell replied, 'As you get older you must have a purpose larger than yourself. That's what makes life meaningful.' Having a sense of purpose in life, and feeling fulfilled, is vital to our overall well-being.

So what is it that gives you a sense of purpose? Of course, your sense of purpose may change at different times in your life; for example, taking care of your family may give you a sense of purpose. But when your children grow up or leave home, what then happens to your sense of purpose? Many people have a sense of purpose through doing work that is important and meaningful. This could be training in a profession, or setting up in business and making it successful. But what happens when you've achieved this? For some, being of service to others gives them a sense of purpose. This could take many forms. It might be service to your children or grandchildren, or to the community. It could include political action, supporting worthy causes that you feel passionate about or simply helping people you meet. Another feeling of purpose can come from having a connection to nature, and doing what you can to nurture the earth – whether it's gardening or recycling, or being involved in environmental issues. For some people, doing everything with love, or with excellence, gives them a sense of purpose. What is it that gives you a sense of purpose? In a moment I'll give you an exercise to help you if you are unclear.

Another purpose can be your own self-development – becoming the best you can be. Sometimes, this is originally motivated through our own desire to be happy and free of emotional pain, but through the process of our own transformation, and learning how to let go of our own limited concepts, negative patterns, selfishness and pettiness, we become more able to be of service to others. For some being of service to the greater good is what gives their life a sense of purpose. Some people practise this by identifying with a figure who represents what they aspire to be – be it the Dalai Lama or perhaps a 'hero' figure.

Changing your purpose through life

Of course, your purpose changes at different times of life. As you get older you may realise your purpose is not so much your job but what you feel 'called' to do – although the two might also be the same.

People who struggle with retirement are often struggling with re-discovering their purpose. A description of increasing maturity could be the expansion of your circle of caring: from yourself, to your family and immediate friends, to the community, and then to the world.

Exercise: discovering your purpose

Ask yourself the following three questions:

1 What do you enjoy doing or love to do? What makes you feel good? What gives you a sense of satisfaction and fulfilment?

2 What are you good at? We all have certain gifts or talents. For some it's the ability to listen; for others having a clear mind. What are your some of your gifts? You are unique and have your own unique gifts, but the secret is knowing what your gifts are and to give them. A sense of fulfilment often comes not from doing great deeds, but from doing small things with love, and to expand your circle of caring. Sometimes we feel we have gifts, but we have no way to give them, or feel that they are not being received. The question then becomes, how can you give your gifts and fulfil your purpose in another context?

3 What do you feel is needed now in the world, in your community or your family?

What purpose would answer these three questions? This could be your purpose.

10 Get in touch with your spiritual side

This chapter would not be complete without consideration of the spiritual dimension of healing, which can encompass many things, including prayer, meditation, energy flow and inner peace. Having some kind of connection to our spiritual side, to nature or to a higher power is what helps us to see the larger context in which we live so that we can live our lives with meaning, purpose and 'connectedness' with others, our family, community or environment. These aspects, of course, are not easily measured in terms of double-blind trials, neither is their direct effect on your biology. However, more and more trials are proving the positive effects of, for example, meditation on both health and happiness. It is important to realise that we are not helpless victims – we can consciously intervene in the healing process.

A complete change

Among the reports of people who have made remarkable recoveries from cancer, we often learn that they have often also made transformations on other fronts – nutritional, psychological and spiritual. The will to live is indeed a powerful part of this equation, and meditation and visualisation techniques have been shown to help. Perhaps best documented is the work of Carl and Stephanie Simonton who have demonstrated the power of visualisation techniques in the healing process. These are described in their book *Getting Well Again* (see Recommended Reading). People faced with a potentially life-threatening diagnosis often go through a stage of denial, followed by anger, fuelled by fear. In working through these issues and emotions, a person may come to accept the reality of their situation and, from that position, they will be better equipped to direct their will towards healing.

Many cancer survivors look back and see that their cancer was a 'turning point' in their lives, which brought them to a deeper, more spiritual understanding about themselves. It not only helped the healing process but also perhaps even inspired them to fulfil an unrealised dream. Lawrence LeShan is a research and clinical psychologist who has worked with cancer patients for over 40 years. In his book *Cancer as a Turning Point*, he explains that when people make certain kinds of psychological and lifestyle changes, they appear to create an inner 'healing climate' that maximises their potential for health.

Making connections

This isn't just talk. There's an increasing body of evidence about how you can induce a greater level of compassion, and in so doing change the brain's ability to connect. One of the first studies to gain

211

an insight into this was carried out at the University of Wisconsin, under the direction of Professor Richard Davidson. Brain activity in volunteers who were new to meditation was compared to that of Buddhist monks who had spent more than 10,000 hours in meditation.[35] The task was to practise 'compassion' meditation, generating a feeling of loving kindness towards all beings. 'We tried to generate a mental state in which compassion permeates the whole mind with no other thoughts,' said Matthieu Ricard, a Buddhist monk at Shechen Monastery in Katmandu, Nepal, who also holds a PhD in genetics.

There was a big difference between the novices and the monks. The monks, during meditation, had a large increase in high-frequency brain activity, which is associated with higher mental activity, such as consciousness, with more connection across the circuits of the brain. MRI brain scans also showed increased activity in the left prefrontal cortex (the seat of positive emotions, such as happiness) and reduced activity in the right prefrontal (the site of negative emotions and anxiety). Their results were also very high on tests for empathy.

Happiness

The more we learn about the impact of emotions on health and hormonal balance the more evident it is that being happy makes a huge difference, not only to your experience of life, but also to your physical health. A number of studies have reported, for example, an increase in DHEA, or a decrease in cortisol in relation to meditation, both of which are measures of less adrenal stress as well as improvements in quality of life (see Chapter 9).[36] Cancer can be conceived of as a communication breakdown between cells; it makes a lot of sense that if you have a communication breakdown with your partner, family and friends, and/or with your self (who you really are and who you need to become) that could be part of the complex picture that leads to cancer, and something you need to deal with to return to health.

PART 4

ANTI-CANCER NUTRIENTS

CHAPTER 24

Exploding the Myths

ancer is complex. In most cases it's due to a variety factors, including exposure to carcinogens that promote cell changes, exposure to cancer cell growth promoters and a poorly functioning immune system. Indeed, these unfavourable circumstances may need to be present for several decades to fuel the process from initiation to diagnosis.

The evidence already shows that we can achieve greater success in the battle against cancer, not only by aggressively treating the disease once it has developed but also by a number of preventative measures: minimising our exposure to carcinogens, limiting cancer promoters, such as excess hormones and hormone-disruptors, and boosting the immune system. The next seven chapters explain this evidence and the importance of optimising your intake of anti-cancer nutrients, such as vitamin C and beta-carotene. Eating foods high in these nutrients and supplementing particular nutrients at higher levels than you are likely to obtain from food alone is associated with a reduced incidence of certain cancers. The evidence for the role of nutritional supplements is already substantial, yet, controversially, supplementation is often reported negatively by the media, and this is what I will look at in this chapter.

Overleaf are just two examples of negative newspaper headlines regarding the use of vitamins:

'Over-use of vitamins may lead to cancer'
(*Financial Times*, May 2003)

'Vitamins A, C and E are a waste of time
and may even shorten your life'
(*Daily Mail*, April 2008)

However, when you look closer at the actual science, you will see that these statements are false.

Beta-carotene myths

There are over 2,000 studies showing a beneficial role for beta-carotene in preventing cancer, yet two studies in which synthetic beta-carotene was given on its own to smokers tend to receive most of the media attention. Such was the case when the *Daily Mail* ran an article headlined 'Cancer alert in vitamin pill probe', which said that there were 28 per cent more cases of lung cancer among a group of smokers supplementing 30mg of vitamin A and 25,000iu of beta-carotene.[1] How could this have happened?

Understanding beta-carotene

Carrots are one of the richest sources of beta-carotene, an antioxidant nutrient found in most orange-coloured foods. It's been well researched: more than 7,000 studies, at least 2,000 of which relate to cancer. There's no doubt that eating foods rich in beta-carotene reduces the risk of cancer.

The World Cancer Research Fund (WCRF), which reviewed hundreds of studies for their 1997 report,[2] concluded that carotenoids (the antioxidants found in fruit and vegetables, of which beta-carotene is one) are highly protective.[3] The WCRF are a little more conservative in their latest report, isolating their optimism for cancers of the mouth, pharynx, larynx and lung for carotenoids generally; oesophagus for beta-carotene; and prostate for lycopene (another carotenoid, which is found in tomatoes: others include lutein and zeaxanthin, both found in green veg). The reason for this is that it is extremely difficult to isolate and study individual nutrients when each food contains a complex mixture of different constituents, all of which may contribute to an effect. Collectively, they are probably more protective than any one in isolation.

There's also no doubt that having a higher beta-carotene level in your bloodstream is good news. In 2005, a ten-year study of several thousand elderly people in Europe, conducted by the Centre for Nutrition and Health at the National Institute of Public Health and the Environment in the Netherlands, found that the higher the beta-carotene level, the lower the overall risk of death, especially from cancer. Eating probably the equivalent of a carrot a day (raising blood level by 0.39mcmol/l) meant cutting the cancer risk by a third.[4]

The controversy about
beta-carotene supplements

All this good evidence has led to trials over the past 20 years in which people have been given beta-carotene supplements, sometimes in combination with other antioxidant nutrients. Many have proven protective; for example, research on 1,954 middle-aged men showed beta-carotene as having a protective effect against lung cancer.[5]

That's the good news. But what about the bad news that tends to make the headlines and stick in people's memories, such as the study mentioned earlier, which found an increased risk of cancer with beta-carotene? If you analyse the studies this scare is based on, you will find that the claim boils down to the fact that one smoker out of a thousand who takes beta-carotene on its own and takes no other antioxidant supplement, and continues to smoke, will have a slightly raised risk of cancer. This illustrates how a very minor risk is whipped up into something alarming. The study, by the National Cancer Institute in the US, gave smokers beta-carotene and reported a 28 per cent increased incidence in lung cancer in those who continued to smoke.[6] Of course, the press had a field day, with headlines such as 'Vitamins cause cancer'. A closer look at the figures, however, shows a rather different picture. In fact, the difference between those getting beta-carotene and those getting the placebo was not big enough to reach 'statistical significance'; it was only what is known as a 'trend'. That's important because it means that the result could have occurred by chance.

The actual figures were 50 cancer cases out of some 10,000 in the placebo group and 65 cases out of 10,000 among those getting beta-carotene. This means that for every five cases of cancer out of 1,000 people taking the placebo, there were 6.5 cases out of 1,000 among those taking the beta-carotene supplement. And remember, both groups involved people who had smoked for years and probably had undetected cancer before starting the trial. But how could such a result be seen as increasing cancer risk by 28 per cent?

Interpreting the results

It's important to know here the difference between 'absolute' risk and 'relative' risk. This way of interpreting results is also regularly used in drug trials to make a very small benefit look much more impressive. Here 64 divided by 50 equals 1.28, or an increased relative risk of 28 per cent. It sounds dramatic put this way but, as we've seen, it is actually not even statistically significant. The absolute risk, remember, is six cases per year in 1,000 for smokers taking beta-carotene, as compared to five cases in 1,000 for smokers on a placebo.

Hidden in the detail

As if this distortion was not unscientific enough, there was another set of findings in the research paper that never made it into the summary, let alone the newspaper headlines. Hidden in the body of the paper, which almost nobody ever reads, because they depend on the summary, was the finding that among those who gave up smoking during the trial and took beta-carotene, there were 20 per cent fewer cases of lung cancer. Again, this was not statistically significant, but if one 'trend' is worth reporting, surely so is another?

The implication of this finding might be that there could be something about smoking that makes it harder for beta-carotene given alone to have an effect.

Being nutritionally aware

There is another shortcoming in the above trial. The researchers were obviously ignorant of basic nutritional principles, and this is a serious failing if you are trying to test supplements. Unlike drugs, which often combine in a harmful way, nutrients, especially antioxidants, usually reinforce each other's effects. As explained in Chapter 2 (see illustration The synergistic action of nutrients in disarming a free radical, on page 14), antioxidants – and indeed most nutrients – work in synergy, so giving an individual nutrient on its own, as if it were a drug, to sick people without changing their diet or lifestyle, bears no relationship to the nutritional medicine approach to disease.

The importance of giving antioxidants together showed up in the other study that contributed to the 'beta-carotene-causes-cancer' scare. This time, male smokers were given either vitamin E, or vitamin E plus beta-carotene, or beta-carotene on its own. The first two groups showed no significant change, but the beta-carotene-only group showed an increased risk.[7] Once again, giving beta-carotene on its own to smokers shows up as very slightly raising the risk of cancer.

More research in 2005 showed this too. A review of all studies giving beta-carotene versus a placebo in relation to lung cancer, involving over 100,000 people concluded: 'For people with risk factors for lung cancer no reduction (*or increase*) in lung cancer incidence or mortality was found in those taking vitamins alone compared with placebo.'[8]

What the risk really is for smokers

So, all this fuss about beta-carotene boils down to a non-significant, tiny increased risk of lung cancer, only in smokers or people at risk, if given on its own. The chances are that it means absolutely nothing. In the worst-case scenario, out of 1,000 smokers supplementing beta-carotene on its own, just one might get lung cancer earlier.

What beta-carotene can do

For people not 'at risk', not smoking and not supplementing beta-carotene *on its own*, the evidence for beta-carotene's protective effect remains highly positive overall.

One large study involving 13,000 people aged between 35 and 60 to investigate the effects of a pill containing a cocktail of antioxidants (beta-carotene and vitamins C and E) found a highly significant 31 per cent reduction in the risk of all cancers in men, plus an overall 37 per cent lower death rate.[9]

Another study found this combination of antioxidants highly protective against colon cancer, but there was no such effect among those who were heavy drinkers and smokers who took only beta-carotene. In fact, for these people there was a very slight increased risk.[10] In response to this the *Daily Mail* ran a headline that read 'Vitamin pills could cause early death' with a subheading that read: 'Vitamins, taken by millions, could be causing thousands of premature deaths'. But it's highly unlikely that a heavy drinker and smoker would be taking beta-carotene on its own!

Looking deeper than the scare stories

If you look at these beta-carotene and cancer studies with a detached scientific eye, they don't actually form the basis for a scare story at all. Instead, they tell you something useful about how antioxidants work and how best to use them. Antioxidant nutrients are team players, as the illustration on page 14 shows. As explained in Chapter 2, their job is to disarm dangerous oxidants, generated by combustion – whether it be a lit cigarette or frying bacon. They do this by passing the oxidant through a chain of reactions involving vitamins E and C, beta-carotene, coenzyme Q_{10}, glutathione and lipoic acid. On their own, these antioxidant nutrients can do more harm than good, by becoming oxidised themselves. This is probably what's happening to beta-carotene among smokers.

Detoxifying cigarettes is a two-step process

One final point is worth mentioning: in the case of smokers, understanding how the liver detoxifies, and the role that beta-carotene plays, provides a logical explanation as to why beta-carotene supplements on their own could increase – not reduce – risk. As explained in Chapter 7, the liver is the major detoxifying organ in the body. It detoxifies harmful substances, including oxidants from tobacco smoke, in a two-step process called Phase 1 and Phase 2 detoxification, as shown in the illustration How the liver detoxifies, on page 51.

You may recall that Phase 1 is dependent on antioxidants such as beta-carotene and vitamin E, but it doesn't actually completely disarm toxins, such as those created from smoking. In fact, it can create toxic 'reactive intermediates'. If you have a toxic diet or lifestyle – for example, by smoking – and then increase your intake of individual antioxidants in supplement form, you can actually create more toxins in a kind of logjam effect. What you need is to support Phase 2 detoxification at the same time as supporting Phase 1, which depends on other nutrients such as B vitamins, selenium, glutathione, glucosinolates and sulphur (see Chapter 7).

What is happening in these trials, where smokers are given only beta-carotene, is that Phase 2 liver detoxification can't cope, or possibly that beta-carotene needs its other 'team players' to work (see illustration The synergistic action of nutrients in disarming a free radical, on page 14). This could certainly explain why studies giving either multivitamins alongside beta-carotene, or an antioxidant complex, don't report a negative result. It would also explain why foods high in beta-carotene seem to be only beneficial. Most of these also contain vital Phase 2 supporting nutrients. (Broccoli and other cruciferous vegetables contain folate and glucosinolates, whereas onions and garlic contain sulphur and glutathione derivatives.) It might also explain why selenium has the most positive effect of all the antioxidants if given singly, because it helps both Phase 1 *and* Phase 2 to work.

The bottom line

The moral of this story is that nutrients work in synergy and are best supplemented as a group, not in isolation. The worst thing a smoker could do is to eat a lousy diet and supplement beta-carotene on its own. So, if you are a heavy smoker or drinker, our advice would be to stop smoking and drinking excessively, and not to supplement beta-carotene on its own. However, even among smokers, a high *dietary* intake of beta-carotene is not associated with increased risk.[11] Therefore, a smoker would probably benefit the most from taking an all-round optimum-nutrition-level multivitamin and a comprehensive antioxidant containing selenium, glutathione and/or N-acetyl-cysteine (NAC), and possibly extra vitamin C – but most importantly, eating antioxidant-rich foods.

Vitamin C myths

Another popular myth is that vitamin C doesn't help reduce cancer risk and could even promote it. No studies have shown this to be the case although research since the 1970s has shown its highly protective effects.

Positive research into vitamin C

Vitamin C was first shown to be a powerful anti-cancer agent in 1971, but it wasn't until 20 years later that it started to be accepted by the medical profession. In 1992, Dr Gladys Block, formerly with the National Cancer Institute, wrote:

> I have reviewed the epidemiologic literature, about 140 studies, on the relationship between antioxidant micro-nutrients or their food sources and cancer risk. The data are overwhelmingly consistent. With possibly fewer than five exceptions, every single study is in the protective direction, and something like 110 to 120 studies found statistically significant reduced risk with high intake.

Vitamin C-rich diets reduce the risk of cancer. High intakes – above 5,000mg a day (the equivalent of 100 oranges) – substantially increase the life expectancy of cancer patients. In Chapter 26, I will give you the very latest evidence on high-dose vitamin C and cancer.

The minority view

Yet, despite the above, one of the most commonly cited studies is that from the University of Leicester, which resulted in newspaper headlines claiming that vitamin supplements cause cancer.[12] The study in question found that one accepted marker for oxidative stress and DNA damage – 8-oxoguanine – decreased with the supplementation of 500mg of vitamin C, indicating a protective effect. Another less accepted marker – 8-oxadenine – increased. On the basis of this latter finding, the authors suggested that vitamin C might have a potentially carcinogenic effect. What the study actually showed was ambiguous. Vitamin C was shown to be both protective and harmful to DNA.

According to vitamin C expert, Dr Balz Frei, Director of the Linus Pauling Institute (a well-respected education and research facility into the study of diet and health), fears about vitamin C are unfounded, both because these results contradict the findings of other research groups and also because poor experimental procedure could easily have led to oxidative damage to DNA, which may have been wrongly blamed on vitamin C. 'Frankly, I question whether this data will hold up when we analyse it further. The value of vitamin C must be considered in its totality, not just one single biological effect,' says Frei.

Nutrients working together

Once again, this work may highlight the importance of nutrient synergy, since sufficient vitamin E, glutathione and flavonoids help to prolong vitamin C's antioxidant effect. With hundreds of studies concluding that high intakes of vitamin C are associated with lowered cancer risk, there is no good reason, on the basis of this one study involving 30 people, to doubt that vitamin C supplementation remains both safe and effective in preventing cancer.

Twisting the statistics

Another way of fuelling scares about supplements is to conduct what is called a 'meta-analysis' or 'systematic review' in a highly selective way. A meta-analysis is a standard way of discovering the real value of a treatment by combining a number of studies and then using statistics to tease out the benefits or problems that may not show up in the individual trials. Done carefully, this can be very useful, but its effectiveness depends heavily on which trials you choose to include and how you do your statistics.

A good example of how not to do it is the systematic review of antioxidants and gastrointestinal cancers published in the prestigious medical journal the *Lancet* in 2004.[13] The abstract (the summary at the beginning) says: 'We could not find evidence that antioxidant supplements can prevent gastrointestinal cancers; on the contrary, they seem to increase overall mortality.'

Apparently another blow for supplements, leading to another round of negative headlines in the press. However, a bit of investigation, including contacting the lead author of the paper who was crucial in producing the negative result, revealed a quite different picture. He told me that he was horrified at the way his results had been distorted.

Partial approaches?

The authors of the review in the *Lancet* looked at seven trials, which, they said, were of high enough scientific quality to be included – that is, they had 'high methodology'. The first hint that the selection might not have been entirely impartial was that they excluded at least one major trial that showed benefit; this had been published by the US National Cancer Institute,[14] so should have shown 'high methodology'.

Even so, six of the trials in the review showed benefits from anti-oxidants. That left just one that came up with an apparently negative result.[15] However, the statistical analysis gave it so much weight that the findings from this one study were enough to outweigh the other six and show that antioxidants increased mortality.

Misrepresenting information

When I looked at this key study, however, it didn't seem to be negative, so I contacted the lead author, Dr Pelayo Correa from the pathology department at the Louisiana State University Health Sciences Center in New Orleans, and asked about the increased risk he had suppos-edly found. Dr Correa was amazed, because his research, far from being negative, had shown clear benefit from taking vitamins.

His study, published in the *Journal of the National Cancer Institute*, had involved giving people with gastric cancer either beta-carotene, vitamin C or antibiotics to kill off the stomach bacterium *Helicobacter pylori*. All three interventions produced highly significantly improve-ments, causing substantial regression of gastric cancer. Correa and his colleagues had concluded: 'dietary supplementation with antioxidant micronutrients may interfere with the precancerous process, mostly

225

by increasing the rate of regression of cancer precursor lesions, and may be an effective strategy to prevent gastric carcinoma'. No evidence of increased mortality there.

In fact, as Correa told me, there was no way the study could show anything about mortality. 'Our study was designed for evaluation of the progress of precancerous lesions,' he said. 'It did not intend, and did not have the power, to study mortality and has no value to examine mortality of cancer.'[16] Without this study, the main conclusion, widely reported in the media, that antioxidants may increase gastrointestinal cancer becomes completely invalid.

Positives ignored

The distortion 'scientific medicine' is capable of didn't stop there. The paper in the *Lancet* did find a highly significant and consistent reduction of overall risk (expressed as 'p.00001' – meaning that if you ran the trials 100,000 times you would get the same result 99,999 times) in four trials giving selenium supplements. These positive results, however, were dismissed on the basis of 'inadequate methodology' in three out of four studies. It's this kind of distorted selection and statistical analysis that, after extensive promotion to the media, adds another brick in the wall designed to keep food medicine out of the mainstream.

How can you get the complete picture?

The moral of these stories is to look at the whole picture and to weigh up the totality of the evidence. Of course, as a lay person, this isn't easy to do. A modicum of common sense is also a good maxim. Despite the fact that no one has ever died from taking a multivitamin, and that most surveys show that those who take supplements, at least high-potency ones, live longer, feel better and are less likely to get sick, vitamin scares aren't about to stop. A few may be valid, but the vast majority are not. Unless you live and breathe this subject as we do, it isn't easy to know when you really need to be concerned. One of the purposes of the 100% Health Club (see Resources, page 381) is so that we can help you sort out the wheat from the chaff in our e-newsletters and blogs. Armed with more in-depth analysis, plus your own common sense, you'll be in a better position to judge for yourself.

As the next chapter shows, there is already enough proof that supplementing antioxidant nutrients and eating antioxidant-rich foods are essential both in preventing cancer and in nutritionally supporting people with the disease.

To dig deeper, and to find out how these vitamin scares have been used to suppress nutritional medicine in favour of drug-based medicine, read my book *Food is Better Medicine than Drugs*, co-authored with Jerome Burne.

CHAPTER 25

The Truth about Antioxidants and Cancer

Great progress is being made in nutritional approaches to cancer. The discovery that vitamins A, C and E can disarm oxidants, the most prevalent carcinogens, is now the subject of mainstream, government-funded research, into both the treatment and the prevention of cancer. To date, results have been very impressive, although we are beginning to understand that the role of a number of anti-cancer agents goes deeper than simply disarming carcinogens.

Vitamin A, for example, not only controls cell growth, but also stimulates communication between cells; vitamin C boosts immune response; vitamin E protects fats from oxidation and recycles vitamin C. These nutrients are best thought of as 'adaptogens' (substances that help us to adapt to a hostile environment), and they are widely available in nature. However, many of today's most significant carcinogens are man-made; in other words, they are a consequence of not respecting our relationship with the environment.

Cancer may be seen as the result of too many carcinogens and too few adaptogens. Tilting the equation back the other way gives us our best hope of preventing or reversing cancer.

Vitamin A and beta-carotene

Both vitamin A, and its precursor, beta-carotene, have anti-cancer properties, as a number of studies have shown.

Lung cancer and others

People with lung cancer have been found to have much lower than normal blood vitamin A and carotenoid levels[17] and there is a strong link between the risk of lung cancer and vitamin A and beta-carotene status. People with low dietary intake of vitamin A have twice the risk of lung cancer as those with the highest vitamin A intake. Similarly, a high intake of beta-carotene from raw fruits and vegetables reduces the risk of lung cancer in smokers[18] and non-smoking men and women,[19] as well as reducing the risk of cancer of the stomach, colon, prostate and cervix.[20]

In a study involving doctors as the volunteers, taking beta-carotene supplements (50mg on alternate days) for 12 years was associated with a 32 per cent decrease in prostate cancer incidence among those with low beta-carotene status at that start of the study.[21]

Breast cancer

Evidence for a link between beta-carotene and breast cancer is less strong. One recent study demonstrated that eating plenty of vegetables (which raise carotenoid levels in the blood, increasing fibre levels and reducing dietary fat) did reduce the risk of the recurrence of breast cancer.[22] In another study, which followed over 7,000 women for up to nine and a half years, high blood levels of lycopene (a carotenoid which is particularly abundant in tomatoes) was linked to a reduced risk of breast cancer. However, the researchers found no evidence of protection from beta-carotene or vitamin A.[23]

Cancers of the head and neck, and leukaemia

One study supplementing beta-carotene (30mg per day) resulted in an improvement in 71 per cent of patients with oral pre-cancer (leuko-plakia), whereas 60,000mcg (200,000iu) of vitamin A a day resulted in complete remission for 57 per cent of patients.[24] Research has also taken place on the cancer 'drug' 13-cis-retinoic acid (isotretinoin) and all-trans-retinoic acid. Dr Huang has shown that all-trans-retinoic acid (the substance the body converts vitamin A into) puts acute myeloid leukae-mia in complete 'remission'.[25] Drs Hong and Lippman have shown that high doses of 13-cis-retinoic acid have effectively 'suppressed' squa-mous cell carcinomas of the head and neck.[26] The researchers noted that 'second primary tumours are the chief cause of treatment failure and death in patients' (with regard to head and neck cancers). After a year of treating 49 patients with 13-cis-retinoic acid and 51 patients with placebos, 4 per cent had second primary tumours in the 13-cis-retinoic acid group, as opposed to 24 per cent in the placebo group.

What the research tells us

These studies are important, not only because they show the value of vitamin A and its metabolites (what vitamin A turns into in the body) in reversing the cancer process but also because they do actu-ally look at the metabolites. Even in a person whose blood level of vitamin A is normal, taking supplements can raise levels of these cancer-protecting metabolites. This is the basis of using large doses of vitamin A as part of an anti-cancer regime.

Supplementing beta-carotene, however, does not appear to affect the recurrence of oral, pharyngeal, or laryngeal squamous cell carci-noma.[27] So this particular benefit relates to derivatives of retinol, the animal-derived source of vitamin A.

Overcoming the problems with vitamin A

Vitamin A and its metabolites are not without toxicity, however. High-dose vitamin A has been shown to increase the risk of birth defects in animals, and for this reason it is unwise to supplement more than 3,000mcg (10,000iu) if you are pregnant or likely to become pregnant. However, the same caution does not apply to beta-carotene. Although it can be converted into vitamin A, the liver converts very little once the body's vitamin A stores are full, so there is a protective mechanism to guard against taking in too much. Since beta-carotene is an antioxidant and anti-cancer agent in its own right, having more of it circulating around the body is definitely good news.

How much should you take?

An ideal daily supplemental intake of vitamin A as a preventative dose is 1,500 to 3,300mcg (5,000–10,000iu) as retinol and 15–25mg as beta-carotene, in addition to eating a diet high in fruits and vegetables. Larger intakes of supplements may be appropriate for people with cancer, but these should be given only with proper guidance by your doctor or a nutritional therapist.

The consistent link between a high dietary intake and sufficient levels in the blood of beta-carotene and vitamin A and a low risk of cancer are good enough reasons to eat foods rich in this key nutrient (as listed below) and to top up with supplements. However, much more research needs to be done to identify the actual role of beta-carotene in the treatment of cancer.

Which foods are best for vitamin A and beta-carotene?

The foods overleaf are listed in order of those that contain the most beta-carotene or vitamin A per calorie of food. The figures in brackets are the amount of beta-carotene or vitamin A, measured in mcg or mcg(RE) in 100g (3½oz), which is roughly equivalent to a cup or a serving.

Beef liver	10,841mcg	Papayas	610mcg
Veal liver	8,049mcg	Pumpkin	485mcg
Carrots	8,523mcg	Broccoli	467mcg
Sweet potatoes	5,168mcg	Tomatoes	343mcg
Apricots (dried)	2,194mcg	Tangerines	279mcg
Squash	2,121mcg	Asparagus	251mcg
Watercress	1,424mcg	Nectarines	221mcg
Mangoes	1,180mcg	Peaches	162mcg
Cabbage	909mcg	Peppers	161mcg
Melon	977mcg	Watermelon	111mcg
Apricots (fresh)	792mcg		

Vitamin C

As with beta-carotene, the overwhelming evidence is that a high intake of vitamin C correlates with a low risk of cancer. In January 1991, Dr Gladys Block, formerly with the National Cancer Institute, published a review[28] of vitamin C research, which concluded that there was very strong evidence of a protective effect of vitamin C for non-hormone cancers. Of the 46 such studies in which a dietary vitamin C index was calculated, 33 found statistically significant protection.

After completing a further review[29] later that year of studies linking vitamin C with cancer prevention, Dr Block reached this conclusion:

> Approximately 90 epidemiologic studies have examined the role of vitamin C or vitamin C-rich foods in cancer prevention, and the vast majority have found statistically significant protective effects. Evidence is strong for cancers of the oesophagus, oral cavity, stomach and pancreas. There is also substantial evidence of a protective effect in cancers of the cervix, rectum and breast. Even in lung cancer there is recent evidence of a role for vitamin C.

Another review of vitamin C research reached similar conclusions: 'Epidemiologic evidence of a protective effect of vitamin C for non-hormone cancers is very strong. Of the 46 such studies in which a dietary vitamin C index was calculated, 33 found statistically sig-nificant protection.'

Early findings

The first ever study in which vitamin C was given to cancer patients was carried out in the 1970s, by Dr Linus Pauling and Dr Ewan Cameron, a cancer specialist, working in Scotland. They gave 100 terminally ill cancer patients 10g (10,000mg) of vitamin C each day (intravenous for ten days, followed by oral doses) and compared their outcome with 1,000 cancer patients given conventional therapy. The survival rate was five times higher in those taking vitamin C and, by 1978, although all of the 1,000 'control patients' had died, 13 of the vitamin C patients were still alive, with 12 apparently free from can-cer.[30] Other studies have backed up these findings. Drs Murata and Morishige of Saga University in Japan showed that cancer patients on 5–30g of vitamin C lived six times longer than those on 4g or less, while those suffering from cancer of the uterus lived 15 times longer on vitamin C therapy.[31] This was also confirmed by the late Dr Abram Hoffer in Canada, who found that patients on high doses of vitamin C survived, on average, ten times longer.

However, Pauling and Cameron's findings were discredited, largely due to an apparent 'replication' of their study by the Mayo Clinic in the US.[32] There was, however, one major difference between the original trial and that of the Mayo Clinic. The 'terminal' patients in the original trial continued to take vitamin C every day, whereas those in the Mayo Clinic trial stopped after an average of 75 days. However, by then, the book was closed and mega-dose vitamin C was considered quackery.

Versatile vitamin C

Of all the antioxidants, vitamin C is the most extraordinary. It is believed to help prevent and treat cancer by enhancing the immune system; stimulating the formation of collagen which is necessary for 'walling off' tumours; preventing metastasis (spreading) by inhibiting a particular enzyme and therefore keeping the ground substance around tumours intact; preventing viruses that can cause cancer; correcting a vitamin C deficiency, which is often seen in cancer patients; speeding up wound healing in cancer patients after surgery; enhancing the effectiveness of some chemotherapy drugs; reducing the toxicity of some chemotherapy; preventing free-radical damage and neutralising some carcinogens.

Numerous studies have found a link between a low intake of vitamin C and the incidence of several different cancers, especially non-hormonal ones.[33] Also, having a high plasma level of vitamin C cuts your risk of dying from cancer.[34] The evidence for the benefits of vitamin C is strongest for cancers of the mouth, oesophagus, stomach, lung, pancreas and cervix. Although one analysis of 12 clinical studies found that, 'Vitamin C intake had the most consistent and statistically significant inverse association with breast cancer risk,'[35] the evidence of an associated decreased risk of breast cancer is not as strong. One study involving 34,000 post-menopausal women reported no association between the intake of vitamins A, C and E and a reduced risk of developing breast cancer.[36]

The World Cancer Research Fund (WCRF) conclude that there is no evidence of a relationship between vitamin C intake and prostate cancer, and insufficient evidence for breast cancer. The studies to date do suggest a big difference between the causes and treatment of hormone-related cancers and those of the lung or digestive tract. These lung and digestive tract cancers may be more related to oxidant carcinogens, and prevented by increasing one's intake of antioxidant nutrients. Having an intake above 100mg a day cuts the risk of lung cancer substantially.[37]

Diet and supplements

Overall, the research to date strongly supports the importance of eating a diet rich in vitamin C (see over). Whereas supplementing 1–5g vitamin C may help prevent some cancers, cancer patients are most likely to benefit from 10g or more a day. These higher levels are best taken with the guidance of your health practitioner.

Which foods are best for vitamin C?

The foods below are listed in order of those that contain the most vitamin C per calorie of food. The figures in brackets are the amount of vitamin C in 100g, which is roughly equivalent to a cup or serving.

Broccoli	(110mg)	Cauliflower	(60mg)
Peppers	(100mg)	Strawberries	(60mg)
Kiwi fruit	(85mg)	Oranges	(50mg)
Lemons	(80mg)	Grapefruits	(40mg)
Papayas	(62mg)	Tangerines	(31mg)
Brussels sprouts	(62mg)	Limes	(29mg)
Watercress	(60mg)	Mangoes	(28mg)
Cabbage	(60mg)	Melons	(25mg)
Tomatoes	(60mg)	Peas	(25mg)

Vitamin E

Whereas vitamin C is a water-based antioxidant, which protects the watery parts of the body, vitamin E is a fat-based antioxidant, protecting cell membranes and structural fats. Having a low level of vitamin E in your blood significantly increases your risk of smoking-related and other cancers, according to a Finnish study of 21,172 men over ten years.[38] Further evidence for vitamin E's potent protective role against cancer was shown in an analysis of 59 clinical studies. The researchers found that there was 'modest' protection from vitamin supplements, but vitamin E supplements were most consistently associated with a reduced risk of cancer.[39]

Low vitamin E and breast cancer

Vitamin E deficiency is most strongly associated with an increased risk of breast cancer. Research in 1984 in Britain, led by Dr Wald at St Bartholomew's Hospital in London, found that 'Those with the lowest vitamin E levels have the highest risk for breast cancer.'[40] A 1996 trial, involving 2,569 women with breast cancer, concluded, 'A diet rich in several micronutrients, especially beta-carotene, vitamin E and calcium, may be protective against breast cancer.'[41] These are but a few examples from a wealth of data that links breast cancer with low vitamin E levels, and the prevention of breast cancer with increased vitamin E intake.

Chemical-family connections

While there is plenty of evidence showing the antioxidant role that vitamin E itself can play in the prevention of breast cancer, a 1998 study confirmed similar benefit from tocotrienols, which are in the same chemical 'family' as vitamin E. Tocotrienols have been found to work in tandem with vitamin E in inhibiting the growth of breast cancer cells in humans. They are found in significant concentrations in palm oil, barley extract and rice oil.[42]

Prostate cancer

Vitamin E supplementation has also been shown to help protect against prostate cancer. A study on Finnish men, published in the *Journal of the National Cancer Institute*, showed a 41 per cent lower death rate from prostate cancer in those supplementing vitamin E. The men who took 50mg of vitamin E daily for five to eight years had a 32 per cent lower rate of symptomatic prostate cancer than men who did not take the supplement. 'This intriguing observation suggests that vitamin E has the potential to prevent one of the most common malignant tumours in the North American and European populations,' wrote Dr Olli Heinonen from the University of Helsinki, who believes that vitamin E's antioxidant properties may help stave off prostate cancer by fighting oxidants and boosting the immune system.[43]

236

Supplements and diet

An optimal supplemental intake for cancer prevention is between 270 and 540mg per day, on top of eating foods rich in vitamin E (see below).

Which foods are best for vitamin E?

Foods are listed in order of those that contain the most vitamin E per calorie of food. The figures in brackets are the amount of vitamin E in 100g, which is roughly equivalent to a cup or serving.

Cold-pressed seed oil	(83mg)	Beans	(7.7mg)
Sunflower seeds	(52.6mg)	Tuna	(6.3mg)
Wheatgerm	(27.5mg)	Sweet potato	(4.0mg)
Almonds	(24.5mg)	Peas	(2.3mg)
Sesame seeds	(22.7mg)	Brown rice	(2.0mg)
Pecans	(19.8mg)	Sardines	(2.0mg)
Walnuts	(19.6mg)	Salmon	(1.8mg)
Peanuts	(11.8mg)	Lentils	(1.3mg)
Cashews	(10.9mg)		

Cutting cancer risk and improving the outcomes for cancer sufferers

In those people not eating an antioxidant-rich diet, supplementing beta-carotene, vitamin E and selenium in combination has been shown to cut risk by 13 per cent.[44] The best action to take is to eat a diet high in antioxidants and to take an all-round antioxidant supplement, rather than taking antioxidants in isolation.

CHAPTER 26

Mega-dose Vitamin C and Cancer

There's a saying about new ideas. First, they say it's not true and not important. Then they say it's true, but not important. Then they say it's true, it's important, but not new. We saw on page 233 that Dr Linus Pauling shocked the medical establishment by claiming that mega-doses of vitamin C could cure cancer. He was ridiculed and attacked – but, according to new research, it appears he was right. As explained in Chapter 25, studies in the 1970s by Pauling and cancer specialist Dr Ewan Cameron were highly criticised at the time, partly because they weren't placebo-controlled trials.[45] While other studies later followed Cameron and Pauling's approach, researchers gave the vitamin C for only a limited period of time or did not include intravenous vitamin C, so the studies didn't get positive results. In short, the idea that high-dose vitamin C could be used for the treatment of cancer was just too controversial and eventually became buried.

New developments

Now, 40 years on, mega-dose vitamin C is finally back on the medical agenda, thanks to a series of detailed studies that have shown that many types of cancer cells simply can't survive in a vitamin-C rich environment and, most recently, that injecting large amounts of vitamin C into lab mice with aggressive and hard-to-treat tumours caused the cancers to shrink by between 41 and 53 per cent.[46] The next stage of this research, headed by Dr Mark Levine from the American National Institutes of Health, is clinical trials on cancer patients using intravenous vitamin C. In fact, they've already published case studies of people with advanced cancer who have responded very well to this treatment.[47]

This might sound like a big breakthrough, but actually the power of mega-dose vitamin C has been known for decades – not only to kill cancer cells but also used to inactivate viruses, from the common cold to HIV. However, this new research is making the medical profession sit up and take note. Also, the research is claiming two things that could make high-dose vitamin C a 'medicine' that would only be prescribed by doctors. The first is that only high doses or intravenous vitamin C work (therefore making it a medical procedure), and second that vitamin C is not working as an antioxidant in these cases, but as a pro-oxidant, so potentially reclassifying it, at least in high doses, as a pharmacological agent rather than a nutrient. (All antioxidants become pro-oxidants in the process of disarming harmful oxidants and these researchers are suggesting that vitamin C, in its oxidised form, is toxic to cancer cells.)

Who is using it so far?

Intravenous vitamin C does work very well for some cancer patients. In the UK, there's a small group of doctors giving intravenous vitamin C. One of these is Dr Julian Kenyon, from the Dove Clinic in Harley Street and Hampshire (www.doveclinic.com), who has treated more than 100 patients over the last ten years with intravenous vitamin C. 'When vitamin C is given intravenously in very high doses it doesn't behave like an antioxidant at all,' says Dr Kenyon. 'What the American study showed is that when you infuse amounts as high as 4 grams per kilo, which means about 75 grams for an average adult, vitamin C has an oxidative effect inside the tumour. It causes a build-up of a chemical called hydrogen peroxide which destroys the tumour.'

Case study

Dennis Vaughan's case is an interesting one. A check-up revealed that his prostate cancer was becoming more active. His prostate specific antigen (PSA) score – which measures how active the tumour is – rose from 13 to 18.5. His oncologist wanted him to have drugs or radiotherapy, but Vaughan, who is a strong believer in a natural approach to health, preferred to try a treatment offered by his London GP that involved infusing vitamin C into the bloodstream. He underwent weekly treatment – with up to 75g of vitamin C at a time. 'It's a very easy treatment,' says Dennis. 'You lie back in a chair and read or listen to music for an hour and a half. There's no discomfort and afterwards you feel fine.' Treatment costs £100 a time, and after seven weeks his PSA score dropped back down to 13, a level described as moderately elevated. At the time of going to press he's back on a strategy of watchful waiting and his oncologist has said that he now doesn't need to see him for another year.

Antioxidant or pro-oxidant?

Vitamin C is a known antioxidant, mopping up dangerous free radicals (see Chapter 2). However, the discovery that, in high doses, it acts like a pro-oxidant – specifically within cancer cells but not in normal cells – opens up a new avenue of understanding for the potential value of mega-dose vitamin C, both for cancer and to eliminate viruses.

To understand how an antioxidant such as vitamin C works, think of it as a 'high energy' particle, or a particle with 'extra information'. Normally, it can disarm harmful oxidants by giving them a free electron so that they become stable and no longer dangerous. At that point the vitamin C becomes an oxidant, called dehydroascorbate. In normal cells it is reloaded back to an antioxidant. In other words, all antioxidants become pro-oxidants if they are doing their job properly, but only temporarily. So you don't get much dehydroascorbate in normal cells. Levine found that even massive levels of intravenous vitamin C were completely non-toxic to normal cells. But something different happens in cancer cells.

Tumour cells are recognised by vitamin C

Vitamin C researcher Dr Steve Hickey, from Manchester Metropolitan University,[48] explains: 'In cancer cells it's quite different. Tumour cells are damaged and have higher levels of unstable metal ions, such as copper or iron. The mixture of free iron and vitamin C generates hydrogen peroxide inside the tumour. As a consequence it poisons the tumour cells or it generates dehydroascorbate which poisons them.' He's careful to point out that this is one mechanism that's thought to explain why vitamin C is so toxic to cancer cells, but there may be other mechanisms. Vitamin C, after all, has about a dozen functions that enhance your body's natural immunity. At one level you can think of a cancer cell as a cell that's lost information, or has low energy. It actually reverts to a primitive way of surviving with disregard for its neighbours. By increasing nutrient intake you are adding energy, or information, into the system to restore health.

Intravenous or oral?

There's little doubt that exposing cancer cells to high-dose vitamin C works, but can you achieve these kinds of levels with oral vitamin C? Dr Mark Levine says that you can't: 'Pharmacological concentrations of plasma ascorbate, from 0.3 mM to 15 mM are achievable only from IV administration. Plasma concentrations achieved from maximal possible oral doses cannot exceed 0.22 mM because of limited intestinal absorption.' But Dr Steve Hickey disagrees: 'We've measured 0.25mM from a single 5 gram dose of vitamin C and recorded 0.42mM with a 36 gram dose of liposomal vitamin C. It looks like you could sustain a level of 0.4, and possibly 0.5 mM in the plasma if you keep taking in vitamin C at a high level.' (Hickey's book *Ascorbate: Science of Vitamin C* is well worth reading if you're contemplating intravenous mega-dose vitamin C treatment for cancer, see Recommended Reading.) In case you are wondering what 'liposomal' vitamin C is, it means that the vitamin C is encased in a liposome, which is a tiny bubble made out of the same material as a cell membrane. This 'capsule' can be filled with drugs, and used to deliver drugs for cancer and other diseases. In this way, the drug – or vitamin C in this case – is able to get directly into the cell itself to do its job.

In Levine's cancer studies, giving enough vitamin C intravenously to achieve a level of 0.28 mM was toxic to cancer cells, and is clearly achievable with oral vitamin C. Hickey's point is that while intravenous treatment might involve one hour of maximising plasma levels to a point not achievable with oral vitamin C, and be more toxic to cancer cells and viruses during that time, if you keep taking high oral doses, with 3g or more every four hours, you can achieve an accumulative build-up of blood levels. So you have a more continuous anti-cancer effect. Of course, doing both, which is what Linus Pauling and Dr Ewan Cameron did back in the 1970s, may be the best strategy.

Why this might work

This makes intuitive sense for a number of reasons. Firstly, there's so much evidence that the higher your intake of vitamin C the lower your cancer risk, and it would be very unusual if low-dose vitamin C, even the levels achieved in a high fruit and vegetable diet, worked in a totally different way from higher doses. We have also seen that high oral doses do clearly work, as Drs Murata and Morishige of Saga University in Japan showed with cancer patients.

> ## Before taking high doses of vitamin C
>
> Remember, if you are interested in having intravenous high doses of vitamin C, contact a clinic that specialises in these treatments, having first spoken to your doctor or oncologist (see Resources). If you are considering taking high dose oral vitamin C you should also speak to your doctor or oncologist first, and I recommend that you also enlist the support of an experienced nutritional therapist.

How much vitamin C to take orally

Advocates of vitamin C have long known that the most therapeutic intake is the 'bowel tolerance' level. This means taking as much as will cause you to have loose bowels, and then reducing the dose slightly. Interestingly, when a person has cancer or a viral infection, they can often tolerate much more vitamin C than usual – often 10 to 50 times their normal amount. Some people with cancer can tolerate 50g a day without getting loose bowels. The main argument for oral vitamin C not working in the way that intravenous vitamin C does is that it can't be absorbed. But if a person isn't getting loose bowels, then it's going somewhere – probably to the cancer cells.

Dangers of too much vitamin C?

Almost everyone has heard rumours that high-dose vitamin C causes kidney stones or might interfere with other cancer treatments. But these are only rumours. Vitamin C has been extensively studied for its potential to cause kidney stones, and has been found not to; even the British government's expert report on vitamin and minerals accepts this. But what about mega doses interfering with other cancer treatments?

According to Jeanne Drisko, Professor of Orthomolecular Medicine at the University of Kansas, who is running human trials to test for safety and tolerability of the treatment, 'We've found no evidence that giving vitamin C orally, along with both chemotherapy and intravenous vitamin C, reduces their effectiveness in destroying a tumour.' She finds it beneficial to give both intravenous and oral vitamin C, and reports that patients feel better. Nor is there any evidence that it interferes with radiotherapy.

Is it appropriate for you?

High-dose intravenous or oral vitamin C therapy works better for some cancers than others. It shouldn't be thought of as a cure-all, however, but, in many cases, is a useful adjunct to other treatment. Also, you do need strong veins, because you would be infusing a couple of litres of liquid several times over the course of a week.

High oral doses of vitamin C shouldn't cause any concerns provided you stick to the bowel-tolerance level. Some people don't tolerate ascorbic acid as well as ascorbate, the alkaline form of vitamin C, and report digestive discomfort. Ascorbate is available as sodium ascorbate, magnesium ascorbate or calcium ascorbate. If you are taking very high amounts, bear in mind that you'll also be getting larger amounts of the minerals it is combined with. For short-term use this is unlikely to be a problem, but for long-term use it's probably better to stick to straight ascorbic acid.

CHAPTER 27

How Vitamin D Protects Against Cancer

Vitamin D, long thought to be only important for bone health, may also help to reduce the risk of certain cancers, including colon, breast and prostate. A person's vitamin D status differs according to latitude and race, with residents in the northern hemisphere and individuals with more skin pigmentation being at increased risk of deficiency. Numerous studies show an association between higher levels of sun exposure, blood levels of vitamin D and intakes of vitamin D (both from diet and supplements) and a lower risk of developing and/or surviving cancer.

A four-year trial involving 1,200 women found those taking vitamin D (27.5mcg, or 1,100iu/day) had a 60 per cent reduction in cancer incidence, compared with those who didn't take it – rising to a 77 per cent reduction for cancers diagnosed after the first year (and therefore excluding those cancers more likely to have originated prior to the vitamin D intervention).[49]

It has long been known that women who live in sunnier countries are less likely to develop breast cancer than women who see little sunshine, but it has also been found that women who have high levels of vitamin D are more likely to survive if they do. Vitamin D is made in the skin in the presence of sunlight, so both diet and exposure of the skin to sunlight play a part.

Halve your risk of colon cancer

This theory, first proposed by Dr Cedrick Garland in 1980, led to research that showed a strong association between risk of colon cancer and dietary intake of vitamin D and calcium.[50] An eight-year study of 25,802 people from the state of Maryland found that those with blood levels of vitamin D equivalent to 10mcg (400iu) or more had half the risk of colon cancer of those with lower levels.[51] This is twice the US RDA of 5mcg (200iu). In the UK, there is no recommended daily dietary intake for vitamin D if you are aged between four and 50 and live a 'normal lifestyle'. However, by 'normal' they mean spending time every day outdoors in the sunshine, which is not always possible given the UK weather and people's lifestyles. For those confined indoors, the experts recommend 10mcg per day.[52]

Since 1980, many researchers have confirmed this association. A scientific review undertaken by the National Cancer Institute in 2007 found that vitamin D was beneficial in preventing colorectal cancer. Although the study found no link between vitamin D status and overall cancer mortality, the study did show that blood levels of 80 nanomoles per litre (nmol/L) or higher were associated with a 72 per cent reduction in colorectal cancer mortality.[53] As you'll see later, to achieve blood levels of 80nmol/L, you would need just over 25mcg (1,000iu) a day.

Similar blood levels and vitamin D intake were found to protect against colon cancer in a study that followed 1,500 people for 25 years. At 80nmol/L the rate was cut by 50 per cent, whereas levels of over 100nmol/L reduced colon cancer incidence by 66 per cent, according to the *American Journal of Preventative Medicine*.

When five studies were 'pooled' together, researchers found that a 50 per cent lower risk of colorectal cancer was associated with a blood level of greater than, or equal to, 83nmol/L, compared to less than or equal to 30nmol/L. They concluded that 1,000–2,000 iu per day of vitamin D could reduce the incidence of colorectal cancer with minimal risk.[54]

Reduce your risk of breast and ovarian cancer by a third

Several teams of researchers have found that adequate levels of vitamin D also lower the chances of developing breast cancer. Low blood levels of vitamin D have been correlated with breast cancer disease progression and the spread of cancer to the bones.[55] Women with advanced breast cancer that had spread to their bones were less likely to die of the disease when they had high amounts of active vitamin D in their blood.[56]

A team of cancer prevention specialists at the University of California, San Diego, found that women with the highest level of vitamin D in their blood had a 50 per cent lower risk of breast cancer than those with the lowest level.[57]

'The results were very clear,' said co-author Dr Cedric Garland, 'the higher your level, the lower the risk.' To have a blood level that would cut your risk by 50 per cent, the researchers said that you would have to take 50mcg (2,000iu) daily and also spend 10–15 minutes in the sun.

Researchers from the same university also reviewed 63 studies, published worldwide between 1966 and 2004, and they found that taking 25mcg (1,000iu) of the vitamin daily could lower an individual's cancer risk by 50 per cent in colon cancer, and by 30 per cent in breast and ovarian cancer.[58] In fact, Dr Garland has estimated that 600,000 cases a year of breast and colorectal cancer could be prevented by adequate intakes of vitamin D.[59]

Protection from prostate cancer

Vitamin D also helps protect men from prostate cancer. A team led by a researcher from Harvard Medical School followed 15,000 men and found that those who had below average levels of the vitamin in their blood had a 'significantly increased risk of aggressive prostate cancer'. In this study, published in *PLOS Medicine*, 50nmol/L counted as deficient and even 80nmol/L was described as 'sub-optimal'.

247

Taking the US Recommended Daily Allowance (RDA) of vitamin D (10mcg, or 400iu/day) was found to reduce the risk of pancreatic cancer by 43 per cent in a sample of more than 120,000 people from two long-term health surveys.[60] They said further work was necessary to determine if consuming vitamin D in the diet, or through sun exposure, might have even more of an effect than taking supplements.

How does vitamin D work?

The anti-cancer activity of vitamin D is thought to result from its role in a wide range of mechanisms central to the development of cancer, such as regulating cell growth, and apoptosis (programmed cell death).[61] Programmed cell death is a normal process that should happen in our bodies if a cell is damaged in any way. This is one of the problems with cancer – the damaged cell continues to replicate. One clinical study of 92 colon cancer patients showed that supplementing the diet with calcium and vitamin D appeared to increase the levels of a protein (called BAX) that controls this process in the colon and might therefore be pushing the pre-cancerous cells into programmed cell death.[62]

Another possible explanation for the cancer-protective effect of vitamin D is that calcium is important for proper immune function (more about calcium in Chapter 29), and vitamin D is needed to enable calcium to be used properly by the body. It is converted into the hormone calcitriol, which works with another hormone, parathormone – produced in the parathyroid gland – to control calcium balance in the body. Calcitriol also plays an important role in the immune system because it is able to suppress pro-inflammatory chemicals that are often implicated in the cancer process. It has been found to kill cancer cells in laboratory and animal studies, and high levels of calcitriol have been shown to be beneficial in patients with advanced prostate cancer.[63]

How much is enough?

Just how much vitamin D is required for optimum health varies depending on where you live in the world (your latitude), the colour of your skin, the time of year, your use of sun block and your level of sun exposure. The amount you need from diet depends on the amount you produce in your skin. Although you make the most vitamin D in the summer, the relative conversion of sunlight, acting on cholesterol, into vitamin D production is apparently at its highest in the autumn; perhaps this is an evolutionary adaptation so that the body can store it for the winter months ahead.

Early humans compared to today

Dr Reinhold Vieth, Associate Professor in the departments of Nutritional Sciences, Laboratory Medicine and Pathobiology at the University of Toronto, and one of the world's top vitamin D experts, estimates that 'humans in a state of nature' probably had about 125 to 150nmol/L of vitamin D in their blood all year long. These levels are only likely to be achieved for a few months a year by the minority of adults: those who spend a lot of time in the sun, such as lifeguards or farmers.

In the remainder of the population, vitamin D levels tend to be lower and crash in winter. In testing office workers in Toronto in winter, Professor Vieth from the University of Toronto found that the average was only about 40nmol/L, or about one-quarter to one-third of the amount humans would have 'in the wild'.

Varying recommendations

Textbooks will tell you that you should be getting between 5 and 10mcg (200–400iu) a day. Some of this we can get from food, notably fatty fish and cod liver oil, and the rest from sunlight, by exposing the face and hands for a few minutes a few times a week (which should be enough to prevent bone-softening that manifests itself as rickets).

If exposure to sunlight is limited, Dr Michael Holick, a top expert on vitamin D, maintains that a minimum of 25mcg (1,000iu) per day from food and/or supplements is required to maintain a

249

healthy concentration in the blood.[64] Most experts now agree that this is the level needed daily to maintain a healthy blood level of 25-hydroxyvitamin D (this is the form of vitamin D measured in the blood, also known as 25(OH)D) of between 75 and 125 nmol/L.[65]

Why levels probably need to rise

In March 2007 Robert Heaney, Professor of Medicine at Creighton University in Nebraska, called for improved levels of vitamin D in the general population on the grounds that this would reduce the risk of bone fractures caused by osteoporosis, as well as protecting against 'various cancers and autoimmune disorders'.[66]

The average UK diet will provide about 3.75mcg (150iu) of vitamin D per day. The low vitamin D intake in several European countries is due to the fact that only a few foods are naturally good sources of vitamin D.[67] Fatty fish such as herring, mackerel, pilchards, sardines and tuna, as well as eggs, are rich sources. There's a little in milk, meat and fortified foods. If you eat these foods regularly *and* expose yourself to natural daylight for half an hour a day, you will achieve the equivalent of about 15mcg (600iu). The ideal intake is at least 30mcg so, to achieve this, you would need to supplement an additional 15mcg of vitamin D each day. A good multivitamin may provide this, but most multis don't. However, if you have cancer and don't get enough sun exposure, for example in winter, I would recommend supplementing 30mcg a day – twice this amount.

Who is at risk of deficiency?

Vitamin D deficiency among the elderly is far from uncommon. According to a survey published in the *New England Journal of Medicine*, 57 per cent of 290 senior citizens in hospital had low blood levels of this vitamin.[68] It's not just the elderly who are at risk. At least 60 per cent of the adult population in the UK do not get enough vitamin D according to the National Diet and Nutrition

Survey for 1995–2004. The survey also showed that 12 per cent were actually deficient. Vitamin D inadequacy is common among post-menopausal women,[69] vegetarians, those eating low-fat diets, and those not getting enough sunlight. Others at risk include people living in urban northerly regions, and immigrants who rarely expose their skin to sunlight. So, for example, an Indian who has dark skin, and remains covered up much of the time, who is also vegan (and therefore does not eat meat, fish, eggs or dairy products) is at risk of vitamin D deficiency. This causes rickets (in children) and osteomalacia (in adults) – diseases in which the bones become malleable. People with dark skin – no doubt due to their high melanin content – are most susceptible to rickets, especially when living in countries with little sunlight.

Experts believe that current recommended levels of vitamin D are too low and that there is an urgent need to recommend a more effective intake.[70] According to Dr Vieth, one of the world's leading authorities on vitamin D:

> Current dietary guidelines for vitamin D in the UK are incorrect in stating that adults below age 50 require no vitamin D and specify too little for older people. Sun avoidance advice makes the vitamin D problem even worse in the UK. The result is an unacceptably high occurrence of what should be regarded as toxic vitamin D deficiency.

The importance of latitude

A study using data on over 4 million cancer patients from 13 countries showed a marked difference in risk of a number of cancers between countries classified as 'sunny' and those classified as 'less sunny'.[71] Research also suggests that cancer patients who have surgery or treatment in the summer have a better chance of surviving their cancer than those who undergo treatment in the winter when they are exposed to less sunlight.[72]

251

To make Vitamin D you need sunlight that contains UVB rays, but these can be blocked by cloud. Fewer and fewer UVB rays reach the ground the further north you go. (It's the UVA rays that age you the most.)

Liverpool in the UK is approximately on the same latitude as Edmonton in Canada (53 degrees north) where it has been found that people's bodies make little vitamin D for up to six months of the year. Furthermore, according to a study by Dr Hypponnen, Scottish people were twice as likely to be vitamin D deficient as those south of the border. Even in Boston in the US – 42 degrees north – you will be unable to make vitamin D from sunlight for four months of the year, from November to February.

In the UK, even in summer you only really get sufficient UVB rays between 10.00 am and 2.00 pm; exposing your hands, face and arms during those hours gives you about 5–10mcg (200–400iu), which isn't nearly enough for the new recommended levels. To get those, the American experts are suggesting you need to expose 50–80 per cent of your skin to the sun's rays for about 20 minutes.

Modern life keeps us indoors away from the sun, which supplies 90 per cent of the vitamin D we need. A billion or more people in Europe obtain insufficient sunlight and vitamin D, putting them at increased risk of many of the common cancers as well as other conditions, including diabetes, arthritis and multiple sclerosis. In fact, some experts believe that the epidemic of chronic disease caused by a lack of vitamin D is probably as large as the epidemics caused by smoking and obesity, but the importance of vitamin D deficiency is still not properly recognised by governments.

The problem with sunscreens

In 2005, a conference was held at the House of Commons to address the issue of 'sunlight, vitamin D and health' and the issue of sun safety. It was pointed out that those regularly using sunscreen at factor 8 or above, or avoiding sunshine, were putting themselves at risk of vitamin D deficiency. This includes women who regularly use foundation cosmetics containing sunscreen. Leading vitamin D campaigner Dr Oliver Gillie, editor of the report, is highly critical of the SunSmart advice put out by Cancer Research UK, which encourages people to stay out of the sun and use sunscreens. 'That programme has probably caused many more deaths from cancer than it has prevented,' claims Gillie. 'It may also be partly responsible for apparent increases in chronic diseases such as multiple sclerosis and diabetes.'[73] Their advice is to sunbathe safely (without burning) at every opportunity, without using sunscreens. 'Safely' means starting slowly (2–3 minutes each side) and gradually increasing from day to day. Only brief full-body exposure to bright summer sunshine – of 10 or 15 minutes a day – is needed to make high amounts of the vitamin.

How do I know if I've got enough?

The vitamin D that you make from sunlight or get from either a supplement or your diet is stored in your blood in a form known as 25(OH)D. A level of 27.5nmol/L of 25(OH)D is what you would make with around 10mcg (400iu) vitamin D a day. 'That's enough to prevent rickets but not enough for your health,' says Dr Heaney. In fact in the latest studies it's a level that counts as deficient; 50nmol/L is considered to be just about acceptable. In a 2007 study, published in the *American Journal of Clinical Nutrition*, the optimum level was 80nmol/L and over.[74]

This is the level that most other studies find of benefit, but to get that you need about 40mcg (1600iu), although this also depends on your age. An average 70-year-old, according to Professor Meir Stampfer, an epidemiologist at Harvard Medical School, can make only about a quarter of the vitamin D from the sun compared to a 20-year-old.

A study of nearly 7,500 middle-aged men and women published in 2007 came to the startling conclusion that most people in Britain have insufficient vitamin D in their blood for at least six months of the year.[75] 'There is now a strong case for fortifying foods with vitamin D', says the author of the study, Dr Elia Hypponen, of the

Institute for Child Health in London. 'You can only make vitamin D from sunlight for about half the year in the UK, so by around Easter 90 per cent of the population are seriously depleted in the amount they have.' She also believes that vitamin D supplements of between 40 and 50mcg (1600 and 2000iu) – four to five times the current recommended daily allowance (RDA) – should be more easily available over the counter.

Heaney calculates that to increase most of the population to a reasonably healthy level of vitamin D would require a daily supplement for everyone that was ten times the current RDA of 5mcg (200iu) – that's 500 mcg (2000iu) – on top of whatever they were already receiving from diet and sunlight. This brings me to a very important question: could you be harmed if you take too much?

Side effects of too much vitamin D

More than 50mcg (2000iu) a day, according to some UK sources, can lead to the body absorbing too much calcium (a condition known as hypercalcaemia), possibly damaging the liver and kidneys. Other side effects of overdosing are said to include increased thirst, nausea, vomiting and the deposit of calcium in blood-vessel walls.

But even among academics there is little agreement on this. The Food and Nutrition Board of the American Institute of Medicine has set the guaranteed safe level per day at 50mcg (2,000iu), whereas many of the North American experts believe that much more is safe.

Reinhold Veith, at the departments of Nutritional Sciences, Laboratory Medicine and Pathobiology, University of Toronto, believes that 1,000mcg (40,000iu) could be a toxic dose, but only if taken over a long time. Campaigners regularly point out that a fair-skinned person with about 80 per cent of their skin exposed to the sun for 20 minutes at midday can produce about 250mcg (10,000iu) with no harm at all.

Further support for higher levels being both necessary and safe comes from a major review of Vitamin D published in July 2007 in the prestigious *New England Journal of Medicine*,[76] which concludes that: 'As long as [someone's] combined total is 30ng per millilitre, the patient has sufficient Vitamin D.' Now, that's an amount that translates to about 65mcg (2,600iu) a day. And as for the dangers, the review comments that: 'Doses of 250mcg (10,000iu) per day for up to 5 months do not cause toxicity.'

In the UK, however, these figures have not filtered through to the Food Standards Agency (FSA). 'Most people can get all the vitamin D they require from a healthy balanced diet and exposure to sunlight,' said a spokesperson. As for supplements, the agency recommends no more than 25mcg (1,000iu) because 'intakes above this amount could be harmful'.

Getting the correct levels for you

To summarise, the evidence clearly shows that we should all be making sure that our vitamin D levels are adequate. In fact, the benefits of vitamin D are now so widely recognised that the pharmaceutical industry is trying to develop a patentable drug version of vitamin D that can be given in high doses without the side effects, namely excess calcium accumulation, which occurs with very high-dose vitamin D. At least that's their story. Personally, I would recommend sticking with the natural vitamin D molecule, and not taking more than 50mcg a day.

In the pursuit of optimum nutrition I recommend eating oily fish three times a week; a serving of salmon or mackerel provides around 8.75mcg (350iu), eating six free-range eggs a week (an egg provides 0.5mcg, or 20iu), exposing your skin to the sun every day (you'll make around 10mcg (400iu) with 20 minutes exposure between 10.00 am and 2.00 pm), and supplementing at least 15mcg (600iu) daily. That will give you around 30mcg (1200iu) a day in total.

If you are mainly vegetarian and don't eat vitamin D-enriched foods, eggs or dairy produce, and do not get substantial exposure to sunlight, I would recommend supplementing your diet with 15–30mcg (600–1200iu) of vitamin D. This level is found in some multivitamins and also in some calcium and magnesium supplements. During the winter months (November to April in the northern hemisphere), it's probably worth supplementing an additional 25mcg (1,000iu) and possibly more, especially if you are older and live in the far north.

If you live in a hot country, however, and are exposed to substantial amounts of sunlight, be careful that you are not getting too much dietary vitamin D, because an excess has a negative effect on calcium balance, as I have explained.

CHAPTER 28

Other Anti-cancer Nutrients

Many other vitamins apart from those discussed in Part 4 are immune boosting and potentially helpful in reducing cancer risk. Of the B vitamins, vitamins B_6, B_{12} and folic acid are vital for the immune system, as discussed in Chapter 8; deficiencies of each have been linked to various cancers, either as part of homocysteine metabolism or independently.

Glutathione

Although not a vitamin, glutathione deserves attention, as it is perhaps the most important antioxidant within cells and has proven to be highly cancer protective. You may remember from Chapter 2 that glutathione is like a protein (made out of three amino acids), and as well as being an antioxidant in its own right, it is also part of key antioxidant enzymes such as glutathione peroxidase and glutathione transferase. It can also recycle vitamin C, multiplying its ability to promote health. It plays a major role in detoxifying the body and protecting it against the harmful effects of carcinogens, especially oxidants and radiation. In addition, it protects DNA and cell growth.[77] In short, it fits the description of an all-round cancer-protective agent, and low levels are often found in cancer patients.

Glutathione helps to kill cancer cells by improving the body's natural immunity.[78] Normally made in the body from the amino acid cysteine, glutathione is also present in a variety of foods (especially garlic). Supplementing it on its own is less effective than taking it with anthocyanidins, found in berry extracts, the problem being that the glutathione sacrifices itself to protect the body from oxidants, thus becoming an oxidant, while anthocyanidins help reload it back to an antioxidant. The discovery that glutathione was effectively recycled back to an antioxidant by anthocyanidins, found in grapes, berries and beetroot, led to a new anti-cancer approach of combining glutathione with anthocyanidins, thereby substantially increasing the power of this key antioxidant.[79]

Coenzyme Q_{10}

The nutrient coenzyme Q_{10} (CoQ_{10}) is not classified as a vitamin, because it can be made in the body. It is a vital antioxidant, helping to protect cells from carcinogens and also helping to recycle vitamin E. There is evidence that CoQ_{10} levels are lower than normal in people with cancer[80] and that the need for CoQ_{10} increases when you have the disease. For this reason, researchers started to consider giving extra to combat cancer. The first cases reported were of women with breast cancer treated in Denmark in 1995. Out of 36 women classified as 'high risk', since their tumours had spread, six patients showed 'apparent partial remission' following the supplementation of 90mg of CoQ_{10}, together with other antioxidants.[81] An additional three women treated with 390mg of CoQ_{10} also showed apparent remission.[82]

There is some evidence that supplementing CoQ_{10} might reduce the toxicity of cancer treatments and help to make them more tolerable. Although this has not been tested by rigorous trials, a systematic review of the evidence carried out in 2004 was promising enough to warrant further investigations.[83] CoQ_{10} has recently been combined with riboflavin (vitamin B_2) and niacin (B_3) in a number of recent trials involving breast cancer patients. (Riboflavin and niacin are two other well-known potent antioxidants and protective agents against many diseases, including cancer.) In 2008, 84 breast cancer patients were given a daily supplement of 100mg CoQ_{10}, 10mg ribo-flavin and 50mg niacin (collectively called CoRN), along with 10mg tamoxifen twice daily. Compared to untreated breast cancer patients and patients treated with tamoxifen alone, those taking the CoRN supplement were found to have a significant increase in DNA repair enzymes, which resulted in tumour reduction.[84] A similar study earlier this year used CoRN alongside tamoxifen for postmenopausal women with breast cancer over a period of 90 days. Once again, the results were promising, showing a statistically significant alteration in certain parameters in the blood, which were favourably reverted back to near normal levels on combined therapy with CoRN.[85]

These results are encouraging and highlight the potential importance of supplementing this nutrient to ensure optimal levels.

Synergy – the whole is greater than the sum of its parts

As explained in Chapter 2, none of these nutrients work in isolation in the body, nor are people ever deficient in just one of them. As good as the results discussed so far appear, they underestimate the power of optimum nutrition in preventing and reversing the cancer process.

Vitamin C, which is water-soluble, and vitamin E, which is fat-soluble, are synergistic vitamins: together they can protect the tissues and fluids in the body. What is more, when vitamin E has 'disarmed' a carcinogen, the vitamin E can be 'reloaded' by vitamin C, so that their combined presence in the diet and the body can continue to have a synergistic effect.

The same is true of selenium (an antioxidant mineral that we will cover more in the next chapter) and vitamin E. When these nutrients are taken together, the level of cancer protection is multiplied considerably; for example, a study from Finland, carried out by Dr Jukka Salonen and colleagues at the University of Kuopio on 12,000 people over several years, found that those whose blood levels were in the top third for both vitamin E and selenium had a 91 per cent decreased risk of cancer compared to those in the bottom third.[86] Having high levels of both these nutrients gave them less than one-tenth the risk of those with sub-optimal levels.

Vitamins C and E are also a powerful anti-cancer combination. A ten-year study on over 11,000 people, completed in 1996, found that those supplementing those two vitamins halved their overall risk of death from all cancers.[87]

One study in Seattle involving over 800 people who took a multi-vitamin supplement daily was associated with halving the risk of developing colon cancer. The nutrients linked to the decreased risk were vitamins A, C, E, folic acid and the mineral calcium. The strongest link was with vitamin E – people who supplemented at least 200iu (134mg) of vitamin E over ten years had 57 per cent less chance of getting colon cancer than those who had taken none.[88] Another study involving over 10,000 adults over 19 years showed that high intakes of vitamins E and C combined with carotenoids were associated with a 68 per cent decrease in the risk of developing lung cancer.[89] An animal study found the combination of beta-carotene, vitamins E and C, and glutathione to be substantially more cancer-protective than any one of these nutrients in isolation.[90]

Supplements and cancer

All in all, these studies strongly suggest that taking supplements providing optimal amounts of vitamin A, beta-carotene, vitamin C and E, plus vitamin D and B vitamins, is likely to substantially reduce your risk of cancer, when combined with an appropriate diet. These findings are confirmed by Dr Richard Passwater, who first identified the synergistic relationship between vitamins C and E. Having spent the past 30 years researching antioxidant nutrients and cancer, Passwater believes that supplementation plus an appropriate diet could cut your risk of cancer to a quarter.

CHAPTER 29

Anti-cancer Minerals – from Selenium to Zinc

L ike vitamins, minerals are essential for the immune system. The key minerals for healthy immunity include calcium, magnesium, zinc and selenium, but of these, selenium is prominent as an important ally in the fight against cancer.

Selenium, like other antioxidant nutrients, has a positive role to play in many stages in the cancer process. It protects genes from damage and helps cells use oxygen efficiently, and it also appears to slow down cell division (resulting in fewer errors as the new cells are made). It can also help detoxify a wide variety of carcinogens by improving liver function, which, as I explained in Chapter 7, is the body's main detoxifying organ.[91]

The role of selenium in protecting against cancer has long been known, and many studies have linked a lower intake of dietary selenium to an increased risk of cancer: in one study conducted on 4,480 men from the US, for example, those who had selenium levels in the lowest fifth at the start of the study were twice as likely to develop cancer as those whose levels fell in the highest fifth.[92] Studies in China confirmed the same finding: that those with low selenium levels in the blood (below 8mcg per dl) had three times the risk of cancer as those with high blood levels (above 11mcg per dl).[93]

Studies on animals have found selenium protected against a number of cancers[94] and, as a result, a number of human trials have now also taken place; their results confirming the importance of this mineral.

In one study, people who lived in areas with low soil selenium supplemented 200mcg of selenium over four and a half years and were found to have a reduced risk of developing cancer. Although the supplementation did not appear to reduce the incidence of skin cancer, total cancers, as well as those of the lung, colon and prostate, were significantly lower.[95] These findings were confirmed by a trial conducted by researchers at Cornel University, in which one group of people were given 200mcg of selenium and another group a placebo. They found a significant reduction in the incidence of lung, colorectal and prostate cancer, as well as reduced mortality from lung cancer in the selenium group.[96]

In the region of Quidong in China, liver cancer rates are among the highest in the world, but studies have found a strong correlation between low selenium intake and cancer risk. Other cancer-risk factors in this area were found to be hepatitis-B infection and exposure to the dietary carcinogen aflatoxin, as well as a genetic predisposition. Scientists then began a large-scale selenium study in which an entire village of 20,000 people supplemented selenium, which was added to their salt. In the years that followed there was a significant drop in the incidence of hepatitis-B and liver cancer.[97]

Not all studies have been positive. One large clinical trial, known as the Selenium and Vitamin E Chemoprevention Trial (SELECT), showed no benefit in the prevention of prostate cancer.[98] However, the most likely explanation is that people with normal selenium status are unlikely to benefit, whereas those that are deficient probably will.

A review of four trials showed a huge 52 per cent reduction in gastrointestinal cancers and a 60 per cent reduced risk of oesophageal cancer.[99] A laboratory study in 2007 found that selenium reduced the risk of lung cancer,[100] while a separate review of epidemiologic studies found that selenium protected against both lung and prostate cancer.[101] However, the amount of selenium you need for this protection is far more than you are likely to get from diet alone.

Supplementing selenium

Few people take in enough selenium from their food and there is evidence that dietary intake and blood levels of selenium are falling in the Western world. In Britain the average intake is about 35mcg a day, compared to 60mcg in 1975. Current low levels of selenium could be a contributing factor to the rise in cancers as well as other health problems such as cardiovascular disease.[102]

Most cancer experts recommend supplementing 100–200mcg of selenium (as selenomethionine or selenocysteine). If you are suffering from cancer, I recommend taking 200 to 300mcg per day, although there is no evidence of benefit in supplementing selenium if you have skin cancer.

For prevention, I recommend 100mcg per day. In addition to this, there is no harm in boosting your selenium intake through diet. Foods rich in selenium include seafood, wholefoods, nuts and seeds (especially Brazil nuts and sesame seeds). If you grind the seeds, the nutrients will become more readily available. Tuna, oysters, mushrooms, herring, cottage cheese, cabbage, courgettes, cod and chicken are other good sources. In practice (with the exception of seafood), the level of selenium in foods reflects the level of selenium in the soil in which they are grown, but it is highly likely that continued intensive farming has led to selenium depletion in the soil and therefore in the plants grown in it.

Other minerals

In the same way as vitamins, minerals work in synergy, and the best disease-prevention strategy is probably an all-round optimal intake of minerals. Zinc, calcium and magnesium, as well as selenium, are especially important for immune function.

Calcium and vitamin D

Particularly when used in conjunction with other micronutrients, calcium has been associated with a reduced risk of cancer, particularly of the breast.[103] Studies on animals have found that a high intake of calcium and vitamin D significantly reduces the risk of breast cancer.[104]

A pooled analysis of ten studies (which found nearly 5,000 colorectal cancer cases among more than 530,000 participants) showed a 22 per cent decreased risk for the groups with the highest calcium intakes.[105]

Vitamin D is known to help the body use calcium, which is a vital nutrient for healthy immunity. Rich sources of calcium are found in seeds and nuts, especially pumpkin seeds and almonds, as well as milk. But, for the reasons discussed in Chapter 12, milk is not the most appropriate source of calcium if you are fighting cancer.

Zinc

Another key immune-boosting nutrient is zinc, and levels of zinc found in people with prostate cancer have been shown to be significantly lower than normal.[106] Zinc deficiency is associated with DNA damage, which can lead to cancer. Also, the toxic element, cadmium, which is a known zinc antagonist, can stimulate the growth of prostate tissue and is therefore considered a carcinogen. Cadmium is found in cigarettes and in exhaust fumes, as well as galvanised pipes and in some household water supplies (this depends of the type of plumbing). Smokers have been found to have a high cadmium-to-zinc ratio, leading to oxidative stress, DNA damage and impaired DNA repair, all part of the carcinogenic process.[107] The best way you can protect yourself against cadmium is by not smoking and by ensuring an optimal zinc intake.

Few studies to date have looked at the therapeutic role of treating cancer with zinc. One showed an increase in risk for prostate cancer with high supplement use.[108] However, the daily dose used was 100mg over a period of ten years – far higher than the maximum nutritional support level of 35mg I would recommend. One recent study used 15mg a day for ten years and reported that, although it didn't prevent prostate cancer completely, it did prevent the disease from progressing to the advanced stage (a 66 per cent decreased risk compared to non-users).[109] An optimal intake of zinc is 15–20mg a day, which is two to three times the average daily intake. Seeds and nuts and other 'seed' foods such as wholegrains, peas, broad beans, lentils and beans are rich in zinc.

CHAPTER 30

Probiotics – Your Immune System's Best Friend

One thing your immune system really needs in order to function at its best is a good supply of beneficial bacteria. We all have billions of bacteria living in our digestive systems – some are good, and some are not so good.

Some bacteria cause disease, but bacteria that play a beneficial role in our life are known as probiotics, which literally means 'for life'. Basically, what probiotics do is help us to maintain a healthy digestive system by maintaining a balance between the harmful and the beneficial bacteria – they actually crowd out the undesirable bacteria by competing with them for nutrients. They also support the friendly bacteria in our digestive tract by secreting certain chemicals (a kind of natural antibiotic) that can break down carcinogens to make them harmless. This, in turn, can help to reduce inflammation that may lead to inflammatory bowel diseases and, potentially, cancer.

Beneficial bacteria are first passed from mother to child through the birth process (passed from mother to baby in the birth canal) and breastfeeding. If you are breastfed this actually decreases your cancer risk, especially if your family has a history of cancer.[110]

Feeding our good bacteria

Keeping the balance right depends on the foods we eat. It is no coincidence that the foods that are beneficial for cancer prevention are also those that are needed to feed our friendly bacteria: wholegrains, and fresh fruit and vegetables – these are also known as prebiotics.

A group of Adventist vegetarians was found to have a higher amount of beneficial bacteria and a lower amount of potentially pathogenic bacteria compared to non-vegetarians on a conventional American diet.[111] The modern diet – high in alcohol, sugar and fat, and low in fibre – wreaks havoc on the digestive tract. As we saw in Chapter 17, there is no question that alcohol is a powerful carcinogen. It damages intestinal bacteria and has been reported to convert gut bacteria into secondary metabolites that increase proliferation of cells in the colon, initiating cancer. Such a diet disrupts the sensitive balance of beneficial bacteria there, inflames the digestive tract wall and disturbs the gut-associated immune system.

The medical profession slow to respond?

Despite mounting evidence that the complex colony of bacteria and microorganisms in our guts is vital to our health in all sorts of ways, most doctors have remained resolutely sceptical about the value of taking probiotics, and very few prescribe them.

The general public, however, aren't so reserved. They clearly believe that probiotics are beneficial – around two million Britons now spend an estimated £135 million on buying drinks, yoghurts and capsules containing probiotics. Meanwhile, the medical mainstream continues to regard the gut largely as a form of plumbing to unblock or solidify, to be treated with drugs to damp down inflammation or acid if either seem too high – and finally to be chopped out if none of that works.

What this fails to take into account is the extraordinary complexity of the gut, not least of the ecosystem of the bacteria inhabiting it. There are more than a thousand species living in our guts, most of which cannot be grown in cultures in the lab, and these are intimately involved in the workings of our immune system, as well as helping us to extract nutrients and to metabolise waste.

The benefits of yoghurt

In February 2008, newspapers carried a story claiming that a 'yoghurt drink could beat hospital superbug'. Patients in a couple of UK hospitals were going to be given yoghurt containing probiotics to reduce the risk of becoming infected with the bug *Clostridium difficile*, which was killing an increasing number of patients. What encouraged doctors at the Royal Sussex County Hospital in Brighton to put patients on probiotics was a randomised controlled trial, published in 2008, which found that a yoghurt containing three probiotics cut down the amount of diarrhoea patients suffered as a result of being put on antibiotics to treat the bug *C. difficile*, which they had picked up in hospital.[112]

As we saw in Chapter 11, the right kind of yoghurt has been found to be significantly protective against colon cancer, since the bacteria *Lactobacillus acidophilus* (found in some, but not most, yoghurts) slows down the development of colon tumours.[113] Lower rates of colon cancer among higher consumers of fermented dairy products have also been observed in some population studies.[114]

How the yoghurt works

Yoghurt and the bacteria that it contains have received much attention as potential cancer-preventing agents in the diet. The yoghurt is usually considered to work by increasing the numbers of beneficial bacteria in the colon, which reduces the ability of the microflora to produce carcinogens. Prebiotics, the food for the probiotics (more about these later), appear to have similar effects by selectively stimulating the growth of beneficial bacteria in the colon. Some studies indicate that combinations of pre- and probiotics are even more effective.[115]

Gathering evidence

Dr Jeremy Nicholson of Imperial College London has been working with other scientists to establish a biochemical evidence base so that probiotics will be able to move into the mainstream, rather than being regarded as some kind of slightly wacky non-drug treatment for conditions that aren't responding well to pharmaceuticals. In a study in January 2008, he showed that taking standard probiotics could, in fact, produce a whole range of beneficial effects in the liver, blood and urine.[116] 'We've established that friendly bacteria can change the dynamics of the whole population of microbes in the gut,' he said.

When it comes to cancer, most research has been done in relation to colon cancer. One laboratory study in 2007 showed that resistant starches (probiotics) are capable of inhibiting the initiation and promotion stages (see Chapter 1) in colon cancer in the test tube.[117]

However, human studies are limited. According to probiotic expert Professor Ian Rowland of Reading University, 'There's good evidence that probiotics can reduce toxic elements in the guts of rats … And pretty convincing evidence they reduce the chance of rats' precancerous cells becoming cancerous. But in humans, we still don't have the full-scale, placebo-controlled trial to show that they actually reduce cancer risk.'

One human trial worth a mention is a 12-week double-blind, placebo-controlled trial involving 37 colon cancer patients and 43 patients who had had polyps removed. It was found that a combination of prebiotics and probiotics significantly reduced colorectal proliferation.[118]

Most human trials have found that the strains tested may exert anti-carcinogenic effects by decreasing the activity of an enzyme called beta-glucoronidase, which is made in excess within a digestive tract in a state of dysbiosis and can generate carcinogens. Having too much beta-glucoronidase is a useful marker for cancer risk, both of the digestive tract and of the breast. It interferes with the liver's ability to break down oestrogen, which results in its continued circulation, thereby contributing to oestrogen dominance, a known risk factor for breast cancer.[119] In the lab, some strains of bacteria (*Lactobacillus bulgaris*) have demonstrated anti-cancer effects thought to be due to their ability to bind with heterocyclic amines, which are carcinogenic substances formed in cooked meat (see Chapter 11).[120]

How can you help yourself?

So, what should you be doing to make the most of all the research indicating that a good balance of friendly bacteria in your gut is essential to your overall health? Of course, you could wait until all the evidence from controlled trials was in, but since there is no evidence that probiotics are harmful, it makes a lot of sense to pay attention to your gut's friendly inhabitants right now.

Prebiotics

The best place to start is with your diet. According to the authors of a recent review of probiotics: 'It's increasingly being recognised that the specific composition of [our gut bacteria], as well as many of its physiological traits, can be modified by relatively small changes in food consumption.'[121] These changes turn out to be familiar healthy-eating advice, because our beneficial bacteria aren't keen on a typical junk-food diet, high in processed and refined foods. What our two main beneficial bacterial species – *Lactobacilli* and *Bifidobacteria* – need us to eat is a diet rich in the fibre found only in fresh, unprocessed fruit, vegetables and grains.[122] These are the hard-to-digest carbohydrates known, rather confusingly, as prebiotics. Both fibre and prebiotics are typically hard-to-digest carbohydrates, and both are typically fermented by gut bacteria. However, a prebiotic differs from fibre in that it can only be used in the gut – as food for the beneficial members of your gut bacteria. However, some manufacturers refer to prebiotics as fibre, because the latter is more familiar to consumers. The best known and most widely tested are called 'oligosaccharides' (oligo = few, and saccharide = sugar). They also come in a supplement form, often shortened to

FOS – fructo-oligosaccharides – (if you see a supplement called inulin, this is a type of FOS). Another is 'resistant starch', which, unlike normal starch, passes through the stomach and can be broken down only in the gut.

Best foods

Other favourite bacterial foods include flavonoids and lignans, found in vegetables, pulses and seeds, such as flaxseeds. *Bifidobacteria* particularly like FOS. Foods rich in prebiotics include chicory, Jerusalem artichokes, leeks, asparagus, garlic, onions, wheat, oats and soya beans. You can also get prebiotic supplements, which can be especially useful for those not getting enough fruit and vegetables. You need to be careful about taking too much, though. Five to eight grams of FOS should be enough – more than that can lead to bloating, flatulence and intestinal discomfort.

Prebiotics can also be useful combined with probiotics if your beneficial bacteria are likely to be under attack. The best probiotic supplements will include some FOS in the capsules. That way you are giving the good-bacteria population a boost along with an added food supply. The number-one situation where this is a good idea is when you've finished a course of antibiotics; that's because *Lactobacilli* and *Bifidobacteria* are sensitive to a wide variety of antibiotics and so their numbers are drastically reduced following therapy.[123] Antibiotic use has also been associated with an increased risk of breast cancer.[124] Although more research is necessary to learn if there is a direct cause-and-effect relationship (it may be that the women involved had compromised immune systems or that other factors were involved), the authors found that the more antibiotics the women in the study had used, the higher their risk of breast cancer. Probiotics are also useful if you have been under a lot of stress – which could be anything from pressure at work, a hangover or even an operation – because stress can shift the balance in your gut in favour of pathogens such as *E.coli* and *Streptococci* and away from *Lactobacilli* and *Bifidobacterium*, which grow more slowly.[125]

When might boosting your probiotics help?

Pre- and probiotics can also help if you've been ill – such as suffering with a bout of cold or flu – and before and after long-distance travel. In addition, you might consider taking them if you are elderly (because good bacteria numbers fall off as we get older) or giving them to a child with an allergy or eczema. A combination of pro- and prebiotics in both these groups has proved beneficial.[126]

Getting the real thing

How can you make sure that you are getting probiotics that are going to actually work? In the past there have been scares about supplements that haven't been properly labelled. One study, for instance, found that eight brands gave the wrong information about either how many bacteria they contained or what strains they were.[127]

As with all supplements, buy from a company you have reason to trust. Look out for the commonest two strains – *Lactobacilli* and *Bifidobacterium* – because more research has been carried out on them. A good place to start is *Lactobacilli acidophilus* and *Bifidobacteria*. This is the 'A and B' of probiotics. Sub-strains from these families, most commonly recognised as safe, include: *L. acidophilus*, *L. rhamnosus*, *L. plantarum*, *L. casei*, *B. bifidum*, *B. infantis* (for babies) and *B. longum*, among others.[128]

It's worth making a distinction between these strains of bacteria and ones that are used for making yoghurt but aren't likely to do much good in the gut, like *Lactobacillus bulgaricus* and *Streptococcus thermophilus*. At the moment, yoghurt is the most familiar way of delivering probiotics, but you can also buy capsules and powder, which are preferable if you are avoiding dairy products. Because you can't get a large amount of beneficial bacteria from just eating live yoghurt, it is best to take a daily supplement and to eat some live yoghurt each day.

How much should I take?

Probiotics are measured in 'CFUs', which stands for colony-forming units – the measure of live microbes in a probiotic. Health benefits have been reported for products ranging from 50 million to more than 1 trillion CFU per day. How much you take will depend on what you are trying to achieve.

According to Gary Huffnagle, Professor of Internal Medicine, Microbiology, and Immunology at the University of Michigan Medical Center, who is an expert on probiotics and author of *The Probiotics Revolution*, the following dosages are recommended:

- 3 to 5 billion as a maintenance dose, if you are not eating the correct level of beneficial foods.

- 6 to 10 billion to improve health or to prevent a problem (Culturelle has 10 billion; Yakult has 6.5 billion per 70 ml bottle – and a lot of sugar. See Chapter 16 for the reasons why sugar is bad news).

- 20 to 30 billion to treat a mild–to-moderate health condition.

- 450 billion to treat severe disease.

Supplements vary in how much bacteria they provide, so check the label carefully.

CHAPTER 31

Herbs and Natural Cancer Remedies

Many plants and plant extracts have powerful immune-boosting properties, which have been found to have beneficial effects on different cancers at various different stages in their development. These include aloe vera, cat's claw, echinacea, garlic, various mushrooms and numerous natural sources of antioxidants, including berry extracts, silymarin from milk thistle, and pycnogenol from pine bark. This is by no means a comprehensive list. However, each of these plants and extracts have been demonstrated either to increase the odds against cancer or to significantly boost the immune system. Unlike vitamins and minerals they are not classified as 'essential nutrients', but they may play an important part in a comprehensive anti-cancer strategy, aimed at supporting the immune system.

As explained in Chapter 1, cancer takes many years to develop and goes through different stages. Cancer is first 'initiated' (the initiation stage) and then 'promoted' (the promotion stage).

Although many of the plants mentioned here are capable of reversing these two stages, they shouldn't be used instead of conventional treatment once the 'progression stage' has been reached (generally the point of diagnosis). Having said that, as you will see, many of these plants have been shown to improve the efficacy/reduce the side effects of various chemotherapy agents.

Most herbs are available as tinctures and/or tablets. In traditional Chinese medicine, many herbs are also used in their natural form (as root or bark for example) and used to make tea or soups. In all cases, make sure you buy them from a reputable supplier (see Resources). For dosage levels and instructions, see page 305. If you have an active cancer, you should consult your doctor or health specialist.

Cat's claw (*Uncaria tomentosa*)

The plant cat's claw is a woody vine that grows in the Peruvian rain-forests, winding its way up through the trees to over 30.5m (100ft) in its attempt to reach the light. Its thorn is shaped like the claw of a cat. Native Indians have long used its bark to treat cancer.

Although human studies regarding the medicinal properties of *Uncaria* are still lacking, early research results have been so convincing that the Peruvian government banned the harvesting and use of the root of the two main species (*U. tomentosa* and *U. guianensis*) to protect the plant from overharvesting, which could endanger the species. Responsible harvesting now takes place and laboratory studies of root extracts have been able to continue by using cultivated plants from experimental university plots in Peru. It appears, however, that the bark contains most or all of the medicinal properties, and active components have also been identified within the leaves.[129]

Components of cat's claw have been shown to increase the ability of white blood cells to carry out phagocytosis (that is, to engulf, digest and so destroy misbehaving cells). It also contains other chemicals that reduce inflammation. It is potentially a super-plant, with immune-stimulating, antioxidant, anti-inflammatory, anti-tumour and anti-microbial properties. Austrian researchers have also identified extracts, which they have been using to treat cancer and viral infections.[130] However, one problem they have come across is that different samples contain different amounts of these therapeutic chemicals, which makes dosages difficult to calculate; it is not yet known whether this is due to location, season or variations in the species.

Cat's claw is available either as capsules, tincture or as tea. For dosages, see the chart on page 305. If you are using the loose tea, boil it for 5 minutes and then add a little blackcurrant and apple juice concentrate to improve the taste if you find it too bitter.

Echinacea

The root of *Echinacea purpurea* (purple coneflower) is probably the most widely used immune-boosting herb. It possesses interferon-like properties and contains special kinds of polysaccharides, such as inulin, which increase macrophage production. These have been shown to destroy cancer cells in test-tube experiments. One study, on a group of healthy men, found that after five days of taking 30 drops of echinacea extract, three times a day, their white blood cells had doubled their 'phagocytic' power.[131] Whether echinacea's immune-boosting properties are maintained over a long period of time is not yet known. Some researchers recommend using it to boost immunity only when your health is actually under threat.

Echinacea is best taken either as capsules of the powdered herb or as drops of a concentrated extract (tincture). For dosages, see the chart on page 305.

Aloe vera

Another source of special polysaccharides is aloe vera. Although it contains numerous beneficial substances, including vitamins, minerals, amino acids, essential fats and enzymes, probably its most potent substance is acemannan. This extract has been proven to improve immune power by increasing the numbers and function of T-cells and macrophages.[132] Aloe vera is usually taken as a concentration of the juice. Check the potency carefully – there's a wide variation. Look for the quantity of MPSs (mucopolysaccharides); reputable companies will provide this information.

Healing mushrooms

Certain kinds of mushrooms have been used for years in China and Japan for their immune-boosting properties. The most popular are ganoderma (reishi), shiitake and maitake.

Shiitake mushrooms contain another special polysaccharide called lentinan, which also boosts immune function. Extracts of the maitake mushroom have shown encouraging results in helping to treat cancer. Researchers in Japan found that giving maitake helped tumours regress in two-thirds of patients with breast, lung and liver cancer. They also found that if maitake was taken in conjunction with chemotherapy, response rates rose from 12 to 28 per cent. In this study, maitake was not shown to be as effective against bone and stomach cancers or leukaemia, however.[133] The immune-boosting benefits of the reishi mushroom (*Ganoderma lucidum*) are becoming increasingly evident. One study in Taiwan showed an extract of the mushroom to have anti-tumour properties[134] and another demonstrated its antioxidant effects.[135]

All these mushrooms are available as powders. For dosages, see the chart on page 305. Many are also included in natural remedies designed to support healthy immunity. However, shiitake mushrooms are now sold fresh in some supermarkets, and dried in most health-food stores. They are delicious and, as a regular part of your diet, can strengthen your immune system. Eat them three or four times a week if you are suffering from cancer.

Astragalus

Another interesting herb that is often used in conjunction with these anti-cancer mushrooms in China is astragalus. Astragalus has been proven to increase T-cell count and function and to protect the immune system from radiation and harmful chemicals including chemotherapy.[136] Astragalus is available in tablet form and as a tincture. For dosages, see the chart on page 305. In traditional Chinese medicine, pieces of the root are boiled in soups and removed prior to serving.

Turmeric

The yellow spice in curry, turmeric is rich in the phytonutrient curcumin, which is a known anti-inflammatory agent and, in animals, has been found to inhibit the growth of cancer.[137] It has been shown to protect against every stage of cancer development: initiation, promotion and progression.[138] It also disarms a wide range of carcinogens. Curcumin has been shown to have antioxidant, anti-inflammatory, anti-viral, antibacterial, anti-fungal and anti-cancer activities[139] and is currently in human clinical trials for a variety of cancers, including multiple myeloma, pancreatic cancer and colon cancer.[140] Dr Bharat Aggarwal, of the M. D. Anderson Cancer Center in Texas, is considered to be the world's leading expert on curcumin and has been researching its benefits for almost 20 years. He has published more than 50 papers on the subject. Hundreds of studies relate specifically to curcumin's anti-cancer effects. These include laboratory tests on human cancer cells and animal studies, which consistently show that curcumin is able to reduce many inflammatory markers that play a role in the cancer process. Curcumin has also been found to exhibit similar activities to many cancer drugs, including Avastin, Erbitux, Erlotinib, Geftinib and Herceptin.[141]

Human trials have shown that curcumin can be used in doses up to 8g daily for up to 18 months without toxicity. There is little doubt that, as research unfolds, curcumin will be seen as an important natural anti-cancer agent.

Anti-angiogenic natural agents

A cancerous tumour can only survive if it has its own blood supply — this is known as angiogenesis. Drugs or natural agents that inhibit this process are therefore called 'anti-angiogenic'. Natural agents that have been found to do this include curcumin, resveratrol and proanthocyanidin (grapeseed extract), green tea, and quercetin.[142]

Plant antioxidants

There are literally hundreds of plant antioxidants, and this is, no doubt, an excellent reason why eating plenty of fruit and vegetables is so strongly connected with significant reductions in cancer risk. Many antioxidants are responsible for the different colours of plants, for example, purple, red, orange, yellow and green. Among these, anthocyanidins and proanthocyanidins are found in fruits with a red/blue hue, including berries and grapes, as well as beetroot. These are especially important, as they increase the powerful effect of glutathione, a key cellular antioxidant (see Chapters 7 and 8). Taken with glutathione, they have proven to be highly cancer-protective.

Grapeseed extract is rich in antioxidants, which have been shown to have a protective effect against cancer. In one study, a particular extract was found to inhibit a key enzyme involved in cell division by up to 50 per cent.[143] Cancer cells spread by dividing rapidly. In animal studies, anthocyanidins have been shown to suppress the growth of tumours.[144]

Carotenoids, such as beta-carotene in carrots and lycopene in tomatoes, are also powerful antioxidants and anti-cancer agents. Other antioxidants known to be cancer-protective include silymarin, a component of the milk thistle plant. One study has shown that it can protect against some forms of cancer in mice.[145] In a test tube experiment on human breast cancer cells, silymarin was shown to inhibit cell growth.[146] Also important are flavonoids, such as those found in citrus fruit, pycnogenol from pine bark and quercetin from cranberry.

We can take in significant amounts of these plant antioxidants simply by eating a diet rich in fruits and vegetables, especially by eating something orange or red every day, such as carrots and tomatoes, and something red or blue, such as berries. Many of these phytonutrients are found in advanced antioxidant supplements and those supplement formulas designed to support the immune system.

Laetrile

An extract from the apricot kernel, laetrile has often been used in aggressive anti-cancer strategies. It acts more like chemotherapy, and is claimed to target only the cancer cells. When laetrile is broken down by the body, one of its components is cyanide. This is not harmful to normal, non-cancerous cells, because they contain an enzyme that converts it to thiocyanate, a non-toxic substance used by the body to make vitamin B_{12} (cyanocobalamin). However, cancer cells lack this enzyme and are effectively poisoned by the cyanide in laetrile.

The California Medical Association was critical of laetrile's effectiveness as an anti-cancer substance, although their report did state: 'All the physicians whose patients were reviewed spoke of an increase in the sense of well-being and appetite, gain in weight and decrease in pain.' It continues to be used, with reported success, as a part of various natural anti-cancer regimes.

Specialised anti-cancer diet regimes

A number of specialised anti-cancer diet strategies have been reported over the years, all applying many of the key dietary principles contained in this book, each with their own combination of supplemental therapies. Most famous is the Gerson diet, based on the work of Dr Max Gerson, who treated hundreds of so-called terminal cases with a reported 50 per cent recovery rate. His regime included taking pancreatic enzymes, administering vitamin B_{12} injections and following a diet, plus enemas designed to detoxify the liver.

Dr W.D. Kelly in the US cured himself of cancer, having been given one month to live and went on to specialise in treating other cancer patients. Like Gerson, his regime also supplemented pancreatic enzymes and emphasised detoxifying the body.

Dr Hans Neiper, a German cancer therapist, also reported success with terminal patients using high doses of enzymes such as bromelain. The reason for using this was that it is a rich source of protein-digesting enzymes that can help to weaken cancer masses. One French study, involving 12 patients with cancer, showed impressive results with 600mg of bromelain a day.[147]

Dr Johanna Budwig emphasised the importance of flax oil for treating cancers, whereas Dr A. Ferenczi in Hungary recommended

1kg of beetroot every day, now known to be an exceedingly rich source of anthocyanidins.

In Britain, the Bristol Cancer Centre pioneered a holistic approach incorporating a mixture of different strategies, including counselling. In Mexico, restrictions on treating cancer are less stringent than in the US and there are a number of clinics using diet and natural therapies. Many clinics advocate very large doses of vitamins, especially vitamin C, and often use laetrile. Some use hydrazine sulphate, a liver enzyme that conserves energy for the patient by converting the lactic acid produced by a tumour back into glucose (normally this is a reaction that takes much more energy from the patient than it generates). Some also use 'oxygen therapy': different ways of helping to oxygenate body tissues.

It is not within the scope of this book to give detailed descriptions or to make judgements on these different approaches. Most have not been proven in extensive medical trials, although many of them report exciting anecdotal results. All focus on detoxifying the body and promoting its ability to fight back. For people with particularly malignant types of cancer, for which conventional treatment has proven unsuccessful, they certainly represent an alternative approach worthy of consideration, with the guidance of your health practitioner.

PART 5

HOW TO AVOID CANCER

CHAPTER 32

The Ideal Diet and Lifestyle Changes

If you have read through the evidence presented in this book, you will now know what you need to eat and drink, and what you should avoid, to minimise your risk of cancer. This chapter spells it out in two ways. First, there's a list of foods and drinks that I recommend you increase and others you should decrease, giving you ideal targets to aim for. This is followed by practical suggestions about which foods to buy.

The suggestions given here can help you to prevent cancer or reduce the risk of recurrence. They can also help to speed up your full recovery if you have, or have had cancer. Depending on your starting point, you may find making all the changes hard at first. But as long as you start making some of these changes, then adding more week by week, you will soon be making good progress.

At the end of the chapter there's a typical day's menu incorporating all the beneficial foods to show how you can enjoy your food and eat yourself to health. All the recipes can be found in the book.

The basics at a glance

There are many different dishes you can concoct using foods that reduce your cancer risk. Of all the principles I've discussed, however, probably the most important ones are:

1 Eat seven servings of fruits and vegetables a day (organic if possible), choosing those with the highest ORAC scores (see page 111).

2 Cut back on meat, choosing fish or vegetarian sources of protein such as beans, lentils and quinoa instead.

3 Avoid alcohol, processed and deep-fried food as much as possible. You can 'steam-fry' instead, by adding a small amount of watery sauce to a panful of, say vegetables and tofu, putting the lid on tightly and steaming in the sauce over a low heat.

The anti-cancer diet

Decrease the following from your diet:

● Avoid, or at least limit, your intake of red meat to a maximum of 310g (11oz) a week, or 150g (5½oz) twice a week –150g (5½oz) is roughly a palm-sized portion.

● Avoid, or rarely eat, burned meat – be it grilled, fried or barbecued – or processed meat products (most pies, burgers, sausages).

● Minimise your intake of fried food. Boil, steam, poach or bake food instead.

● Limit your intake of dairy food, choosing organic whenever possible. Ideally, avoid it if you have any cancer, but certainly avoid it completely if you have breast, prostate or colorectal cancer.

● Don't drink alcohol and, if you do, certainly limit your intake to one drink a day if you are male, or one drink four times a week if you are female. Ideally, limit your intake to three drinks a week, preferably choosing organic red wine.

Increase the following in your diet

● If you eat meat, choose organic low-fat varieties, game or free-range and organic chicken.

- Eat fish, such as herring, mackerel and salmon, instead of red meat, as well as white fish. Arctic cod and halibut are the least polluted.

- Eat plenty of fruit and vegetables – seven or more servings a day (organic whenever possible).

- Have a variety of colours in your selection of fruits and vegetables, including something red/orange every day (such as carrots, sweet potato, tomatoes, peaches or melons) and something blue/purple (such as berries, cherries, grapes or beetroot) and something yellow (mustard or turmeric) most days.

- Have a serving of cruciferous vegetable every day. This includes broccoli, Brussels sprouts, cabbage, cauliflower and kale.

- Eat a clove or two of garlic every day.

- Choose shiitake mushrooms and spice up dishes with turmeric. These contain anti-cancer agents.

- Have some soya milk or tofu, or a bean dish, every other day.

- Add flaxseeds to your breakfast and use flaxseed oil in salad dressings. Generally avoid refined vegetable oils – use only cold-pressed oils.

- Eat wholefoods, such as wholegrains, lentils, beans, nuts, seeds and vegetables, all of which contain fibre. Some of the fibre in vegetables is destroyed by cooking, so it's good to eat something raw every day.

- Drink green tea and 'red' herb teas, rich in antioxidants, or regular tea, in preference to coffee. However, for general health, don't drink excessive amounts of any caffeinated tea.

- Have a shot of CherryActive every day (see Resources).

- Drink six glasses of water each day, or herb or fruit teas if you prefer, perhaps with a glass of diluted juice or cherry concentrate. An excellent choice for immune boosting would be cat's claw tea sweetened with blackcurrant and apple concentrate.

Shopping list

Fruit and vegetables:
Fresh, low-GL fruits (preferably organic), such as apples, melon, pears, cherries, plums, apricots, berries
Other fruits (higher GL, but eat in moderation) bananas, dried fruits such as raisins, apricots and dates
Frozen mixed berries
Fresh vegetables (preferably organic), such as lettuce, rocket, watercress and spinach, cherry tomatoes, cucumber, spring onions, alfalfa sprouts or cress, artichoke, asparagus, avocado, beetroot, Brussels sprouts, carrots, cauliflower, courgettes, red onions, shallots, leeks, mushrooms, Tenderstem broccoli (or purple-sprouting or normal broccoli), cabbage, aubergine, peppers
Baby new potatoes (these have the lowest GL of all potatoes, as they are younger and smaller so have not developed such high sugar levels)
Sweet potatoes
Fresh herbs, such as basil, coriander and chives
Garlic
Fresh root ginger

Fresh products:
(from the chiller cabinet)
Organic skimmed milk or ideally a dairy-free alternative such as soya milk, nut milk (such as almond or hazelnut) or quinoa milk. Note that all these contain protein, lowering the GL, whereas rice milk is very high in carbohydrates and has a high GL
Live natural yoghurt, or ideally soya yoghurt
Tofu (soya bean curd) or tempeh (fermented soya beans)
Anchovies in olive oil (canned, in a jar or fresh from the deli)
Fresh or canned sardines
Organic or wild salmon, kippers, mackerel

Storecupboard staples:
Organic and/or free-range eggs; look out for omega-3 eggs from chickens fed on flaxseeds

Dried or canned legumes and pulses (such as lentils, chickpeas, borlotti beans, red kidney beans and flageolet beans, plus canned mixed pulses. Choose pulses canned in water, and always drain and rinse before use

Rye bread (pumpernickel-style or sourdough)

Rough oatcakes (Nairn's are best)

Wholemeal pasta (try a gluten-free variety, such as brown rice or buckwheat pasta)

Brown basmati rice

Soba noodles (made from buckwheat)

Quinoa

Whole organic oats

Cornflour (for thickening sauces and puddings)

Coconut butter oil,* extra virgin olive oil or Essential Balance or Udo's Choice Oil blends (for salad dressings)

Tamari (wheat-free soy sauce)

Tahini (ground sesame seed paste)

Canned chopped tomatoes

Tomato purée

Sun-dried tomato paste

Mixed antipasti (for example, roasted peppers, sun-blush tomatoes or mushrooms)

Marinated artichoke hearts in oil and canned artichoke hearts

Olives

Xylitol

Vanilla extract (natural)

Almond extract (natural)

Good-quality dark chocolate (about 70 per cent cocoa solids)

Unsalted, unroasted nuts and seeds for snacking and cooking, such as walnuts, almonds, Brazil nuts, hazelnuts, pumpkin seeds, sunflower seeds

Black peppercorns

Solo low-sodium salt

Vegetable bouillon powder

Dried herbs and spices

* Although coconut butter oil has received some negative press because of its high saturated fat content, it is very heat stable (it doesn't create any harmful by-products when heated), so is excellent for cooking and frying.

A typical anti-cancer menu

(For recipes, see Chapter 33.)

Breakfast:
Immune Berry Booster: a delicious, textured blend of yoghurt, berries, wheatgerm and seeds
or
Oat Muesli with Berries: a hearty, healthy breakfast full of variety – oats, berries, yoghurt and more
or
Super Oats: filling and full of flavour – oats with fruit and seeds

Mid-morning snack:
A piece of fruit with a small handful of nuts

Lunch:
Winter Warmer Soup: a chunky vegetable soup
or
Carrot Soup in the Raw: carrots and other ingredients, blended raw and heated gently to serve
or
Rainbow Root Salad: a wonderfully colourful mixture of carrot, cabbage, parsnip and beetroot in a tangy vinaigrette
or
Recovery Soup: vegetables and tofu, seasoned and blended cold, then heated to serve
or
Carrot and Sweet Potato Soup: flavoured with a hint of coconut, this soup is warming and delicious

Mid-afternoon snack:
Watermelon Protection: a refreshing shake
or
Berry Juice Cocktail: vibrant and tasty

Dinner:

Thai-style Buckwheat Noodles with Shiitake Mushrooms: shiitake mushrooms and tofu sautéed in spices and served on nutritious noodles

or

Salmon in a Hummus and Mushroom Sauce with Sweet Potato: the title speaks for itself – a gourmet meal

or

Fish Stew with Artichokes and Oyster Mushrooms: a delicious, thick stew, brimming with goodness too

Lifestyle changes

The combination of changing your diet, taking protective nutritional supplements and making a few lifestyle changes designed to reduce your exposure to carcinogens is likely to reduce your overall risk of developing cancer by at least 50 per cent, and even as high as 90 per cent. In real terms this could mean adding 10–20 years to your life (as well as adding life to your years). Your greatest chance of reducing your risk is by starting early – it is never too soon for prevention.

Top ten lifestyle tips

Listed below are the top ten lifestyle tips for reducing your exposure to potential carcinogens. Some are relatively easy to put into effect. Others, such as cutting down your exposure to exhaust fumes, depend on where you choose to live and work, and how you get from home to work, and vice versa. Such factors should be part of your long-term plan. Your health is your greatest asset. It is worth protecting.

1 Don't smoke, and minimise the time you spend in smoky environments.

2 Minimise the time you spend in traffic jams, breathing in exhaust fumes, and, if possible, live in a less polluted area.

3 Minimise your exposure to very strong sun and use a good sunscreen, ideally containing vitamin A (such as Environ's RAD), which protects your skin from damage but doesn't stop you making vitamin D. A sunscreen is especially important if you have fair hair, light eyes and many moles. Don't combine alcohol and strong sunlight.

4 Use natural alternatives to drugs whenever possible. Don't have oestrogen- or progestin-containing HRT and have an X-ray only if it is absolutely essential.

5 If you use a mobile phone, use it infrequently and use an earphone attachment.

6 Don't heat food in plastic, and reduce the amount of drinks and fatty foods you buy that are packaged in direct contact with soft plastics.

7 Switch to natural detergents and check that your bathroom and household products don't contain known carcinogens (see Chapters 4 and 22).

8 Don't use pesticides in your garden or on your indoor pot plants.

9 Control the level of stress in your life. Prolonged stress depletes your immune strength.

10 Get enough sleep. It is vital for the immune system.

CHAPTER 33

Anti-cancer Recipes

Breakfast

Get Up & Go

Healthy Get Up & Go is a powdered breakfast drink, which is blended with skimmed milk or soya milk and banana or berries. Nutritionally speaking, it is the ultimate breakfast: each serving gives you more fibre than a bowl of porridge, more protein than an egg, more iron than a cooked breakfast and more vitamins and minerals than a whole packet of cornflakes. In fact, every serving of Get Up & Go gives you at least 100 per cent of every vitamin and mineral and a lot more of some key nutrients. For example, you get 1,000mg of vitamin C – the equivalent of more than 20 oranges.

Get Up & Go is made from the best-quality wholefoods, ground into a powder. The carbohydrate comes principally from apple powder, the protein comes from quinoa, soya and rice flour, the essential fats from ground sesame, sunflower and pumpkin seeds, the fibre from oat bran, rice bran and psyllium husks, and additional flavour from almond meal, cinnamon and natural vanilla.

It contains no sucrose, no additives, no animal products, no yeast, wheat or milk, and it tastes delicious. Each serving, with half a pint of skimmed milk or soya milk and some fruit, provides fewer than 300 calories and, when mixed up, only 10 GLs, making it ideal as part of a low-GL diet to keep your blood sugar balanced. It is nutritionally super-ior to any other breakfast choice and is totally suitable for adults and children alike. It is fine to have this for breakfast every day, if you choose.

It is widely available in health-food shops (see Resources).

Make Get Up & Go with berries such as strawberries, raspberries or blueberries, or a soft pear. If you use a banana have a small, less ripe one or use half a larger banana.

Serves 1
300ml (10fl oz/½ pint) skimmed milk or soya milk
1 small banana or a serving of other fruit, such as berries or a peach
1 serving Get Up & Go powder

Blend the milk, fruit and Get Up & Go powder, and serve.

Immune Berry Booster

Fresh-tasting and brightly coloured.

Serves 1
150g (5½oz) low-fat live yoghurt
115g (4oz) berries, such as strawberries, blueberries, raspberries, blackcurrants
1 tbsp wheatgerm
1 tbsp mixed ground seeds, such as sesame seeds, pumpkin seeds, flaxseeds, sunflower seeds

Mix all the ingredients together and serve.

Oat Muesli with Berries

The slow-releasing carbohydrate in oats makes them an ideal breakfast to keep you going and to avoid blood sugar highs and lows. Apple, hazelnuts and berries add flavour and nourishment to the muesli.

Serves 4
4 tbsp rolled oats
1 tbsp oat germ and bran

125ml (4fl oz) warmed soya milk

150g (5½oz) plain yoghurt

2 tbsp honey

2 tbsp lemon juice

1 red apple and 1 green apple, washed, cored and grated, but not peeled

4 tbsp chopped hazelnuts

2 tbsp blueberries or blackcurrants, plus a few whole berries

4 mint sprigs

1 Soak the rolled oats, oat germ and bran in the soya milk in a bowl overnight or for at least two hours.
2 Stir in the yoghurt, honey and lemon juice, then add the grated apples and the hazelnuts, followed by the berries or blackcurrants just before serving. Decorate each portion with a sprig of mint and a few whole berries.

You can buy oat-based and gluten-free muesli in health food stores but get one that doesn't have lots of hidden sugar in the form of raisins or dates. Have with soya milk and some fresh fruit.

Super Oats

This sustaining oat breakfast includes omega-3 and 6 oils from the ground seeds and vitamin E from the wheatgerm.

Serves 1

25g (1oz) oat flakes

1 tbsp wheatgerm

125ml (4fl oz) soya milk, rice milk or oat milk

1 tbsp mixed ground seeds, such as sesame seeds, pumpkin seeds, flaxseeds, sunflower seeds

1 handful of berries

1 apple, washed and chopped

Mix the oat flakes, wheatgerm and milk together. Add the seeds, berries and apple, and serve.

Lunch

Super Greens Mix

This pesto-style blend of dark green leaves and herbs is a brilliant way to dramatically increase your intake of these flavonoid and vitamin C-rich ingredients without having to wade through buckets of salad. Simply blend it all together with some oil and serve in soups, or with pasta, salads or main meals. I recommend you have a serving of this on at least one of your meals each day, but ideally add it to both to give your liver a helping hand. You can vary the leaves and herbs used according to taste and availability. Add avocado (rich in vitamin E and protein) for a thicker consistency, or cucumber (a very cleansing vegetable) for a thinner texture. Equally, you can ring the changes by adding raw garlic, sun-blush tomatoes or roasted peppers, marinated artichoke hearts, pumpkin seeds or pine nuts.

Serves 1

¼ bag (a good handful) watercress, rinsed and dried

¼ bag (a good handful) baby leaf spinach, rinsed and dried

a good handful of basil leaves

a good drizzle of extra virgin olive oil, or an omega-rich seed oil, such as hemp or flaxseed oil (the mixture should hold together a little like pesto)

Whiz the leaves and herbs together in a blender or food processor, or finely chop using a sharp knife. Stir in the oil.

Winter Warmer Soup

Here's a wonderfully warming and easy-to-make meal in itself.

Serves 4

1 tbsp olive oil

1 medium onion, peeled and chopped

2 garlic cloves, peeled and crushed

680g (1½lb) fresh seasonal vegetables, such as potatoes, swede, celeriac, leeks, celery, carrots, broccoli, cabbage, prepared and chopped

400g (14oz) can tomatoes
1 tsp vegetable stock concentrate, such as Vecon

1 Heat the olive oil in a pan and briefly sauté the onion and garlic. Add the vegetables, tomatoes, and enough water to cover.
2 Add the vegetable stock. Simmer for 20–25 minutes or until the vegetables are cooked.

Variations

- This soup can be liquidised if you prefer.

- Use potatoes in moderation if you don't want a particularly thick soup.

- Add lentils for a thicker, more filling version.

- For vegetable stew, use less water.

Patrick's Primordial Soup

I designed this soup to help my wife Gaby get over a bug, and it is now a renowned health tonic for my readers! It is so-called because it contains foods that provide the key nutrients to ensure good health. It's incredibly rich in vitamin E and beta-carotene, as well as anti-inflammatory onions, garlic and ginger. The coconut milk not only gives a rich, creamy flavour but it also contains medium-chain triglycerides – special kinds of saturated fat that are not stored as fat but are used to give you energy. Coconut is also thought to help thyroid function and to fight infection.

Serves 2–3
1 tbsp coconut butter oil or medium (not extra virgin) olive oil
½ red onion, roughly chopped
1 garlic clove, crushed
1 large carrot or 2 small–medium ones, peeled and chopped
1 large sweet potato, or 2 small–medium ones, unpeeled, chopped to the same size as the carrot to ensure even cooking

1 heaped tsp grated fresh root ginger
¼ tsp turmeric
2 tsp Marigold Reduced Salt Vegetable Bouillon powder
½ red pepper, diced
75ml (2½fl oz) coconut milk

1 Heat the oil in a large pan and gently sauté the onion and garlic for a few minutes until they start to soften but do not brown.
2 Add the carrot, sweet potato, ginger, turmeric and bouillon powder. Just cover with boiling water, bring to the boil, then put the lid on and simmer for 15 minutes or until the vegetables are soft.
3 Add the pepper and coconut milk, then blend until smooth and thick.

Carrot Soup in the Raw

Ever had a hot, raw soup? This soup is made cold and then heated gently, which keeps all the vitamin and mineral content intact. It's also full of fibre. Be careful not to overheat it.

Serves 4
450g (1lb) organic carrots, washed and cut into chunks
85g (3oz) ground almonds
300ml (10fl oz/½ pint) soya milk
1 tsp vegetable stock concentrate, such as Vecon
1 tsp dried mixed herbs

Put the carrots into a food processor or blender and process to a purée. Add the other ingredients and process until well combined. Warm very gently in a pan.

Rainbow Root Salad

This colourful combination of carrots, cabbage and beetroot is more filling than you may think. Go easy on the beetroot as its strong taste can overpower the carrots.

Serves 4
3 medium organic carrots, washed and grated
¼ red cabbage, washed and grated

¼ white cabbage, washed and grated
1 beetroot, peeled and grated
2 tbsp extra virgin olive oil or Essential Balance or Udo's Choice Oil
1 tsp Dijon mustard
2 garlic cloves, peeled and crushed
lemon juice

1 Mix together all the vegetables in a large salad bowl.
2 Put the oil into a small bowl and add the mustard, garlic and lemon juice to taste. Pour over the vegetables and toss well.

Recovery Soup

This soup is blended raw, then heated to serve. You can use the same principle to invent other instant, high-energy soups. Serve with oatcakes.

Serves 1
2 organic carrots, washed and cut into chunks
85g (3oz) broccoli, washed and broken into florets
1 bunch watercress, washed
85g (3oz) tofu
125ml (4fl oz) soya milk
2 tsp Vecon or Bouillon vegetable concentrate
tomato purée, spices or freshly chopped herbs, to taste

Blend all the ingredients together in a food processor or blender. Serve hot or cold, with oatcakes.

Carrot and Sweet Potato Soup

Sweet potatoes are rich in carotenoids and vitamin E. This simple soup takes only a short time to prepare and tastes delicious.

Serves 2
4 medium sweet potatoes, peeled and chopped into small pieces
4 large organic carrots, washed and chopped into small pieces
⅓ × 400ml (14fl oz) can coconut milk
1 garlic clove, peeled and crushed
ground black pepper

1 Put the sweet potatoes and carrots in a pan with just enough water to cover, and boil until soft.
2 Purée in a blender or food processor, then add the coconut milk, garlic and black pepper to taste.

Variation
Use butternut squash instead of the sweet potato.

Mid-afternoon snack

Watermelon Protection

The flesh of watermelon is rich in beta-carotene and vitamin C. The seeds are a great source of essential fats, vitamin E, zinc and selenium. If you blend the seeds with the flesh, the husk (the black part) of the seed sinks to the bottom and the seeds blend with the flesh to make an incredibly immune-boosting fruit drink. It provides enough glucose for energy, some protein from the seeds and plenty of immune-boosting nutrients.

Serves 1
1 medium slice of watermelon, about 200g (7oz) rindless weight
ice (optional)

Blend the watermelon flesh, seeds and all, until smooth. Serve with ice, if you like, or blend the ice with the watermelon for an instant chilled juice.

Berry Juice Cocktail

This cocktail is nectar for the immune system, with plenty of vitamin C and anthocyanidins.

Serves 1
300ml (10fl oz/½ pint) apple juice
350g (12oz) mixed berries, such as blueberries, blackberries, strawberries

Put the ingredients into a blender and whiz up.

Shopping tip

There's also an ever-increasing variety of fruit and berry juices available to buy. See what's available in your local health-food store. Choose pure juices with no added sugar. Particularly good are loganberries, blueberries and blackcurrants. Bought juices are often best diluted half and half with water to dilute the natural fruit sugars.

Dinner

Thai-style Buckwheat Noodles with Shiitake Mushrooms

Buckwheat is a wheat-free food with a good protein content. However, most buckwheat noodles also contain wheat, which makes them easier to cook than pure buckwheat noodles, which fall apart if cooked too long. They are best boiled for five minutes, drained, then boiled again.

Serves 2
200g (7oz) buckwheat noodles
1 tbsp olive oil
2 garlic cloves, peeled and chopped
115g (4oz) shiitake mushrooms, or 15g (½oz) dried and soaked (see Cook's tip overleaf)
2 organic carrots, washed and thinly sliced lengthwise into 5cm (2in) pieces
115g (4oz) broccoli, washed and broken into florets
115g (4oz) marinated tofu pieces
1 tsp Thai spices
2 tbsp coconut milk or 1 tbsp soy sauce

1 Cook the noodles according to the pack instructions. Meanwhile, heat the olive oil in a wok or deep frying pan. Sauté the garlic for 3 minutes, then add the mushrooms and toss briefly.
2 Add the remaining vegetables with the tofu, spices and coconut milk or soy sauce. Pour in 4 tbsp water for the ingredients to 'steam-fry'. Cover and turn down the heat until the vegetables are cooked but remain crunchy. Serve over a nest of cooked buckwheat noodles.

Cook's tip

If using dried shiitake mushrooms, put them into a small bowl and pour over some lukewarm water. Leave for 2 minutes, then drain and quickly rinse to remove any grit. Soak in warm water for 30 minutes. Drain. Cut off the stalks and discard.

Salmon in a Hummus and Mushroom Sauce with Sweet Potato

Shiitake mushrooms have a good, rich flavour, which goes very well with hummus to make a simple sauce to serve with poached salmon, mashed sweet potato and Brussels sprouts.

Serves 2

2 pieces salmon fillet or 2 salmon steaks

2 tsp vegetable stock concentrate, such as Vecon

600ml (20fl oz/1 pint) boiling water

2 large sweet potatoes, peeled and cut into chunks

225g (8oz) shiitake mushrooms, or 25g (1oz) dried, soaked (see Cook's tip above)

1 tbsp olive oil

225g (8oz) Brussels sprouts, trimmed and washed

115g (4oz) hummus

ground black pepper

1 Wash the salmon and pat dry with kitchen paper. Dilute the vegetable stock concentrate in the boiling water in a large pan. Leave to cool until just warm.

2 Boil the sweet potatoes until tender. Put the salmon in the stock and bring gently up to a simmer. Poach for a few minutes until the fish flakes easily when lifted gently with a knife. (Alternatively, grill the salmon under a medium heat for a few minutes on each side until just cooked.)

3 Sauté the mushrooms in the oil for 2 minutes, then add 2 tbsp water, cover and reduce the heat. Simmer for 5 minutes until tender and juicy. Meanwhile, boil or steam the Brussels sprouts for 5 minutes.

4 Purée the mushrooms in a blender and return to the pan. Stir in the hummus and warm through gently. Mash the sweet potatoes, adding black pepper to taste.

5 Put the salmon, mashed sweet potatoes and Brussels sprouts on a plate, pour the sauce over the fish and serve.

Fish Stew with Artichokes and Shiitake Mushrooms

Salmon and mackerel are both healthy oily fish and taste very good in this full-flavoured and nutritious stew. Serve with brown rice.

Serves 4
450g (1lb) thick-cut, skinless salmon fillet
450g (1lb) thick-cut mackerel fillet
3 tbsp cornflour
2 tbsp olive oil
2 onions, peeled and cut into 8 wedges, retaining the root to hold the layers together
2 garlic cloves, peeled and chopped
300ml (10fl oz/½ pint) white wine
175ml (6fl oz) fish stock
225g (8oz) shiitake mushrooms
1 bay leaf
12 artichoke hearts in oil, drained and halved
1 lemon, thinly sliced
2 tbsp chopped fresh basil
ground black pepper

1 Cut the fish into bite-size chunks, removing any bones. Season with black pepper and dust with cornflour. Heat the olive oil in a deep pan. Add the chunks of fish and cook until sealed all over. Remove the fish with a slotted spoon and set aside.
2 Add the onions to the pan and cook until softened. Add the garlic and cook for 2 minutes. Stir in the wine and stock, the mushrooms and bay leaf. Bring to the boil and simmer for 5 minutes. (Boiling evaporates the alcohol content of the wine.)
3 Add the fish and artichokes to the sauce, then lay the lemon slices on top. Cover and cook for 10–15 minutes. Stir in the chopped basil. Serve immediately with brown rice.

Find out more

For more delicious and healthy recipes, see:

The Optimum Nutrition Cookbook, Patrick Holford and Judy Ridgway, Piatkus (2000)

The Holford Low-GL Diet Cookbook, Patrick Holford and Fiona McDonald Joyce, Piatkus (2005)

Food GLorious Food, Patrick Holford and Fiona McDonald Joyce, Piatkus (2008)

CHAPTER 34

Supplementary Benefit

In addition to eating an immune-boosting anti-cancer diet, there's definite value in taking supplements of certain vitamins, minerals and herbs. The ideal intake depends very much on your particular needs – a consequence of genetic factors, your diet, lifestyle and environment. The 'basic' recommendations given below are therefore only a general guide for people wanting to minimise their risk of getting cancer and other nutrition-related diseases. They are your 'insurance policy'.

In practical terms, the easiest way to achieve these levels is to supplement:

- A good all-round multivitamin and mineral

- Vitamin C (ideally with bioflavonoids or anthocyanidins)

- An antioxidant complex (with A, C, E, zinc and selenium, plus other antioxidant nutrients such as glutathione or N-acetyl-cysteine, alpha lipoic acid and coenzyme Q_{10})

The levels needed for these nutrients to exert their most positive effect far exceed the amounts needed for basic prevention. Such levels are given in the table below under 'maximum nutritional support'. They do not cover requirements during chemotherapy, radiation or surgery. Nutritional needs under these circumstances are discussed in Chapter 36.

A further argument for micronutrient supplementation is that many cancer patients suffer from malabsorption and may not be getting the micronutrients they need from their food, even if their diet is good.

Seek professional nutritional help

If you have been diagnosed with cancer you should not undertake a nutritional strategy on your own. Seek the guidance of a nutritional therapist who can work with your doctor to devise the most appropriate strategy for you. Just because a substance is 'natural' it doesn't mean it is never harmful. Very high doses of nutrients can have adverse effects and this is why you need a nutritional therapist to advise you and run tests to find out what you need.

Ideal supplementary nutrient intake to protect against cancer

Nutrient	Basic prevention	Maximum nutritional support
Vitamins		
Vitamin A	6,000mcg	10,000mcg
as retinol	2,500mcg	5,000mcg*
as beta-carotene	3,300mcgRE	10,000mcgRE†
Vitamin C	2,000mg	10,000mg
Vitamin D	15mcg (600iu)	30mcg (1,200iu)
Vitamin E	150mg (200iu)	300–600mg (400–800iu)
B_1 (thiamine)	25mg	–
B_2 (riboflavin)	25mg	–
B_3 (niacin)	25mg	100mg
B_5 (pantothenic acid)	25mg	50–300mg
B_6 (pyridoxine)	25mg	50–100mg
B_{12}	10mcg	50–1,000mcg
Folic acid	200mcg	400–800mcg**
Biotin	50mcg	–

cont ▶

Nutrient	Basic prevention	Maximum nutritional support
Minerals		
Calcium	350mg	800mg
Magnesium	200mg	500mg
Zinc	15mg	25–35mg
Iron	10mg	–
Manganese	5mg	10mg
Chromium	50mcg	100mcg
Selenium	100mcg	200mcg
Other nutrients		
Glutamine	1,000mg	5,000mg
CoQ_{10}	30mg	90mg
Reduced glutathione***	50mg	300mg
Lipoic acid	10mg	20–200mg
Anthocyanidins	20mg	50mg
Resveratrol	10mg	40mg
Bioflavonoids	100mg	300mg
N-acetyl-cysteine	50mg	100–500mg
Herbs		
(Best divided into three daily doses)		
Cat's claw caps	4.5–6g per day	
Cat's claw tincture	4–10 ml per day	
Echinacea caps	2.4–5g per day	
Echinacea tincture	3–6 ml per day	
Astragalus caps	2.5–3.4g per day	
Astragulus tincture	12–24 ml per day	
Milk thistle caps	30–60g per day	
Milk thistle tincture	4–8 ml per day	
Mushrooms (Ganoderma)	1500mg	
Aloe vera	as instructed	

cont ▶

Optional extras include: curcumin, bromelain and garlic, which are all available as supplements. There are many different sources of bioflavonoids and anthocyanidins such as pycnogenol, quercetin and grapeseed extract. Supplements containing a complex of anthocyanidins and bioflavonoids are becoming widely available. Best of all are supplements of salvestrols (see Chapter 14). Also of interest for hormone-related cancers are extracts from soya, which are rich in genistein, daidzein and other isoflavonoids.

† Retinol equivalent

* Do not take this amount of retinol, the non-vegetable form of vitamin A, if you are pregnant or likely to conceive.

** Do not supplement more than 200mcg per day if you have cancer unless your homocysteine level is high or you have been recommended to do so by your doctor or oncologist.

*** Glutathione must be enteric-coated to prevent degradation in the stomach. It must also be combined with anthocyanidins, which recycle glutathione, making it much more powerful. Alternatively, supplement 500 to 1,000mg of N-acetyl-cysteine (NAC) from which the body can make glutathione.

PART 6

WHAT TO DO IF YOU HAVE CANCER

CHAPTER 35

Conventional and Alternative Treatment

If you have been diagnosed with cancer, and offered specific treatment by your oncologist, and yet you are interested in complementary approaches, how do you make a decision regarding the best way forward? Your anti-cancer strategy needs to consist of three angles of attack.

1   Look at what you can do right now to deal with the existing cancer mass and cancer cells.

2   Think about your post-treatment strategy, to minimise further cancer cells developing and growing.

3   Plan the strategy that you can adopt to change your diet, lifestyle and attitude so that you can strengthen your body's immune system and reduce your exposure to carcinogens – switching your body's chemistry away from cancer promotion.

These three strategies are likely to involve a combination of conventional and alternative approaches. I call this an integrated approach. At the extremes I would be wary of any health practitioner who either says that all conventional treatments are unnecessary – meaning chemotherapy, radiation and surgery – and also any oncologist whose only focus is on a combination of these three, disregarding the factors that may have led you to develop cancer in the first place.

The different ways of treating cancer

The effectiveness of surgery depends on the nature of the tumour and the skills of the surgeon. Athough surgery may remove the immediate problem – the tumour – it does nothing to address the underlying factors that led your intelligent body to produce cancer cells. If this is recommended for you, there are constructive things you can do to speed up your recovery, and we will talk about these in the next chapter.

Radiotherapy is another local treatment, and is performed by skilled radiotherapists who specialise in targeting the radiation beam onto the tumour so that damage to neighbouring healthy cells will be minimal. It does not cause nausea or hair loss but can leave you feeling pretty wiped out, and it can burn the skin. There may also be long-term side effects. One study found that child cancer survivors had increasing risk of developing diabetes with increasing amounts of radiotherapy.[1] There are things you can do to minimise these side effects and maximise your recovery, which I will be discussing.

Chemotherapy is the use of specific drugs to target and destroy cancer cells. Recent developments in chemotherapy are focused on targeting cancer cells, rather than healthy cells, more successfully. Chemotherapy is associated with a host of side effects, such as nausea and hair loss, but this depends on the specific chemotherapeutic agent. Some, such as intravenous vitamin C and salvestrols, don't have any side effects. Salvestrols have not yet been subjected to clinical trials so, despite a clear mechanism for their anti-cancer action, supported by some impressive case histories, this is not a proven approach.

There are other chemotherapeutic approaches; for example, photodynamic therapy (PDT), which relies on tumour-killing drugs that are activated by light. In the case of skin cancer, the drug is rubbed on in the form of a cream; with internal cancers, the patient swallows the drug, which is then activated by a light at the end of an endoscope (a flexible tube). It is licensed by NICE (National Institute for Health and Clinical Excellence) for use on the skin, head, neck and oesophagus. PDT has been used for a number of years at the National Medical Laser Centre based at University College Hospital, London. However, in spite of the fact that it is less invasive and is cheaper than many conventional therapies, it is not widely available, and most cancer patients will need to ask for it. For further information, see Resources.

Keep informed

My advice is to get as much information as possible, ideally working with an oncologist and/or doctor specialising in cancer treatment that is open to, and informed about, natural approaches. I also recommend you work with a nutritional therapist to support you in developing an appropriate diet and lifestyle, and a personalised supplement programme to minimise the risk of recurrence.

You may also be offered drug treatments as part of your 'prevention' strategy, such as tamoxifen and other drugs designed to block oestrogen receptors for oestrogen-positive breast cancer (most breast cancer cells are oestrogen responsive). I will tell you much more about breast cancer (currently the most common cancer in women in many countries, including the UK and the US), and how to reduce your risk of recurrence, in Chapter 37. I will also tell you how to prevent and reverse prostate cancer, the most common cancer in men. Whether you choose to take these drugs, and for how long – perhaps in conjunction with natural approaches aimed at achieving the same thing – is something for you to discuss with your team of experts.

CHAPTER 36

Maximising Recovery from Chemotherapy, Radiation and Surgery

As explained in the last chapter, if you have been diagnosed with cancer you will probably have been offered one or more of three treatments: surgery, chemotherapy or radiotherapy. There are advantages and disadvantages to each of these treatments, the disadvantages of which can often be counteracted by specific nutritional strategies.

The purpose of this chapter is to give you information about different forms of cancer treatment and how optimum nutrition can improve your body's response to them. You should consider carefully what course of action to take, in consultation with both your doctor and a nutritional therapist, who can advise you on the most appropriate nutritional support.

Surgery

This procedure is most effective when a tumour is interfering with the body's ability to function, but surgery leaves cancer cells behind in about a quarter of cancer patients, allowing malignant growth to reoccur, as numerous studies have shown. It is not a cure as such, because the tumour is the symptom rather than the cause of the underlying disease process. As surgery is naturally traumatic to the body, it is wise to increase your intake of vitamins A, C and E, zinc and glutamine before and after surgery, which help the body to heal. They are particularly important after surgery, especially glutamine – 10 grams or two heaped teaspoons per day.

Radiotherapy

Although radiation is used to slow down certain cancers, it rarely provides a cure. Some damage will also occur to healthy cells and organ tissue. Radiation is a carcinogen itself, and it greatly weakens the immune system. Nutritional support during radiation is important, especially using antioxidant nutrients (vitamins A, C and E, CoQ_{10}, zinc and selenium) and possibly glutathione.

Chemotherapy

The administration of drugs that are toxic to cancer cells is called chemotherapy. The problem with this treatment is that many of the drugs also harm healthy cells and are carcinogens in their own right. This applies to both powerful chemotherapeutic agents and to mild ones such as tamoxifen. As ever, researchers are trying to develop more specifically targeted chemotherapeutic drugs that won't damage healthy cells.

Despite being the most commonly prescribed breast cancer drug, tamoxifen is a double-edged sword. Chemically related to DES (a drug that caused cancer in people exposed to it during foetal development), it is a weakly oestrogenic chemical that acts as an oestrogen blocker, much like plant oestrogens in soya. It is only likely to be effective in post-menopausal women who have oestrogen-sensitive breast cancer, and even then the protective effects wear off after five years. Although some studies have shown that it reduced their chances of developing cancer in the other breast by 30 to 50 per cent,[2] others show marginal benefit. A review of a number of studies involving 30,000 breast cancer patients, published in the *Lancet* medical journal, found only a 3.5 per cent difference in survival after five or six years in those taking the drug compared to those taking a placebo.[3]

However, there is a dark side to tamoxifen. While it might slightly reduce the risk of breast cancer, it has repeatedly been shown to increase the risk of liver cancer and double the risk of endometrial cancer,[4] as well as carrying side effects ranging from eye damage and risk of blood clots to menopausal symptoms. As such, it is a known carcinogen. Despite all this, tamoxifen is now being licensed to be given to women without breast cancer on the grounds that it will prevent it. This is lunacy, in the light of the known disadvantages of this drug and the overwhelming evidence on non-toxic dietary strategies that provide significantly more protection. See Chapter 37 for more information on tamoxifen and how to reduce your risk of breast cancer recurrence.

Nutritional support for chemotherapy and radiotherapy

If you are receiving chemotherapy or radiotherapy it is useful to know that numerous clinical studies have shown that making dietary and lifestyle changes can help improve general well-being, increase life expectancy and help reduce the effects of the therapies. It is best to start an immune-boosting programme a month before treatment (see Chapter 6) and then to follow a detoxification programme after treatment to help the body rid itself of toxins (see Chapter 7). A nutritional therapist can help you to do this. Factors involved in immune boosting include reducing your intake of fats, eating more vegetables, taking vitamin and mineral supplements and minimising your exposure to pollution.[5]

Vitamin and mineral support

Although some people advise not to take vitamin or mineral supplements during chemotherapy or radiotherapy, several studies have shown that antioxidants may not only protect against the toxicity of the drugs and radiation but can also enhance their cancer-killing effects.[6] My advice is certainly to supplement before and after treatment and, in the case of chemotherapy, discuss any specific nutrient contraindications for the specific type of chemotherapy you are getting, and ask for actual evidence to support their recommendation to help you understand how to maximise benefit from the treatment. Don't accept a blanket dismissal. Supplementing vitamin B_6 can prevent nausea and vomiting caused by radiotherapy. (Other ways to help nausea include drinking peppermint or ginger tea – made by adding a walnut-sized piece of peeled ginger root, crushed, to boiling water – or drinking good quality ginger beer or ale. Most importantly, keep hydrated.)

One common chemotherapeutic agent, Adriamycin, has the unfortunate side effect of inducing heart problems. Because it is known to deplete levels of CoQ_{10} – which is essential for heart function – a group of patients were given 100mg of CoQ_{10} daily during chemotherapy and compared to other patients given chemotherapy alone. Those on CoQ_{10} did not experience the increase in cardiac problems that occurred in the group not supplementing CoQ_{10}.[7]

Another nutrient worth supplementing during chemotherapy is bromelain, a protein-digesting enzyme found in pineapple. In one study conducted in Germany giving bromelain alongside chemotherapy produced significant tumour regression. The researchers found that up to 2g of bromelain a day was needed for optimal effects.[8]

Glutamine helps you heal

In addition to the nutrients recommended in Chapter 34, the amino acid glutamine can greatly help recovery after surgery and during chemotherapy. Glutamine is the primary nutrient for the lining of the small intestine and may be useful for healing a variety of inflammatory gut conditions. It is also a precursor for the key antioxidant glutathione (glutamine participates in the chemical reaction that produces glutathione). Patients receiving chemotherapy frequently suffer from nausea, vomiting and diarrhoea, probably because the chemotherapy attacks and destroys the fast-growing intestinal cells. In one study, 11 patients undergoing chemotherapy for acute leukaemia received 6g of oral glutamine three times a day for three days prior to therapy, and then for between 11 and 39 days afterwards. Compared to the 22 subjects in the control group, the glutamine group experienced less severe diarrhoea, for a significantly shorter period of time.[9]

Other studies have shown that glutamine speeds up recovery from chemotherapy and reduces the incidence of infection,[10] a common occurrence following these powerful drugs. Likewise, animal studies have shown that chemotherapy is more effective when glutamine is also given.[11] It also reduces mouth sores,[12] and injury from radiation.

Cancer patients may not feel like eating and may absorb fewer calories from the foods they eat. This can cause severe weight loss, known as cachexia, which is why dietary advice is generally aimed at preventing it. If lack of appetite is a problem, it is best to eat light snacks, little and often, and to drink plenty to avoid becoming dehydrated. If chewing and swallowing is a problem, try nutritional-supplement drinks, particularly those that contain a source of protein (see Resources). There's a good variety, and they also provide a source of calories. Or you could try juicing fruits and vegetables such as carrots, apples, strawberries, mangoes, and so on.

Herbs such as astragalus, cat's claw, and echinacea can all be taken after treatment is finished to restimulate the immune system.

Natural cancer strategies

Should you choose to pursue a nutritional approach to cancer, this is best done with the guidance of a nutritional therapist. In any event it is wise to supplement a good multivitamin, vitamin C and probably additional antioxidants (see Chapter 34). He or she can work out the most appropriate strategy for you, based on a complete assessment of your nutritional needs. This assessment is likely to include:

- **Blood and urine tests** to determine your current health status. These can include using what is known as DNA assays (which can also be used to assess your genetic risk of cancer occurring in the first place), as well as tests to show which antioxidants may be lacking and how well your detoxification processes are working in the liver. These advanced tests help to pinpoint the best course of action.

- **A detoxifying diet**, aimed at giving your body the maximum nutrients with the minimum ingestion of toxic substances.

- **A nutritional supplement programme**, with high levels of anti-oxidants and key nutrients known to boost your immune system and stack the odds in your favour. This is likely to include large amounts of vitamins A and C, and selenium, as well as glutathione and anthocyanidins.

- **Looking at appropriate natural anti-cancer agents** for your type of cancer. For hormone-related cancers this might involve phytoestrogens such as genistein and daidzein from soya. There are a number of other anti-cancer agents that your nutritional therapist can advise you about.

- **Providing support**. This is an important part of the process and there are a number of support groups for people with cancer and for those who choose non-conventional treatments.

- **Education**. The more you know, the greater your ability to make informed choices.

To find a nutritional therapist in your area, see Resources, page 381. Some have more experience of working with people with cancer so it's worth asking around before making your choice.

Get the best out of both

Pursuing a nutritional strategy is not an alternative to medical treatment. In fact, the two together may produce the best outcome (this is known as integrated medicine). That's not just what I believe; it is also the opinion of many cancer specialists, including Dr Keith Block, director of the Integrative Cancer Care Center in Evanston, Illinois. Block and his colleagues combine cautious amounts of chemotherapy, radiotherapy and surgery with generous amounts of supplements, diet advice and psychological support. In the same way, your nutritional therapist and doctor, together with whoever else you choose to employ, should be viewed as members of a team whose purpose is to provide you with the best possible strategy for restoring health.

CHAPTER 37

Reducing the Risk
of Recurrence

I f you've been diagnosed with cancer, you've had to make some
tough decisions about what treatment to pursue. Now you want
to do whatever you can to minimise the likelihood of recurrence
after the tumour has gone. This chapter highlights the dietary and
lifestyle choices that you can make to give yourself the best possible
chance.

Arguably, one of the most important questions to address is why
your cancer occurred in the first place. If you haven't already con-
sulted a nutritional therapist, now may be the time to do so, as he
or she can help you to assess any diet or lifestyle factors that may
reduce your risk of recurrence. It may be recommended that you take
certain tests to help your nutritional therapist tailor a programme
for you; for example, in Chapter 8 I explained the importance of
knowing your homocysteine level. Homocysteine is a natural substance in your blood and is a marker of your ability – or inability – to
perform a vital biochemical process called methylation. It's important that you can do this well, because one in four gene mutations is
caused by faulty methylation. So, check your homocysteine level (see
Resources) and, if necessary, supplement a cocktail of homocysteine-
lowering nutrients – including vitamins B_2, B_6 and B_{12}, folic acid, a
nutrient called TMG, zinc and magnesium (see chart on page 75 for

relevant dosage levels) – to bring yours down to below 7. (Ideally you want to achieve a homocysteine level of about one-tenth of your age.)

In this chapter I'm going to talk you through how to reduce the risk of two of the most common cancers: breast and prostate. Much of the advice applies to *all* cancers, so pay particular attention to the summary at the end of the chapter. Part 7 gives you more information on other types of cancer.

Breast cancer drugs used for preventing recurrence

The drugs most often prescribed for breast cancer patients are tamoxifen, raloxifene, Arimidex, and the newest and most controversial kid on the block, Herceptin. But how effective are they? What are their side effects, and how do they compare with treatment approaches that focus on diet, nutritional supplements and lifestyle changes? Let's take a look at them.

Tamoxifen, raloxifene and Arimidex: the anti-oestrogens

Tamoxifen, the market leader, is potentially effective only for patients with oestrogen-positive breast cancer. It also does not appear to be effective when the cancer has spread to the lymph nodes. Trials have shown that, with oestrogen-positive breast cancer, the longer a woman takes tamoxifen, the more she reduces her risk of a recurrence. Reviews typically report that 10 per cent more women survive longer than ten years when they take tamoxifen for five years. However, these reviews also indicate that tamoxifen significantly increases the incidence of endometrial cancer, quadrupling it after those same five years of use. This is because tamoxifen causes the uterus to quickly thicken in virtually all test subjects, doubling their risk of endometrial cancer in the first year or two of use.

Other side effects of tamoxifen include a tripling of the risk of potentially fatal blood clots in the lungs, increased risk of stroke, blindness and liver dysfunction. In consideration of these potential problems, tamoxifen's overall reduction in risk of mortality is considerably less than 10 per cent.

The National Cancer Institute (NCI) admits that tamoxifen is indicated for preventive use only in women with increased risk of breast cancer as determined primarily by family history, now identifiable by inheriting specific genes such as BRCA. The NCI estimates that only about 0.3 per cent of women aged 39 or younger would be candidates for tamoxifen treatment, yet it used to be common practice to put most women with breast cancer on the medication.

Raloxifene is the major rival for tamoxifen. It hasn't been so extensively studied in long-term trials, but the general consensus is that it reduces recurrence in oestrogen-positive breast cancer only slightly better than tamoxifen, but with less risk of endometrial cancer and no real difference in risk of stroke or cardiovascular problems. Some have claimed that raloxifene might reduce cardiovascular risk because, like tamoxifen, it appears to lower LDL (bad) cholesterol and raise HDL (good) cholesterol. But a recent trial, which studied the effects of raloxifene in women who had a history of heart disease, or who were at high risk of heart disease, showed that after five years of follow-up, participants experienced no real improvement in heart problems.[13]

This trial also found that taking raloxifene put some women at greater risk of dangerous blood clots, although the risk of stroke was found to be the same in women taking raloxifene as those taking the placebo. However, among women who had strokes during the time of the study, more women in the raloxifene group had fatal strokes than in the placebo group.

Arimidex is a second rival to tamoxifen. Although the survival rates of patients taking Arimidex don't appear to be any different from the survival rates of patients taking tamoxifen, there are quite a few studies that focus on symptoms affecting 'quality of life'; for example, one study says that women who took Arimidex reported less vaginal bleeding and thromboembolic events than women taking tamoxifen, but more hot flushes and vaginal dryness.[14] Another study reported more loss of libido with Arimidex, but less dizziness.[15]

Over-hyped Herceptin

Herceptin works by targeting the human epidermal growth factor receptor 2 (HER2) protein, which can fuel the growth of breast cancer tumours in women with HER2-positive breast cancer. However, this accounts for only 25 per cent of breast cancer cases.

Herceptin proponents tout clinical trials, which show a 46 per cent decrease in recurring breast cancer when the drug is prescribed to late-stage breast cancer patients. But one of the main studies cited in support of Herceptin, called the Hera trial,[16] saw 34 deaths in the control group (2 per cent of the participants) and 23 deaths (1.4 per cent) in the group treated with Herceptin. This is a 0.6 per cent absolute reduction in deaths.

There are problems, however. A study carried out by the University of Texas, published in the *Journal of Clinical Oncology*, found that a significant number of patients using Herceptin for at least a year suffered cardiac problems.[17] In this study of 173 patients, 28 per cent of those treated with Herceptin experienced a cardiac event after taking the drug for an average of 21 months – and this included one cardiac-related death. At £30,000 a year, given its risks and benefits, Herceptin hardly seems good value for money when you consider what you could do with that money by way of reducing your risk naturally.

Natural ways to reduce your risk

To put natural solutions in perspective, a survey of more than 44,000 twins determined that no more than 15 per cent of breast cancer cases are the result of genetic predisposition.[18] Therefore, 85 per cent of cases are likely to be a consequence of environmental factors, including diet and lifestyle. It makes sense to look at what these factors might be. One logical place to start is in China.

According to research quoted by Professor Jane Plant, cancer sur-
vivor and author of *The Plant Programme*, age-standardised data from
the year 2000 showed that women living in China had an incidence of
breast cancer of 16.4 per 100,000, compared to an incidence of 91.4 per
100,000 for women living in the US (so it's more than five times lower in
China).[19] Because Chinese women living in the US have a risk compar-
able to other women in the country, the difference must lie in a quality or
practice in China that doesn't exist in the US (or vice versa). As suggested
by Professor Plant, one explanation is that the Chinese don't consume
dairy products and they eat phytoestrogen-rich beans every day.

Furthermore, there is convincing evidence that lactation protects
against breast cancer at all ages thereafter.[20] So breastfeeding is not
just important for babies, it also has many benefits for the mother.

Natural anti-growth foods

The drugs I've discussed above work by blocking growth signals to
breast cancer cells. Two key growth hormones for cancer cells are
oestrogen and IGF-1 (insulin-like growth factor). IGF-1 is made in
the body, but it is also found in milk. (You can read much more about
this in Chapter 12.) A woman who drinks one pint of milk a day has
substantially higher IGF-1 levels and a three times greater risk of
breast cancer than a woman who drinks no milk.[21]

Although it's not possible to be certain how much your risk
would be reduced by cutting out all dairy products, it would definitely appear to be a wise precaution. The odd bit of butter isn't likely
to stimulate cancer by itself. However, drinking milk and eating
yoghurt and cheese on a regular basis might well do. My advice is to
avoid all dairy products except for unavoidable butter; for example,
when eating out in a restaurant.

Pulses and vegetables for health

Phytoestrogens in beans, especially soya beans, but also in chickpeas, lentils, nuts, seeds and rye, help block oestrogen receptors from

323

powerful hormone-disrupting chemicals that mimic oestrogen, such as PCBs, dioxins and some pesticides. Eat some beans, lentils, raw nuts or seeds every day, but don't rely only on soya. When you do eat soya, choose fermented soya products, such as natto or tempeh, as the protective components are more active. In terms of seeds, flax-seeds and pumpkin seeds are the best anti-cancer varieties.

Broccoli is especially rich in di-indolylmethane (DIM), which mops up excess oestrogens. All the cruciferous vegetables – including kale, cabbage, cauliflower and Brussel sprouts – are good sources of this. So, making these vegetables a daily part of your diet is essential to help avoid recurrence. You might also look into boosting your levels of DIM by taking supplements, although, in the UK, they can be obtained only through a nutritional therapist.

Natural progesterone

One of the most potent anti-oestrogenic substances is the hormone progesterone. If your progesterone level is low, taking it in amounts equivalent to what your body would naturally produce is likely to greatly reduce your risk of cancer recurrence. You can do this with a transdermal progesterone cream; however, I strongly recommend that you read Dr John Lee's book, *What Your Doctor May Not Tell You About Breast Cancer* (Warner, 2002), to explore this approach fully.

Antioxidants support the immune system

Researchers at the National Cancer Institute of Canada have found that diet and vitamin intakes are key factors in surviving breast cancer.[22] Their study analysed the dietary habits of 678 women who were diagnosed with breast cancer between January 1982 and June 1992, 76 of whom died from the cancer during the study period. After reviewing the dietary habits of the women prior to their diagnosis, the researchers found that the women who had a relatively high intake of beta-carotene (greater than 4.6mg daily) had half the risk of dying from breast cancer compared to the women with a low intake of beta-carotene (less than 2.2mg daily). Similar results were found for vitamin C. Women who consumed more than 210mg daily had a 57 per cent lower risk of dying from breast cancer than women consuming less than 110mg daily. Vitamin E also showed a slight protective effect, despite the fact that the amounts consumed by the women were very small. Vitamin C has tremendous cancer-fighting properties, but less so for breast cancer. Even so, I would recommend 4g a day, i.e. 2g twice a day. Garlic has similar properties so add a clove, or preferably two, to your cooking every day.

Reducing saturated fat reduces risk

The researchers also concluded that the risk of dying from breast cancer increases by 50 per cent for every 5 per cent increase in saturated fat in overall calories. Other studies have found that omega-3 fats – and fish consumption in general – reduce risk, but I would urge that you be extremely careful about the source of fish. PCB contamination in the ocean is high. There's less contamination in smaller fish from the Pacific, but I would stick to, and possibly favour, supplementing the purified fish oil instead and eating more protein from vegetables such as quinoa.

Other studies clearly show that reducing your intake of fat and increasing your intake of fibre cause substantial positive changes in many measures known to increase breast cancer risk, including reductions in IGF-1 levels. Reducing your intake of sugar does the same thing.

Keeping your body lean

In reality, eating a diet with a low glycemic load (see Chapter 16), which is the best way to lose fat, is also the best way to reduce your risk of breast cancer recurrence. One of the simple reasons for this is that oestrogen is not only made in the ovaries it's also made in fat cells. The fewer fat cells you have, the less oestrogen you tend to make. In post-menopausal women especially, losing weight and eating less sugar can make a big difference in cancer survival, as does taking regular exercise and staying relaxed. Evidence suggests that you can improve your chances of surviving breast cancer and reduce recurrence by achieving a healthy weight post-treatment. The best way to lose weight is to choose healthy, low-GL, and low-fat meals made up of legumes (peas, beans and lentils), wholegrains, vegetables and fruit, and to incorporate moderate physical activity into your lifestyle.[23]

Recognise the role of stress

Reducing stress also has a profound effect on surviving cancer, which is itself a stressful experience. So, it's extremely important to know your priorities and to take care of yourself. I would recommend working with a psychotherapist, if sorting this out seems overwhelming.

Prostate cancer

Prostate cancer has become the single most common cancer among men, and the second most common cause of death. The incidence has quadrupled since the 1970s, and this is not just because of improved screening. In 2009 in the US a man's lifetime risk of a diagnosis was one in six, and predictions are that the risk of men in the UK will be the same within a decade. Currently, nearly 35,000 British men are diagnosed with prostate cancer every year, and 10,000 die from it.

So what can you do to make sure you, or the men in your life, never suffer from what I believe to be a preventable disease, caused by a combination of diet and lifestyle factors? There is also growing evidence that these same principles, when applied in the early stages of prostate cancer, may also reverse the condition.

While drug companies search for the perfect pill, a consistent picture is emerging that suggests that prostate cancer is caused by a combination of factors, the most significant being:

- Exposure to carcinogens

- Lack of antioxidants

- Inflammation

- Excess hormonal growth signals

These factors are remarkably similar to the emerging story for breast cancer. This is not surprising, since the cells that make up prostate tissue are under hormonal control. During adolescence, hormones trigger the prostate to grow from the size of a pea to the size of a walnut; in a similar way they trigger female breast growth.

Problems with your prostate?

If the prostate swells (inflammation) or enlarges (overgrowth of cells) it can act like a clamp, making it harder to urinate. This is very common in men later in life. Sometimes overgrowth of cells can be benign. This is called benign prostatic hyperplasia (BPH) and affects one in three men over the age of 60. Although there is no clear link between BPH and prostatic cancer, other than difficulty peeing, too many men avoid going to their doctor. In both cases, the earlier you know what's happening the better.

Traces of prostate cancer are commonly found in older men who have died from other causes. According to Professor Jonathan Waxman of Imperial College London, little spots of cancer occur in 70 per cent of 70-year-olds, 60 per cent of 60-year-olds and 50 per cent of 50-year-olds, but their relationship with the development of aggressive cancer is unknown. A non-aggressive type of prostate cancer is known as prostatic intra-epithelial neoplasia or PIN. Some doctors regard PIN as being a precursor of cancer; however, not all agree.

The most commonly used screening test for prostate health is a blood test measuring PSA (prostate-specific antigen). This is produced by the prostate gland. High levels of PSA may be an early indicator of prostate cancer – but it is also raised in BPH, so a high level doesn't mean you are going to develop cancer. Generally, having a PSA below 2.5 if you're under 60, or 4 if you are over 60, is consistent with good health. Doctors can also carry out a digital rectal examination (DRE), however, this is also prone to false positives. I recommend having more than one PSA test over a period of months if the initial test is high. If your level is above 10, combined with a positive DRE, you will probably be recommended to have a needle biopsy. This identifies if there are any cancerous cells present, and the degree of abnormality.

If you are diagnosed with prostate cancer, one of the most interesting and non-invasive treatments is HIFU (high intensity focused ultrasound). This is targeted at the cancer cells only. Another is PDT (photodynamic therapy), which uses a laser light to activate chemotherapy drugs. If done well this means that the drugs designed to kill cancer cells don't end up damaging other healthy cells, which is the fundamental problem with chemotherapy, and part of the reason why the side effects are so bad. But none of these address the underlying cause. What you can do to make sure you never get this far.

What causes prostate cancer?

To search answers to these questions I went to meet Professor Jane Plant, who became an expert on certain hormonal cancers after reversing her own breast cancer at the stage when treatment was considered a waste of time. She has written the highly informative book *Prostate Cancer: Understand, Prevent and Overcome Prostate Cancer*. I also contacted Dr Emily Ho from the Linus Pauling Institute, and studied the work of Colin Campbell in his book *The China Diet*. This is especially relevant since prostate cancer is virtually unknown in rural China (the incidence is one in 25,000).

The general view is that there are three contributory sets of conditions. First, there is initiation, whereby prostate cells get damaged in some way so that they become cancerous. Second, there is generalised inflammation, which itself increases oxidants, which, in turn, damage cells. And last, there is growth, encouraged by certain hormones and growth factors.

Limiting your exposure to herbicides, pesticides, hormone-disrupting chemicals and toxic elements, such as cadmium, will put your body in a stronger position to avoid it becoming an environment that is favourable for cancers to occur. I recommend a diet high in organic fresh fruit, vegetables and wholefoods, low in meat, but including anti-inflammatory omega-3-rich oily fish to minimise the risk of chronic inflammation. Dr Ho believes that chronic inflammation may be the cause for as much as one-third of all cancers.[24]

Two key antioxidants are zinc and selenium. Zinc is found to be deficient in prostate cancer patients, and low levels are a good predictor of risk. Zinc is both antioxidant and anti-inflammatory, as well as helping to repair damaged DNA. Most of us don't get anything like enough. I recommend supplementing 10–20mg and eating zinc-rich foods (seeds and nuts, and butters made from them, such as tahini).

I recommend anyone to supplement 30–80mcg of selenium a day, and 100–200mcg if you have had cancer or have a high PSA. Seafood is rich in selenium.

Lycopene in tomatoes, quercetin in red onions, and vitamins C and E are all important antioxidants with good evidence suggesting an anti-prostate-cancer effect both from foods and isolated nutrients. A recent study found that a glass of pomegranate juice helps lower PSA levels,[25] while a diet high in vegetables lowers risk of BPH.[26] Spices are amazing antioxidants, especially turmeric, cinnamon, chilli and ginger. I recommend you maximise your use of all these foods in your diet.

Milk makes prostate cancer cells grow rapidly

Cancer develops only if cancer cells grow. Their growth is under the influence of hormones and growth factors. Professor Plant and Colin Campbell are convinced that the single major cancer growth promoter is dairy products. Milk is naturally high in oestrogen, as well as insulin-like growth factor (IGF). This is hardly surprising since milk's job is to make cells grow. Milk consumption is the second most predictive risk factor, with age being the first. According to the National Cancer Institute (NCI), 19 out of 23 studies have shown a positive association between dairy intake and prostate cancer. 'This is one of the most consistent dietary predictors for prostate cancer in the published literature,' reports NCI. 'In these studies, men with the highest dairy intakes had approximately double the risk of total prostate cancer, and up to fourfold increase in risk of metastatic or fatal prostate cancer relative to low consumers.'[27] Another piece of research published in their journal concludes that 'Men with high IGF-1 have more than five times the risk of advanced prostate cancer.'[28]

There's no question that milk, and all dairy products, contain both oestrogens and IGF, and raise IGF levels in your blood if you consume them. Most people don't realise the scale of the problem. You can literally predict a country's incidence and mortality rate from prostate cancer just from knowing the average dairy intake. Switzerland, for example, has the highest dairy intake and the highest numbers of deaths from prostate cancer, whereas rural China has the least. I therefore consider it safest to avoid all dairy products. Industrialised meat is also high in hormones. The only meat I would generally recommend is wild game or organic lamb although any lean, organic meat is not so bad. I have not eaten any meat for 30 years.

Middle-aged men (aged around 50) naturally have lower levels of testosterone, oestrogens and IGF. But the average intake of milk and meat changes this. It basically creates a hormonal environment similar to puberty, so it's no surprise that this would cause cell growth. Many of the drugs used to treat prostate cancer attempt to block the growth signals of hormones. Yet some of these are less effective after a couple of years as the cancer is said to become 'drug resistant'. This is hardly surprising if you don't change your intake of growth factors.

Protect with fish

Fish and fish oils, on the other hand, may be protective against prostate cancer. A study published in the *Lancet* followed more than

6,000 Swedish men aged 55 for up to 30 years.[29] Its conclusion: eating fatty fish, such as salmon, sardines, herring and mackerel, could reduce the risk of prostate cancer by a third. Supplementing purified omega-3 fish oils (EPA and DHA) provides a guaranteed PCB-free source of these powerful anti-inflammatory agents. If you're suffering from BPH or prostatitis, supplementing the equivalent of 1,000mg of EPA a day can have an anti-inflammatory effect.

Essential sunlight

One of the most potent anti-cancer vitamins is vitamin D, which is made in the skin in the presence of sunlight. Having enough can halve your risk of prostate and other cancers (see Chapter 27). If you live in the northern hemisphere, especially in winter, you just won't make sufficient. Nor will diet alone give you enough – oily fish being the best source. Interestingly, a diet high in meat protein and one high in calcium, which is what you get from dairy products, blocks the ability to create active vitamin D. Most experts agree we should all be supplementing somewhere between 15 and 50mcg a day. The pharmaceutical industry have cottoned on to this and are trialling a vitamin D-derived drug for prostate cancer.

Soya is a superfood

The dietary antidote to an overload of growth-promoting hormones is soya, the staple source of protein for the Chinese. The evidence consistently shows that a regular intake of soya and other phytoestrogen-rich foods such as beans, lentils and peas, greatly reduces the risk of both breast and prostate cancer, as well as menopausal problems.

Phytoestrogens, from plant foods, are about 1,000 times less oestrogenic than other oestrogens, but bind more effectively to hormone receptors on cells, hence they lower the oestrogen load by protecting your cells from too many growth signals. Phytoestrogen levels are high in many fruits and vegetables – from strawberries to oats.

A plant-based diet, deriving protein from these foods, is consistent with a much lower cancer risk and may help to reverse the condition.

Another superfood is broccoli, which is high in DIM, a phytochemical that mops up excess growth hormones. Growth hormones stop cancer cells 'committing suicide', a process called 'apoptosis'. DIM switches this suicide signal back on.[30] One study involving 12 men (two with PIN) taking 100mg of DIM as a supplement, found that PSA levels dropped in 11 of them and PIN had disappeared in both cases. I recommend eating lots of broccoli and possibly supplementing a concentrate containing DIM (in the UK this is obtainable only through a nutritional therapist).

Dr Dean Ornish put this kind of diet to the test on a group of people with early prostate cancer. There was clear evidence of a reversal of all the indicators of prostate cancer. 'Intensive lifestyle changes', he concludes, 'may affect the progression of early, low grade prostate cancer in men.'[31]

Professor Jane Plant agrees. 'If you cut your growth factors right back I think you can reverse the cancer process. I always tell people to continue their conventional medicine but radically change their diet. A man came to see me four years ago with a terrible prognosis, and was considered not worth treating. He changed his diet and is now alive and well. His PSA dropped from above 100 to about 0.1.' You can see other success stories on Professor Jane Plant's website www.cancersupportinternational.com.

Helpful herbs

The most consistently helpful herbs are saw palmetto and pygeum. Saw palmetto has been proven to help inhibit cancer growth and to reduce inflammation. This makes it the perfect herb for both BPH, prostatitis and prostate cancer. Studies have shown reduction in enlargement of the prostate with daily supplementation. It also inhibits an enzyme, called 5-alpha reductase, which turns testosterone into DHT – the form of testosterone that promotes prostate cancer.[32] It has also been shown to inhibit the growth-promoting effects of IGF in milk.[33] I think there's enough evidence now to recommend that any man over 50, or at risk, supplements saw palmetto. It's the fatty acids in this herb that seem to be the most biologically active, so choose a supplement that is standardised to 45 per cent fatty acids. This means it's high quality. Take 120mg a day for prevention and 360mg a day if you have BHP or prostate cancer.

The other prostate-friendly herb that shows many similar beneficial properties is the African bark pygeum. When supplementing pygeum it's worth getting high quality standardised extract with up to 5 per cent B-sitosterol. I recommend 40mg a day for prevention and 120mg a day if you have BPH or prostate cancer. It also lessens the harmful effect of too much IGF and, in animal studies, is profoundly anti-cancer.[34]

Checklist of natural ways to prevent recurrence

There are many options that can help prevent a recurrence of most cancers, including breast and prostate, and they are all things you can do without drugs. Here they are for easy reference:

- Follow a low-GL diet, emphasising omega-3 fats instead of saturated, burned or fried fats. Avoid sugar and stimulants.

- Eat eight servings of fruit and vegetables a day, especially carrots, tomatoes and cruciferous vegetables such as broccoli.

- Supplement additional all-round antioxidants, plus 4g of vitamin C a day.

- Eat beans, lentils, nuts or seeds every day. Have fermented soya products.

- Have a tablespoon of flax or pumpkin seeds a day.

- Avoid dairy products and minimise red meat and burned meat or fish.

- Eat organic where possible and be very selective about the meat or fish you eat, choosing lean meat and fish from unpolluted waters.

- Supplement a high-strength multivitamin with plenty of B vitamins, zinc and selenium plus vitamins A and D.

- Have two cloves of garlic every day.

- Keep fit and active, but don't over-stress yourself.

- Consult a nutritional therapist (see Resources) about supplementing DIM and other nutritional assistance, and consider laboratory testing to assess any other dietary and lifestyle factors that need to be addressed.

In addition, for breast cancer:

- Consider natural progesterone.

And for prostate cancer:

- Take 120–360mg of saw palmetto daily if you have BHP or prostate cancer.

The next section of this book identifies which dietary factors and nutritional supplements have the most prevention power for each type of cancer.

PART 7

THE A–Z OF NUTRITIONAL HEALING

Strategies for Each Type of Cancer

W hat follows is a summary of the associated risk factors and prevention strategies for each type of cancer. As explained in Part 1, although some people have attributed their recovery from cancer to dietary changes, nutritional therapy is never claimed to 'cure' cancer. Rather, it can create the best possible conditions within the body for its own anti-cancer mechanisms (primarily the immune system) to restore health.

This part details nutrients that have been found to be of particular benefit both for prevention and for recovering cancer patients (see the chart on pages 304–5 for 'basic prevention' and for 'maximum nutritional support' levels for each nutrient).

If you are a cancer patient undertaking, or about to undertake, treatment such as surgery, chemotherapy or radiotherapy, nutritional support before and after (and sometimes during) these treatments can reduce side effects and speed up recovery (see Chapter 36). However, you must not undertake an extensive nutritional strategy on your own.

Breast

Breast cancer is the most prevalent cancer among women, and it can also occur in men. Around 80 per cent of breast cancers are termed oestrogen-receptor positive. There is a high likelihood that hormone-disrupting chemicals play a part in such cancers (see Chapters 3 and 20). If your diet is high in meat and saturated fat this may mean that you have greater exposure to such chemicals, which can be stored in fat tissue.

Associated risk factors Oral contraceptive use; hormone replacement therapy (HRT) containing oestrogens or synthetic progestins; high body-fat percentage and waist-to-hip ratio; sedentary lifestyle; rapid early development and early menstruation; high-fat diet; high saturated fat and excess calorie intake; alcohol consumption above one drink a day; smoking; high meat consumption; low intake of fruit and vegetables; exposure to pesticides, hormone-disrupting chemicals, radiation (including mammograms); presence of the genes BRCA1 and 2-oncogenes; low dietary fibre.

Prevention Follow the general advice in Part 5. Particularly important nutrients (often contained within a high quality daily multivitamin-mineral) are vitamins D and E, and the minerals selenium and calcium (to be prescribed by a nutritional therapist – see Chapter 34 for details of dosages for prevention and treatment). Avoid dairy products if you have, or have had, breast cancer. If you eat meat, don't eat too much of it, especially red, and be careful of the type you buy and how you cook it (see Chapter 11). Eating fish lowers risk, especially mackerel, herring and salmon, which are rich in omega-3 fats. Flaxseeds and their oil are the best vegetarian source of omega-3 fats. If you are a vegetarian or vegan, make sure you read Chapters 8, 11, 15 and 27 carefully. Regular consumption of soya (such as tempeh or tofu) and other phytoestrogens also lowers risk (see Chapter 13). Tomatoes, rich in lycopene, and garlic are also recommended. Eat organic foods wherever possible. Eat low-GL foods; ensure your homocysteine level is optimal by having it tested (see Chapter 8). Lactation decreases the risk of both pre- and post-menopausal breast cancer. Physical activity of at least 30 minutes a day is recommended.

Nutritional support Recommended are maximum support levels (see page 304) of vitamin C, E and calcium (as prescribed by a nutritional therapist).

Cervical

Cancer of the cervix can be diagnosed early with pap smears. The pre-invasive form of cervical is almost always curable, and early diagnosis has led to a 70 per cent reduction in death rate.

Associated risk factors Infection with human papillomavirus (HPV) – many sexual partners increase risk of this; oral contraceptives; smoking; low carotenoids; low vitamin C; low intake of fruit and vegetables providing carotenoids (carrots are thought to decrease risk) and vitamin C; exposure to hormone-disrupting chemicals.

Prevention Follow the general advice in Part 5. Particularly important nutrients (often contained within a high quality daily multivitamin-mineral) are vitamins D and E, and the minerals selenium and calcium (to be prescribed by a nutritional therapist – see Chapter 34 for details of dosages for prevention and treatment). If you eat meat, don't eat too much of it, especially red, and be careful of the type you buy and how you cook it (see Chapter 11). Eating fish lowers risk, especially mackerel, herring and salmon, which are rich in omega-3 fats. Flaxseeds and their oil are the best vegetarian source of omega-3 fats. If you are a vegetarian or vegan, make sure you read Chapters 8, 11, 15 and 27 carefully. Regular consumption of soya (such as tempeh or tofu) is also likely to lower risk (see Chapter 13). Eat organic foods wherever possible. Ensure your homocysteine level is optimal by having it tested (see Chapter 8).

Nutritional support Pre-malignant changes in cervical cells, called cervical dysplasia, respond well to vitamin C and folic acid. These are recommended at maximum support levels (see page 304), together with antioxidant vitamins A, beta-carotene and E (as prescribed by a nutritional therapist).

Colorectal

Cancers of the colon or rectum are some of the most common cancers, particularly in the Western world. They are strongly linked to diet and there is little doubt that dietary carcinogens, caused by putrefying food, and created by microorganisms in an unhealthy gut, play a big part. A high-fibre diet shortens the time food takes to pass through the digestive tract and reduces carcinogen exposure.

Associated risk factors A high-fat (especially saturated fat) and high-sugar diet; high meat consumption (especially grilled, barbecued or burned meat); high processed-meat consumption; low fibre intake; history of polyps; smoking; alcohol consumption above one drink a day for women and two drinks a day for men; lack of exercise; adult weight gain; abdominal fatness; total body fatness; lack of vegetables; high calories; prolonged stress.

Prevention Diet is the major prevention factor. Follow the general advice in Part 5. Follow a high-fibre diet with plenty of non-starchy vegetables and fruit. Avoid, or limit, red and processed meat. Foods that are particularly important to include are those containing folate, beta-carotene, vitamin C, vitamin D, calcium and selenium, such as greens, orange foods, berries, seafood, including some oily fish, nuts and seeds. Regular garlic consumption reduces risk, as does live yoghurt, which provides beneficial bacteria to improve intestinal health. Ensure your homocysteine level is optimal by having it tested (see Chapter 8). Stay as lean as possible within the healthy weight range. Exercise for at least 30 minutes per day.

Nutritional support Recommended are maximum support levels (see page 304) of beta-carotene, vitamin C, folic acid (see page 304), vitamin D, calcium and selenium, and a strict dietary regime (as prescribed by a nutritional therapist).

Endometrial (uterine)

The endometrium is the lining of the womb (the uterus). Endometrial cancer is very much on the increase – it is a hormone-sensitive cancer that shares many risk factors with breast cancer. There is a high likelihood that hormone-disrupting chemicals play a part in such cancers (see Chapters 3 and 20).

Associated risk factors Obesity; high intake of saturated and animal fats; high red meat intake; low intake of fruit and vegetables high in carotenoids and vitamin C; exposure to hormone-disrupting chemicals; oral contraceptive use; HRT containing oestrogen or synthetic progestins; tamoxifen.

Prevention Follow the general advice in Part 5. Particularly important nutrients (often contained within a high quality daily multivitamin-mineral) are vitamins D and E, and the minerals selenium and calcium (to be prescribed by a nutritional therapist – see Chapter 34 for details of dosages for prevention and treatment). If you eat meat, don't eat too much of it, especially red, and be careful of the type you buy and how you cook it (see Chapter 11). Eating fish lowers risk, especially mackerel, herring and salmon, which are rich in omega-3 fats. Flaxseeds and their oil are the best vegetarian source of omega-3 fats. If you are a vegetarian or vegan, make sure you read Chapters 8, 11, 15, and 27 carefully. Regular consumption of soya (such as tempeh or tofu) also lowers risk (see Chapter 13). Tomatoes, rich in lycopene, are also recommended. Eat organic foods wherever possible. Exercise for 30 minutes per day.

Nutritional support Recommended are maximum support levels (see page 304) of vitamin C, E and calcium (as prescribed by a nutritional therapist).

Kidney and bladder

The kidneys filter the blood, removing toxic material and passing it on to the bladder. It is very likely that a poor diet, plus exposure to toxins and carcinogens, increases the risk of either of these types of cancer. Smoking is a risk factor for bladder cancer. Improving detoxification potential may reduce risk (see Chapter 7).

Associated risk factors Low intake of fruit and vegetables; high intake of dairy produce; obesity.

Prevention Follow the general advice in Part 5. Particularly important nutrients (often contained within a high quality daily multivitamin-mineral) are all antioxidants, especially selenium in the case of bladder cancer (to be prescribed by a nutritional therapist – see Chapter 34 for details of dosages for prevention and treatment).

Nutritional support Recommended are maximum support levels (see page 304) of vitamins A, C and E, beta-carotene and selenium (as prescribed by a nutritional therapist).

Liver

The liver is the primary organ of detoxification and liver cancer is highly indicative of over-exposure to carcinogens and/or an inability to detoxify them. Improving your detoxification potential may reduce your risk (see Chapter 7).

Associated risk factors Alcohol consumption above one or two drinks a day; tamoxifen; possibly long-term use of other prescribed medical and recreational drugs used in excess.

Prevention Follow the general advice in Part 5. Particularly important nutrients (often contained within a high quality daily multivitamin-mineral) are all antioxidants, including selenium (to be prescribed by a nutritional therapist – see Chapter 34 for details of dosages for prevention and treatment). Also cruciferous vegetables such as broccoli, cauliflower, kale, cabbage and Brussels sprouts.

Nutritional support Recommended are maximum support levels (see page 304) of vitamins A, C and E, beta-carotene and selenium, which help the liver detoxify (as prescribed by a nutritional therapist). The herb milk thistle may also be beneficial. Nutritional therapists can test which pathways in the liver are most overloaded and devise a nutritional strategy to ease the load.

Lung

Cancer of the lung is the most prevalent cancer in men and is also exceedingly common in women. Although smoking is a major factor, diet plays an important role too. In countries where smoking is on the decrease, so too is lung cancer (see Chapter 21).

Associated risk factors Smoking; alcohol; excess fat and saturated fat; high intake of red and processed meat; lack of fruit and vegetables, especially carotenoids; high pollution or diesel fuel, or radon exposure.

Prevention Follow the general advice in Part 5. Particularly important nutrients (often contained within a high quality daily multivitamin-mineral) are all antioxidants, including selenium, quercetin, and beta-carotene (to be prescribed by a nutritional therapist – see Chapter 34 for details of dosages for prevention and treatment). Eat a carrot every day and don't smoke.

Nutritional support Recommended are maximum support levels (see page 304) of vitamins A, C and E, beta-carotene and selenium (as prescribed by a nutritional therapist). Do not take beta-carotene supplements if you are a smoker or heavy drinker.

Lymphoma (Non-Hodgkin's) and leukaemia

Non-Hodgkin's lymphoma and leukaemia are less common cancers, although the incidence of non-Hodgkin's lymphoma is on the increase.

Associated risk Although little is known about the risk factors for these cancers, pesticide exposure appears to be a risk factor for both, and radiation is a risk factor for leukaemia.

Prevention Follow the general advice in Part 5. Important nutrients (often contained within a high quality daily multivitamin-mineral) are all antioxidants, including selenium and beta-carotene (to be prescribed by a nutritional therapist – see Chapter 34 for details of dosages for prevention and treatment), which help to detoxify the body. Eating a diet high in organic fruit and vegetables, especially cruciferous vegetables, such as broccoli, cauliflower, kale, cabbage and Brussels sprouts, and low in red meat and dairy, may decrease toxic load and risk. Ensure your homocysteine level is optimal by having it tested (see Chapter 8).

Nutritional support Recommended are maximum support levels (see page 304) of vitamins A, C and E, beta-carotene and selenium (as prescribed by a nutritional therapist).

Mouth, throat and oesophagus

The location of these cancers is strongly suggestive of ingested or inhaled carcinogens.

Associated risk factors Alcohol consumption above one drink per day for women or two drinks per day for men; smoking; high intake of red or processed meat; lack of fruit and vegetables; high intake of maté tea, or very hot drinks. The combination of smoking and drinking increases the risk of oesophageal cancer.

Prevention Follow the general advice in Part 5. Important nutrients (often contained within a high quality daily multivitamin-mineral) are folate, the antioxidants vitamins C and A, and selenium (to be prescribed by a nutritional therapist – see Chapter 34 for details of dosages for prevention and treatment). Also, follow a diet high in fruit and non-starchy vegetables and low in alcohol. Avoid smoking and very hot drinks.

Nutritional support Recommended are maximum support levels (see page 304) of vitamins A and C, plus selenium (as prescribed by a nutritional therapist).

Ovarian

Cancer of the ovary is one of the less common cancers, and its prevalence does not appear to be increasing significantly. Little is known about its cause, but problems with ovulation, coupled with exposure to hormone-disrupting chemicals, may possibly play a part. It is probably good logic to follow the recommendations for breast cancer.

Associated risk factors Exposure to hormone-disrupting chemicals; oral contraceptive use; and HRT containing oestrogen or synthetic progestins.

Prevention Probably the same as for breast cancer, namely to follow the general advice in Part 5. Important nutrients, in addition to a daily multivitamin-mineral, may be vitamins D and E, and the minerals selenium and calcium (to be prescribed by a nutritional therapist – see Chapter 34 for details of dosages for prevention and treatment). If you eat meat, don't eat too much of it, especially red, and be careful of the type you buy and how you cook it (see Chapter 11). Eating fish lowers risk, especially mackerel, herring and salmon, which are rich in omega-3 fats. Flaxseeds and their oil are the best vegetarian source of omega-3 fats. If you are a vegetarian or vegan, make sure you read Chapters 8, 11, 15, and 27 carefully. Regular consumption of soya (such as tempeh or tofu) also lowers risk (see Chapter 13). Tomatoes, rich in lycopene, are also recommended. Eat organic foods wherever possible. Lactation is thought to help protect women from ovarian cancer.

Nutritional support Recommended are maximum support levels (see page 304) of vitamins C and E, and calcium (as prescribed by a nutritional therapist). Consider a supplemental source of genistein and daidzein, the protective factors found in soya.

345

Pancreas

As well as producing hormones, the pancreas produces enzymes to digest foods. Pancreatic cancer is a less common type of cancer that interferes with digestion, often impeding optimal nutrition.

Associated risk factors Low intakes of fruit and vegetables; low intake of fibre; high consumption of red and processed meat; alcohol; smoking; and possibly excessive coffee consumption; although not all studies agree.

Prevention Follow the general advice in Part 5. Important are foods containing folate, the antioxidants vitamins C, A, E and selenium, plus a diet high in fruit and vegetables and low in meat and alcohol. Avoid smoking and excessive coffee consumption. Exercise for at least 30 minutes per day.

Nutritional support Recommended are maximum support levels (see page 304) of the antioxidants vitamins A, C and E, and selenium (as prescribed by a nutritional therapist). Digestive enzymes and specially prepared food, soups and juices may be necessary to assist digestion and absorption of nutrients.

Prostate

This is the most rapidly increasing cancer in men; it is predicted to become the most common within 20 years, possibly affecting as many as one in four men at some point during their life. Its causes and nutritional approach are very similar to breast cancer. There is a high likelihood that hormone-disrupting chemicals play a part in this (see Chapters 3 and 20).

Associated risk factors High-fat and a high saturated-fat diet; regular consumption of dairy products (avoid if you have, or have had, prostate cancer) and processed meat; diets high in calcium; a low intake of fibre; obesity; smoking; high cadmium levels; exposure to hormone-disrupting chemicals and pesticides; high levels of testosterone.

Prevention Follow the general advice in Part 5. Particularly important nutrients (often contained within a high quality daily multivitamin-mineral) are vitamins A, D and E and beta-carotene and the minerals selenium and zinc (to be prescribed by a nutritional therapist – see Chapter 34 for details of dosages for prevention and treatment). If you eat meat, don't eat too much of it, especially red, and be careful of the type you buy and how you cook it (see Chapter 11). Eating fish lowers risk, especially mackerel, herring and salmon, which are rich in omega-3 fats. Flaxseeds and their oil are the best vegetarian source of omega-3 fats. If you are a vegetarian or vegan, make sure you read Chapters 8, 11, 15, and 27 carefully. Regular consumption of soya (such as tempeh or tofu) and pulses (peas, beans and lentils) also lowers risk (see Chapter 13). Foods rich in lycopene, such as tomatoes, are also recommended. Eat organic foods wherever possible.

Nutritional support Recommended are maximum support levels (see page 304) of vitamins A, C and E, and beta-carotene, and the minerals selenium and zinc (as prescribed by a nutritional therapist). Consider a supplemental source of the herb saw palmetto, which helps benign prostatic hyperplasia. **WARNING** Calcium supplements should be avoided by prostate cancer patients (as they may reduce the amount of vitamin D activated by the kidneys).

Skin

There are two main kinds of skin cancer: basal or squamous cell carcinoma and melanoma. Skin carcinoma is both common and relatively easy to treat. Melanoma is rare and highly malignant, and hence represents more of a risk. Excessive exposure to strong sunlight is the main risk factor (see Chapter 19).

Associated risk factors Excessive exposure to ultraviolet light, especially in fair-skinned people with red or blonde hair and those with a lot of moles; use of sunbeds, especially by young people, increases the risk of skin cancer.

Prevention Follow the general advice in Part 5, especially avoiding exposure to strong sunlight without wearing an appropriate sunblock. Particularly important nutrients (often contained within a high quality daily multivitamin-mineral) are vitamins A and E, and beta-carotene (to be prescribed by a nutritional therapist – see Chapter 34 for details of dosages for prevention and treatment), although all antioxidants help to protect against skin damage.

Nutritional support Recommended are maximum support levels (see page 304) of the antioxidants vitamins A, C and E, and beta-carotene (as prescribed by a nutritional therapist).

Stomach

Cancer of the stomach is very strongly linked to dietary carcinogens. It can be prevented both by avoiding high-risk foods and having a good intake of nutrients, which can disarm carcinogens in food. Infection with the bacterium *Helicobacter pylori* increases the risk of stomach cancer. However, as millions of people are infected with these bacteria and most of them do not get stomach cancer, there must be other factors at work.

Associated risk factors Salt and salted foods; processed meat; grilled, fried, smoked, barbecued or burned meat; lack of refrigeration, introducing pathogens; low intake of fresh fruit and vegetables; exceptionally high intake of chillies may increase risk.

Prevention Follow the general advice in Part 5. Particularly important nutrients (often contained within a high quality daily multivitamin-mineral) are the antioxidants beta-carotene, vitamin

C and selenium (to be prescribed by a nutritional therapist – see Chapter 34 for details of dosages for prevention and treatment). Regular consumption of non-starchy vegetables, allium vegetables such as onions, leeks and garlic, fruits, pulses (beans, peas and lentils) – including soya and soya products, are also protective.

Nutritional support Recommended are maximum support levels (see page 304) of the antioxidant vitamins A, C and E, beta-carotene and selenium (as prescribed by a nutritional therapist).

Testicular

This is the most common type of cancer in men under 35. Although testicular cancer is still quite rare, with just over 1,500 new cases a year in the UK, it is a matter of concern that the incidence has doubled in the last 20 years. It is, however, the most curable of all cancers: over 90 per cent of sufferers make a complete recovery. Early detection is crucial, so men are encouraged to check their testes monthly for any changes, such as lumps, swelling or hardening.

Associated risk factors Men who are born with an undescended testicle are five times more likely to develop the disease. Other risk factors are a family history of the disease, early puberty and low levels of exercise. Early exposure to chemicals, such as pesticides, has also been implicated (see Chapter 20).

Prevention Follow the general advice for minimising your cancer risk given in Part 5. Minimise your intake of meat and dairy products. Eat plenty of fruit, vegetables and fibre, and eat organic foods as much as possible. Avoid alcohol, recreational drugs and smoking, and limit coffee consumption. Ensure a good intake of antioxidants.

Nutritional support Follow the same recommendations as for prostate cancer.

References

Introduction

1. R. Waller, 'The Diseases of Civilisation', *Ecologist*, 1970;1(2)
2. P. Lichtenstein, et al., 'Environmental and heritable factors in the causation of cancer-analyses of cohorts of twins from Sweden, Denmark, and Finland', *New England Journal of Medicine*, 2000 July 13;343(2):78–85
3. S. Epstein, 'Winning the War Against Cancer? . . . Are they even fighting it?' *Ecologist*, 1998;28(2):69–80
4. S. Gapstur and M. Thun of the American Cancer Society, Atlanta, presented the commentary at a media briefing of the *Journal of the American Medical Association* in March 2010.

Part 1

1. 'Third of breast cancer harmless', BBC News online, 10 July 2009.
2. R.B. Shekelle, et al., 'Dietary vitamin A and risk of cancer in the Western Electric study', *Lancet*, 1981 Nov. 28;2(8257):1185–90
3. S. Epstein, 'Winning the War Against Cancer? . . . Are they even fighting it?' *Ecologist*, 1998;28(2):69–80
4. Typescript of interview with Simon Wolff by Andrew Baron, 13 May 1993, cited in: M. Walker, 'Sir Richard Doll: A questionable pillar of the cancer establishment', *Ecologist*, 1998;28(2):82–92
5. National Cancer Institute, 'Bioassay of chloradane for possible carcinogenicity', Carcinogenesis Technical Report Series No. 8 (1977)
6. J.D. Scribner and N.K. Mottet, 'DDT acceleration of mammary gland tumors induced in the male Sprague-Dawley rat by 2-acetamidophenanthrene', *Carcinogenesis*, 1981;2(12):1235–9
7. J.B. Westin and E. Richter, 'The Israeli breast-cancer anomaly', *Annals of the New York Academy of Sciences*, 1990;609:269–79

8. M. Wassermann, et al., 'Organochlorine compounds in neoplastic and adjacent apparently normal breast tissue', *Bulletin of Environmental Contamination and Toxicology,* 1976 Apr.;15(4):478–84

9. A.M. Soto, et al., 'p-Nonyl-phenol: An estrogenic xenobiotic released from "modified" polystyrene', *Environmental Health Perspectives,* 1991 May;92:167–73

10. Official Journal of the European Union: Directive 2003/53/EC of the European Parliament and of the Council of 18 June 2003 amending for the 26th time Council Directive 76/769/EEC relating to restrictions on the marketing and use of certain dangerous substances and preparations (nonylphenol, nonylphenol ethoxylate and cement), 17.7.2003. See http://eur-lex.europa.eu/LexUriServ/LexUriServ.do?uri=OJ:L:2003:178:0024:0027:EN:PDF

11. K.J. Chang, et al., 'Influences of percutaneous administration of estradiol and progesterone on human breast epithelial cell cycle in vivo', *Fertility and Sterility,* 1995 Apr.;63(4):785–91

12. A.L. Herbst, et al., 'Adenocarcinoma of the vagina: Association of maternal stilbestrol therapy with tumor appearance in young women', *New England Journal of Medicine,* 1971 Apr. 15;284(15):878–81

13. W.B. Gill, 'Effects on human males of in utero exposure to exogenous sex hormones', in T. Mori and H. Nagasawa (eds), *Toxicity of Hormones in Perinatal Life,* CRC Press Inc., 1988; see also: W.B. Gill, et al., 'Structural and functional abnormalities in the sex organs of male offspring of mothers treated with diethylstilbestrol (DES)' *Journal of Reproductive Medicine,* 1976 Apr;16(4):147–53

14. C.M. Antunes, et al., 'Endometrial cancer and estrogen use. Report of a large case-control study', *New England Journal of Medicine,* 1979 Jan. 4;300(1):9–13. A. Paganini-Hill et al., 'Endometrial cancer and patterns of use of oestrogen replacement therapy: a cohort study', *British Journal of Cancer,* 1989 Mar.;59(3):445–7. P.K. Green, et al., 'Risk of endometrial cancer following cessation of menopausal hormone use (Washington, United States)', *Cancer Causes and Control,* 1996 Nov.;7(6):575–80

15. S.A. Beresford, et al., 'Risk of endometrial cancer in relation to use of oestrogen combined with cyclic progestagen therapy in postmenopausal women', *Lancet,* 1997 Feb. 5;349(9050):458–61. E. Weiderpass, et al., 'Risk of endometrial cancer following estrogen replacement with and without progestins', *Journal of the National Cancer Institute,* 1999 July 7;91(13):1131–7

16. L. Bergkvist, et al., 'The risk of breast cancer after estrogen and estrogen-progestin replacement', *New England Journal of Medicine,* 1989 Aug. 3;321(5):293–7

17. G.A. Colditz, et al., 'The use of estrogens and progestins and the risk of breast cancer in postmenopausal women', *New England Journal of Medicine,* 1995 June 15;332(24):1589–93

18. S.A. Beresford, et al., 'Risk of endometrial cancer in relation to use of oestrogen combined with cyclic progestagen therapy in postmenopausal women', *Lancet,* 1997 Feb. 5;349(9050):458–61

19. No authors listed, 'Breast cancer and hormone replacement therapy: Collaborative reanalysis of data from 51 epidemiological studies of 52,705 women with breast cancer and 108,411 women without breast cancer. Collaborative Group on Hormonal Factors in Breast Cancer', *Lancet*, 1997 Oct. 11;350(9084):1047–59

20. V. Beral, 'Breast cancer and hormone-replacement therapy in the Million Women Study', *Lancet*, 2003 Aug. 9;362(9382):419–27

21. R.T. Chlebowski, et al., 'Breast cancer after use of estrogen plus progestin in postmenopausal women', *New England Journal of Medicine*, 2009 Feb. 5;360(6):573–87

22. C. Rodriguez, et al., 'Estrogen replacement therapy and fatal ovarian cancer', *American Journal of Epidemiology*, 1995 May 1;141(9):828–35

23. P.P. Garg, et al., 'Hormone replacement therapy and the risk of epithelial ovarian carcinoma: a meta-analysis', *Obstetrics and Gynecology*, 1998 Sept.;92(3):472–9

24. S.S. Coughlin, et al., 'A meta-analysis of estrogen replacement therapy and risk of epithelial ovarian cancer', *Journal of Clinical Epidemiology*, 2000 Apr.;53(4):367–75

25. J.V. Lacey, Jr., et al., 'Menopausal hormone replacement therapy and risk of ovarian cancer', *Journal of the American Medical Association*, 2002 July 17;288(3):334–41

26. Dr J. Lee, 'Oestrogen dominance is the major cause of breast cancer', 30 October 2002, Pauling Lectures, London

27. A. Fournier, et al., 'Unequal risks for breast cancer associated with different hormone replacement therapies: Results from the E3N cohort study', *Breast Cancer Research and Treatment*, 2008 Jan.;107(1):103–11

28. M. Messina and S. Barnes, 'The role of soy products in reducing risk of cancer', *Journal of the National Cancer Institute*, 1991 Apr. 17;83(8):541–6; W. Troll, et al., 'Soybean diet lowers breast tumor incidence in irradiated rats', *Carcinogenesis*, 1980 June;1(6):469–72

29. S. Barnes, 'Soybeans inhibit mammary tumor growth in models of breast cancer', *Mutagens and Carcinogens in Diet*, Pariza, M. (ed), Wiley, New York (1990); see also: S. Barnes, et al., 'Soybeans inhibit mammary tumors in models of breast cancer', *Progress in Clinical and Biological Research*, 1990;347:239–53

30. S. Epstein, 'Winning the War Against Cancer? . . . Are they even fighting it?' *Ecologist*, 1998;28(2):69–80

31. V. Howard, 'Synergistic effect of chemical mixtures: Can we rely on traditional toxicology?' *Ecologist*, 1997;27(5)

32. J.G. Hogervorst, et al., 'Dietary acrylamide intake and the risk of renal cell, bladder, and prostate cancer', *American Journal of Clinical Nutrition*, 2008 May;87(5):1428–38

33. P. Watson, et al., 'Prognosis of BRCA1 hereditary breast cancer', *Lancet*, 1998 Jan. 31;351(9099):304–5

34. P. Murphy and W. Bray, 'How cancer gene testing can benefit patients', *Molecular Medicine Today*, 1997 Apr.;3(4):147–52

35. S.K. Katiyar, et al., 'Protective effects of silymarin against photocarcinogenesis in a mouse skin model', *Journal of the National Cancer Institute*, 1997 Apr. 16;89(8):556–66

36. P. Lichtenstein, et al., 'Environmental and heritable factors in the causation of cancer: Analyses of cohorts of twins from Sweden, Denmark, and Finland', *New England Journal of Medicine*, vol. 343(2), pp. 78–85 (2000)

37. R.W. Pinner, et al., 'Trends in infectious diseases mortality in the United States', *Journal of the American Medical Association*, 1996 Jan. 17;275(3):189–93

38. 'The Health of Adult Britain 1841–1994', Office of National Statistics

39. *Daily Mail*, 15 April 1997, p. 11

40. H. Kaya, et al., 'The protective effect of N-acetyl-cysteine against cyclosporine A-induced hepatotoxicity in rats', *Journal of Applied Toxicology*, 2008 Jan.;28(1):15–20; R. Ruffmann and A. Wendel, 'GSH rescue by N-acetyl-cysteine', *Klinische Wochenschrift*, 1991 Nov. 15;69(18):857–62; O.F. Woo, et al., 'Shorter duration of oral N-acetyl-cysteine therapy for acute acetaminophen overdose', *Annals of Emergency Medicine*, 2000 Apr.;35(4):363–8; S.J. Flora, 'Arsenic-induced oxidative stress and its reversibility following combined administration of N-acetyl-cysteine and meso 2,3-dimercaptosuccinic acid in rats', *Clinical and Experimental Pharmacology and Physiology*, 1999 Nov.;26(11):865–9; A.J. Makin, et al., 'A 7-year experience of severe acetaminophen-induced hepatotoxicity (1987–1993)', *Gastroenterology*, 1995 Dec.;109(6):1907–16; P. Villa and P. Ghezzi, 'Effect of N-acetyl-L-cysteine on sepsis in mice', *European Journal of Pharmacology*, 1995 Mar. 16;292(3–4):341–4

41. C. Weber, et al., 'Effect of dietary coenzyme Q10 as an antioxidant in human plasma', *Molecular Aspects of Medicine*, 1994;15 Suppl:s97–102

42. M. G. Wohl, et al., *Modern Nutrition in Health & Disease,* 8th Revised edition (1 Sep 1993); Lea & Febiger, U.S.; pp. 432–48 and E. Schwedhelm, et al., 'Clinical pharmacokinetics of antioxidants and their impact on systemic oxidative stress', *Clinical Pharmacokinetics*, 2003;42(5):437–59

43. M. G. Wohl, et al., *Modern Nutrition in Health & Disease,* 8th Revised edition (1 Sep 1993); Lea & Febiger, US; pp. 326–41; and E. Schwedhelm, et al., 'Clinical pharmacokinetics of antioxidants and their impact on systemic oxidative stress', *Clinical Pharmacokinetics*, 2003;42(5):437–59; and R.I. van Haaften, et al., 'Effect of vitamin E on glutathione-dependent enzymes', *Drug Metabolism Reviews*, 2003 May;35(2–3):215–53

44. E. Schwedhelm, et al., 'Clinical pharmacokinetics of antioxidants and their impact on systemic oxidative stress', *Clinical Pharmacokinetics*, 2003;42(5):437–59

45. E. Schwedhelm, et al., 'Clinical pharmacokinetics of antioxidants and their impact on systemic oxidative stress', *Clinical Pharmacokinetics*, 2003;42(5):437–59

46. M. Touvier, et al., 'Dual association of beta-carotene with risk of tobacco-related cancers in a cohort of French women', *Journal of the National Cancer Institute*, 2005 Sept. 21;97(18):1338–44 and J. Virtamo, et al., 'Incidence

of cancer and mortality following alpha-tocopherol and beta-carotene supplementation: A postintervention follow-up', *Journal of the American Medical Association*, 2003 July 23;290(4):476–85

47. J.M. Gaziano, 'Vitamin E and cardiovascular disease: Observational studies', *Annals of the New York Academy of Sciences*, 2004 Dec.;1031:280–91 and M.J. McQueen, et al., 'The HOPE (Heart Outcomes Prevention Evaluation) Study and its consequences', *Scand. J. Clin. Lab Invest Suppl*, 2005;240:143–56

48. M. Yoshida, et al., 'Dietary indole-3-carbinol promotes endometrial adenocarcinoma development in rats initiated with N-ethyl-N'-nitro-N-nitrosoguanidine, with induction of cytochrome P450s in the liver and consequent modulation of estrogen metabolism', *Carcinogenesis*, 2004 Nov.;25(11):2257–64

49. Y.J. Moon, et al., 'Dietary flavonoids: Effects on xenobiotic and carcinogen metabolism', *Toxicology In Vitro*, 2006 Mar.;20(2):187–210 and P. Hodek, et al., 'Flavonoids-potent and versatile biologically active compounds interacting with cytochromes P450', *Chemico-Biological Interactions*, 2002 Jan. 22;139(1):1–21

50. G. Mazza, et al., 'Absorption of anthocyanins from blueberries and serum antioxidant status in human subjects', *Journal of Agricultural and Food Chemistry*, 2002 Dec. 18;50(26):7731–7

51. M. Athar, et al., 'Multiple molecular targets of resveratrol: Anti-carcinogenic mechanisms', *Archives of Biochemistry and Biophysics*, 2009 June 15;486(2):95–102

52. C. Morand, et al., 'Plasma metabolites of quercetin and their antioxidant properties', *American Journal of Physiology*, 1998 July;275(1 Pt 2):R212-R219 and H. de Groot and U. Rauen, 'Tissue injury by reactive oxygen species and the protective effects of flavonoids', *Fundamental and Clinical Pharmacology*, 1998;12(3):249–55

53. V. Cody, et al., *Plant Flavonoids in Biology and Medicine*, Alan R. Liss, N.Y. (1988), pp. 135–8

54. K. Hruby, et al., 'Chemotherapy of Amanita phalloides poisoning with intravenous silibinin', *Human Toxicology*, 1983 Apr.;2(2):183–95, and H.A. Salmi and S. Sarna, 'Effect of silymarin on chemical, functional, and morphological alterations of the liver: A double-blind controlled study', *Scandinavian Journal of Gastroenterology*, 1982 June;17(4):517–21, and C.G. Wu, et al., 'Protective effect of silymarin on rat liver injury induced by ischemia', *Virchows Archive B – Cell Pathology Including Molecular Pathology*, 1993;64(5):259–63, and A. Pietrangelo, et al., 'Antioxidant activity of silybin in vivo during long-term iron overload in rats', *Gastroenterology*, 1995 Dec.;109(6):1941–9, and K. Kropacova, et al., 'Protective and therapeutic effect of silymarin on the development of latent liver damage', *Radiatsionnaia Biologiia, Radioecologiia*, 1998 May;38(3):411–5, and R. Campos, et al., 'Silybin dihemisuccinate protects against glutathione depletion and lipid peroxidation induced by acetaminophen on rat liver', *Planta Medica*, 1989 Oct.;55(5):417–9

55. C.D. Mann, et al., 'Phytochemicals as potential chemopreventive and chemo-therapeutic agents in hepatocarcinogenesis', *European Journal of Cancer Prevention*, 2009 Feb.;18(1):13–25

56. C. Dwivedi, et al., 'Effect of calcium glucarate on beta-glucuronidase activity and glucarate content of certain vegetables and fruits', *Biochemical Medicine and Metabolic Biology*, 1990 Apr.;43(2):83–92; and W.A. Nijhoff, et al., 'Effects of consumption of brussels sprouts on plasma and urinary glutathione S-transferase class-alpha and -pi in humans', *Carcinogenesis*, 1995 Apr.;16(4):955–7

57. M. Khashab, et al., 'Epidemiology of acute liver failure', *Current Gastroenterology Reports*, 2007 Mar.;9(1):66–73

58. G.P. Biewenga, et al., 'The pharmacology of the antioxidant lipoic acid', *General Pharmacology*, 1997 Sept.;29(3):315–31; and S. Khanna, et al., 'Alpha-lipoic acid supplementation: Tissue glutathione homeostasis at rest and after exercise', *Journal of Applied Physiology*, 1999 Apr.;86(4):1191–6; and D. Han, et al., 'Lipoic acid increases de novo synthesis of cellular glutathione by improving cystine utilization', *Biofactors*, 1997;6(3):321–38; and J. Bustamante, et al., 'Alpha-lipoic acid in liver metabolism and disease', *Free Radical Biology and Medicine*, 1998 Apr.;24(6):1023–39

59. T. Remer and F. Manz, 'Potential renal acid load of foods and its influence on urine pH', *Journal of the American Dietetic Association*, 1995 July;95(7):791–7

60. H.G. Linhart, et al., 'Dnmt3b promotes tumorigenesis in vivo by gene-specific de novo methylation and transcriptional silencing', *Genes and Development*, 2007 Dec. 1;21(23):3110–22; and C. Lengauer, 'Cancer: An unstable liaison', *Science*, 2003 Apr. 18;300(5618):442–3; and C.D. Davis and E.O. Uthus, 'DNA methylation, cancer susceptibility, and nutrient interactions', *Experimental Biology and Medicine* (Maywood, N.J.), 2004 Nov.;229(10):988–95

61. S.E. Vollset, et al., 'Plasma total homocysteine and cardiovascular and non-cardiovascular mortality: the Hordaland Homocysteine Study', *American Journal of Clinical Nutrition*, 2001 July;74(1):130–6

62. L.L. Wu and J.T. Wu, 'Hyperhomocystenemia is a risk factor for cancer and a new potential tumor marker', *Clinica Chimica Acta*, 2002 Aug.;322(1–2):21–8

63. A. Cortelezzi, et al., 'Hyperhomocysteinemia in myelodysplastic syndromes: Specific association with autoimmunity and cardiovascular disease', *Leukemia and Lymphoma*, 2001 Mar.;41(1–2):147–50

64. S.W. Thomson, et al., 'Correlates of total plasma homocysteine: Folic acid, copper, and cervical dysplasia', *Nutrition*, 2000 June;16(6):411–6

65. R. Prinz-Langenohl, et al., 'Beneficial role for folate in the prevention of colorectal and breast cancer', *European Journal of Nutrition*, 2001 June;40(3):98–105

66. B. Shannon, et al., 'A polymorphism in the methylenetetrahydrofolate reductase gene predisposes to colorectal cancers with microsatellite instability', *Gut*, 2002 Apr.;50(4):520–4

67. J.B. Mason, et al., 'A temporal association between folic acid fortification and an increase in colorectal cancer rates may be illuminating important

biological principles: A hypothesis', *Cancer Epidemiology, Biomarkers and Prevention*, 2007 July;16(7):1325–9

68. B. Van Guelpen, et al., 'Low folate levels may protect against colorectal cancer', *Gut*, 2006 Oct.;55(10):1461–6

69. J. Kim, et al., 'Folate intake and the risk of colorectal cancer in a Korean population', *European Journal of Clinical Nutrition*, 2009 June 24 [Epub ahead of print]

70. M. Ebbing, et al., 'Cancer incidence and mortality after treatment with folic acid and vitamin B12', *Journal of the American Medical Association*, 2009;302(19):2119–26

71. U. Ericson, et al., 'High folate intake is associated with lower breast cancer incidence in postmenopausal women in the Malmo Diet and Cancer cohort', *American Journal of Clinical Nutrition*, 2007 Aug.;86(2):434–43

72. J.E. Goodman, et al., 'COMT genotype, micronutrients in the folate metabolic pathway and breast cancer risk', *Carcinogenesis*, 2001 Oct.;22(10):1661–5

73. K. Koyama, et al., 'Efficacy of methylcobalamin on lowering total homocysteine plasma concentrations in haemodialysis patients receiving high-dose folic acid supplementation', *Nephrology, Dialysis, Transplantation*, 2002 May;17(5):916–22

74. D.O. McGregor, et al., 'Betaine supplementation decreases post-methionine hyperhomocysteinemia in chronic renal failure', *Kidney International*, 2002 Mar.;61(3):1040–6

75. D. Goleman, *Emotional Intelligence*, Bloomsbury paperbacks (1996)

76. M.E. Kemeny, et al., 'Psychological and immunological predictors of genital herpes recurrence', *Psychosomatic Medicine*, 1989 Mar.;51(2):195–208

77. J.M. Scanlan, et al., 'Lymphocyte proliferation is associated with gender, caregiving, and psychological variables in older adult', *Journal of Behavioural Medicine*, 2001 Dec.;24(6):537–559

78. J.K. Kiecolt-Glaser, et al., 'Distress and DNA repair in human lymphocytes', *Journal of Behavioral Medicine*, 1985 Dec.;8(4):311–20

79. J.G. Courtney, et al., 'Stressful life events and the risk of colorectal cancer', *Epidemiology*, 1993 Sept.;4(5):407–14

80. G.E. Miller, et al., 'Chronic psychological stress and the regulation of pro-inflammatory cytokines: A glucocorticoid-resistance model', *Health Psychology*, 2002 Nov.;21(6):531–41

81. S. Malhotra, et al., 'The therapeutic potential of melatonin: A review of the science', *Medscape General Medicine*, 2004;6(2):46

82. E. Mills, et al., 'Melatonin in the treatment of cancer: a systematic review of randomized controlled trials and meta-analysis', *Journal of Pineal Research*, 2005 Nov.;39(4):360–6

83. J.L. Glaser, et al., 'Elevated serum dehydroepiandrosterone sulfate levels in practitioners of the Transcendental Meditation (TM) and TM-Sidhi programs', *Journal of Behavioral Medicine*, 1992 Aug.;15(4):327–41; see also L.E. Carlson, et al., 'Mindfulness-based stress reduction in relation to quality of

life, mood, symptoms of stress and levels of cortisol, dehydroepiandrosterone sulfate (DHEAS) and melatonin in breast and prostate cancer outpatients', *Psychoneuroendocrinology*, 2004 May;29(4):448–74; H. Wahbeh, et al., 'Binaural beat technology in humans: a pilot study to assess psychologic and physiologic effects', *Journal of Alternative and Complementary Medicine*, 2007 Jan.;13(1):25–32

84. M.A. Rosenkranz, et al., 'Affective style and in vivo immune response: neuro-behavioral mechanisms', *Proceedings of the National Academy of Sciences*, 2003 Sept. 16;100(19):11148–52

85. C.L. Hart, et al., 'Effect of conjugal bereavement on mortality of the bereaved spouse in participants of the Renfrew/Paisley Study', *Journal of Epidemiology and Community Health*, 2007 May;61(5):455–60; see also N.A. Christakis and P.D. Allison, 'Mortality after the hospitalization of a spouse', *New England Journal of Medicine*, 2006 Feb. 16;354(7):719–30

86. H. Tindle, et al., American Psychosomatic Society Annual Meeting, March 5 2009 University of Pittsburgh (see http://www.reuters.com/article/lifestyleMolt/idUSTRE5247NO20090305)

Part 2

1. World Cancer Research Fund/American Institute for Cancer Research, *Food, Nutrition, Physical Activity, and the Prevention of Cancer: A Global Perspective*. Washington, DC: AICR, 2007

2. U. Nothlings and L.N. Kolonel, 'Risk factors for pancreatic cancer in the Hawaii-Los Angeles Multiethnic Cohort Study', *Hawaii Medical Journal*, 2006 Jan.;65(1):26–8

3. E.F. Taylor, et al., 'Meat consumption and risk of breast cancer in the UK Women's Cohort Study', *British Journal of Cancer*, 2007 Apr. 10;96(7):1139–46

4. E. Cho, et al., 'Red meat intake and risk of breast cancer among premeno-pausal women', *Archives of Internal Medicine*, 2006 Nov. 13;166(20):2253–9

5. B.D. Cox and M.J. Whichelow, 'Frequent consumption of red meat is not risk factor for cancer', *British Medical Journal*, 1997 Oct. 18;315(7114):1018

6. P. Lindblad, et al., 'Diet and risk of renal cell cancer: A population-based case-control study', *Cancer Epidemiology, Biomarkers and Prevention*, 1997 Apr.;6(4):215–23

7. T.J. Key, et al., 'Cancer incidence in British vegetarians', *British Journal of Cancer*, 2009 July 7;101(1):192–7

8. T.J. Key, et al., 'Cancer incidence in vegetarians: Results from the European Prospective Investigation into Cancer and Nutrition (EPIC-Oxford)', *American Journal of Clinical Nutrition*, 2009 May;89(5):1620S–6S

9. D. Ganmaa, et al., 'Incidence and mortality of testicular and prostatic cancers in relation to world dietary practices', *International Journal of Cancer*, 2002 Mar. 10;98(2):262–7

10. J.C. van der Pols, et al., 'Childhood dairy intake and adult cancer risk: 65-y follow-up of the Boyd Orr cohort', *American Journal of Clinical Nutrition*, 2007 Dec.;86(6):1722–9

11. J.L. Stanford, et al., 'Prostate cancer trends 1973–1995', SEER Program, *National Cancer Institute*. NIH Pub. No. 99–4543. Bethesda, MD, 1999

12. P.V. Krogh, 'Meat, eggs, dairy products, and risk of breast cancer in the European Prospective Investigation into Cancer and Nutrition (EPIC) cohort', *American Journal of Clinical Nutrition*, 2009 June 2; [Epub ahead of print]

13. D. LeRoith and C.T. Roberts, Jr, 'The insulin-like growth factor system and cancer', *Cancer Letters*, 2003 June 10;195(2):127–37; see also S.E. Hankinson, et al., 'Circulating concentrations of insulin-like growth factor-I and risk of breast cancer', *Lancet*, 1998 May 9;351(9113):1393–6

14. M.H. Wu, et al., 'Relationships between critical period of estrogen exposure and circulating levels of insulin-like growth factor-I (IGF-I) in breast cancer: Evidence from a case-control study', *International Journal of Cancer*, 2009 July 7; [Epub ahead of print]

15. J.M. Chan, et al., 'Plasma insulin-like growth factor-I and prostate cancer risk: a prospective study', *Science*, 1998 Jan. 23;279(5350):563–6

16. E. Giovannucci, et al., 'Calcium and fructose intake in relation to risk of prostate cancer', *Cancer Research*, 1998 Feb. 1;58(3):442–7; J.M. Chan, et al., 'Dairy products, calcium, and prostate cancer risk in the Physicians' Health Study', *American Journal of Clinical Nutrition*, 2001 Oct.;74(4):549–54

17. J.M. Chan, et al., 'Dairy products, calcium, and prostate cancer risk in the Physicians' Health Study', *American Journal of Clinical Nutrition*, 2001 Oct.;74(4):549–54

18. S.C. Larsson, et al., 'Milk, milk products and lactose intake and ovarian cancer risk: A meta-analysis of epidemiological studies', *International Journal of Cancer*, 2006 Jan. 15;118(2):431–41

19. 'National Diet and Nutrition Survey: Adults aged 19 to 64', volume 2, *Food Standards Agency*, UK, July 2003

20. M. de Lorgeril, et al., 'Mediterranean dietary pattern in a randomized trial: Prolonged survival and possible reduced cancer rate', *Archives of Internal Medicine*, 1998 June 8;158(11):1181–7

21. P.N. Mitrou, et al., 'Mediterranean dietary pattern and prediction of all-cause mortality in a US population: results from the NIH-AARP Diet and Health Study', *Archives of Internal Medicine*, 2007 Dec. 10;167(22):2461–8

22. B. Buijsse, et al., 'Plasma carotene and alpha-tocopherol in relation to 10-y all-cause and cause-specific mortality in European elderly: The Survey in Europe on Nutrition and the Elderly, a Concerted Action (SENECA)', *American Journal of Clinical Nutrition*, 2005 Oct.;82(4):879–86

23. E. Giovannucci, et al., 'Intake of carotenoids and retinol in relation to risk of prostate cancer', *Journal of the National Cancer Institute*, 1995 Dec. 6; 87(23):1767–76; see also M.S. Ansari and S. Ansari, 'Lycopene and prostate cancer', *Future Oncology*, 2005 June;1(3):425–30; E.C. Miller, et al., 'Tomato products, lycopene, and prostate cancer risk', *Urologic Clinics of North America*, 2002 Feb.;29(1):83–93

24. T. Hirayama, 'A large-scale cohort study on cancer risks by diet with special reference to the risk reducing effects of green-yellow vegetable consumption', *Princess Takamatsu Symposia*, 1985;16:41–53

25. 'Food, Nutrition and the Prevention of Cancer', World Cancer Research Fund/American Institute for Cancer Research, pp. 239–42 (1997)

26. B.L. Pool-Zobel, et al., 'Consumption of vegetables reduces genetic damage in humans: First results of a human intervention trial with carotenoid-rich foods', *Carcinogenesis*, 1997 Sept.;18(9):1847–50

27. K. Irani, et al., 'Mitogenic signaling mediated by oxidants in ras-transformed fibroblasts', *Science*, 1997 March 14, 275;(5306):1649–52

28. A.B. Weitberg and D. Corvese, 'Effect of vitamin E and beta-carotene on DNA strand breakage induced by tobacco-specific nitrosamines and stimulated human phagocytes', *Journal of Experimental and Clinical Cancer Research*, 1997 Mar.;16(1):11–4

29. S. Zhang, et al., 'Dietary carotenoids and vitamins A, C, and E and risk of breast cancer', *Journal of the National Cancer Institute*, 1999 Mar. 17;91(6):547–56

30. D.C. Schwenke, 'Does lack of tocopherols and tocotrienols put women at increased risk of breast cancer?', *Journal of Nutritional Biochemistry*, 2002 Jan.;13(1):2–20

31. J.M. Chan, et al., 'What causes prostate cancer? A brief summary of the epidemiology', *Seminars in Cancer Biology*, 1998 Aug.;8(4):263–73; and World Cancer Research Fund/American Institute for Cancer Research, *Food, Nutrition, Physical Activity, and the Prevention of Cancer: a Global Perspective*. Washington, DC: AICR, 2007

32. R.K. Peters, et al., 'Diet and colon cancer in Los Angeles County, California', *Cancer Causes and Control*, 1992 Sept.;3(5):457–73

33. N. Tawfiq, et al., 'Dietary glucosinolates as blocking agents against carcinogenesis: Glucosinolate breakdown products assessed by induction of quinone reductase activity in murine hepa1c1c7 cells', *Carcinogenesis*, 1995 May;16(5):1191–4

34. V.A. Kirsh, et al., 'Prospective study of fruit and vegetable intake and risk of prostate cancer', *Journal of the National Cancer Institute*, 2007 Aug. 1;99(15):1200–9

35. L. Tang, et al., 'Consumption of raw cruciferous vegetables is inversely associated with bladder cancer risk', *Cancer Epidemiology, Biomarkers and Prevention*, 2008 Apr.;17(4):938–44

36. C.J. Grubbs, et al., 'Chemoprevention of chemically-induced mammary carcinogenesis by indole-3-carbinol', *Anticancer Research*, 1995 May;15(3):709–16; M.N. Preobrazhenskaya, et al., 'Polyfunctional indole-3-carbinol derivatives: 1-(indol-3-yl)glycerols and related compounds, beta-hydroxytryptamines and ascorbigens. Chemistry and biological properties', *Farmaco*, 1995 June;50(6):369–77

37. H. Adlercreutz, et al., 'Plasma concentrations of phyto-oestrogens in Japanese men', *Lancet*, 1993 Nov. 13;342(8881):1209–10

359

38. W.H. St Clair and D.K. St Clair, 'Effect of the Bowman-Birk protease inhibitor on the expression of oncogenes in the irradiated rat colon', *Cancer Research*, 1991 Sept. 1;51(17):4539–43; W.H. St Clair, et al., 'Suppression of dimethylhydrazine-induced carcinogenesis in mice by dietary addition of the Bowman-Birk protease inhibitor', *Cancer Research*, 1990 Feb. 1;50(3):580–6

39. A.R. Kennedy, 'Chemopreventive agents: protease inhibitors', *Pharmacology and Therapeutics*, 1998 June;78(3):167–209

40. L.J. Lu, et al., 'Altered time course of urinary daidzein and genistein excretion during chronic soya diet in healthy male subjects', *Nutrition and Cancer*, 1995;24(3):311–23

41. D. Ingram, et al., 'Case-control study of phyto-oestrogens and breast cancer', *Lancet*, 1997 Oct. 4;350(9083):990–4; M. Messina, et al., 'Phyto-oestrogens and breast cancer', *Lancet*, 1997 Oct. 4;350(9083):971–2

42. W.H. Xu, et al., 'Soya food intake and risk of endometrial cancer among Chinese women in Shanghai: Population based case-control study', *British Medical Journal*, 2004 May 29;328(7451):1285

43. J.T. Dwyer, et al., 'Tofu and soy drinks contain phytoestrogens', *Journal of the American Dietetic Association*, 1994 July;94(7):739–43

44. W.C. You, et al., 'Allium vegetables and reduced risk of stomach cancer', *Journal of the National Cancer Institute*, 1989 Jan. 18;81(2):162–4

45. K.A. Steinmetz, et al., 'Vegetables, fruit, and colon cancer in the Iowa Women's Health Study', *American Journal of Epidemiology*, 1994 Jan. 1;139(1):1–15

46. A.T. Fleischauer, et al., 'Garlic consumption and cancer prevention: meta-analyses of colorectal and stomach cancers', *American Journal of Clinical Nutrition*, 2000 Oct.;72(4):1047–52

47. Y.Y. Yeh and S.M. Yeh, 'Homocysteine-lowering action is another potential cardiovascular protective factor of aged garlic extract', *Journal of Nutrition*, 2006 Mar.;136(3 Suppl):745S–9S

48. Environmental Working Group (EWG), 'Shoppers Guide to Pesticides' (The Shopper's Guide to Pesticides ranks pesticide contamination for 47 popular fruits and vegetables based on an analysis of 87,000 tests for pesticides on these foods, conducted from 2000 to 2007 by the US Department of Agriculture and the Food and Drug Administration), see http://www.foodnews.org/methodology.php. Read more: http://www.thedailygreen.com/healthy-eating/eat-safe/Dirty-Dozen-Foods#ixzz0S0sJGMTX [Accessed 24 September 2009]

49. Read more: http://www.thedailygreen.com/healthy-eating/eat-safe/Dirty-Dozen-Foods#ixzz0S0uEGTSH (Page 18) [Accessed 24 September 2009]

50. Read more: http://www.thedailygreen.com/healthy-eating/eat-safe/Dirty-Dozen-Foods#ixzz0S0uEGTSH (Page 17) [Accessed 24 September 2009]

51. M.D. Burke and G. Potter, 'Salvestrols: Natural plant-derived anticancer agents?', *British Naturopathic Journal*, 2006;23(1):10–13

52. G.A. Potter and M.D. Burke, 'Salvestrols – Natural Products with Tumour Selective Activity', *Journal of Orthomolecular Medicine*, 2006; 21(1):34–6

53. Dr John Briffa, '20 Big Ideas', *Observer Magazine*, 2 January 2005

54. G.I. Murray, et al., 'Tumor-specific expression of cytochrome P450 CYP1B1', *Cancer Research*, 1997 July 15;57(14):3026–31

55. H.L. Tan, et al., 'Salvestrols: A new perspective in nutritional research', *Journal of Orthomolecular Medicine*, 2007;22(1):39–47

56. L. Nadler, '*Cytochrome P450 1B1 is a Universal Tumor Antigen Eliciting Cytotoxic T Cell Responses*', 2008, Dana-Farber Cancer Institute, USA. [Accessed at: http://www.dana-farber.org/res/technology/printable.asp?case_number=641 8 July 2009].

57. Gray Cancer Institute [Accessed at: http://www.gci.ac.uk/newsite/research/groups/free_radicals/index.htm 8 July 2009]

58. H.L. Tan, et al., 'Salvestrols: A new perspective in nutritional research', *Journal of Orthomolecular Medicine*, 2007;22(1):39–47

59. G.A. Potter and M.D. Burke, 'Salvestrols: Natural products with tumour selective activity', *Journal of Orthomolecular Medicine*, 2006; 21(1):34–6

60. G.A. Potter, et al., 'The cancer preventative agent resveratrol is converted to the anticancer agent piceatannol by the cytochrome P450 enzyme CYP1B1', *British Journal of Cancer*, 2002 Mar. 4;86(5):774–8

61. G.A. Potter, et al., 'The cancer preventative agent resveratrol is converted to the anticancer agent piceatannol by the cytochrome P450 enzyme CYP1B1', *British Journal of Cancer*, 2002 Mar. 4;86(5):774–8

62. S. Chanvitayapongs, et al., 'Amelioration of oxidative stress by antioxidants and resveratrol in PC12 cells', *Neuroreport*, 1997 Apr. 14;8(6):1499–502; and L. Belguendouz, et al., 'Interaction of transresveratrol with plasma lipoproteins', *Biochemical Pharmacology*, 1998 Mar. 15;55(6):811–6; and M. Jang, et al., 'Cancer chemopreventive activity of resveratrol, a natural product derived from grapes', *Science*, 1997 Jan. 10;275(5297):218–20; and D. Bagchi, et al., 'Benefits of resveratrol in women's health', *Drugs Under Experimental and Clinical Research*, 2001;27(5–6):233–48; and M. Jang and J.M. Pezzuto, 'Cancer chemopreventive activity of resveratrol', *Drugs Under Experimental and Clinical Research*, 1999;25(2–3):65–77; and Y. Schneider, et al., 'Antiproliferative effect of resveratrol, a natural component of grapes and wine, on human colonic cancer cells', *Cancer Letters*, 2000 Sept. 29;158(1):85–91; and K. Bove, et al., 'Effect of resveratrol on growth of 4T1 breast cancer cells in vitro and in vivo', *Biochemical and Biophysical Research Communications*, 2002 Mar. 8;291(4):1001–5

63. W.R. Ware, 'Nutrition and the prevention and treatment of cancer: association of cytochrome P450 CYP1B1 with the role of fruit and fruit extracts', *Integrative Cancer Therapies*, 2009 Mar.;8(1):22–8

64. B.A. Schaefer, et al., 'Nutrition and Cancer: Salvestrol Case Studies', *Journal of Orthomolecular Medicine*, 2007;22(4):1–6

65. World Cancer Research Fund/American Institute for Cancer Research, *Food, Nutrition, Physical Activity, and the Prevention of Cancer: A Global Perspective*. Washington, DC: AICR, 2007

66. E. Cho, et al., 'Premenopausal fat intake and risk of breast cancer', *Journal of the National Cancer Institute*, 2003 July 16;95(14):1079–85

67. W.C. Willett, et al., 'Dietary fat and the risk of breast cancer', *New England Journal of Medicine*, 1987 Jan. 1;316(1):22–8

68. R. Uauy-Dagach and A. Valenzuela, 'Marine oils: The health benefits of n-3 fatty acids', *Nutrition Reviews*, 1996 Nov.;54(11 Pt 2):S102–S108

69. E.L. Wynder, et al., 'Breast cancer: Weighing the evidence for a promoting role of dietary fat', *Journal of the National Cancer Institute*, 1997 June 4;89(11):766–75; L. Hilakivi-Clarke, et al., 'Breast cancer risk in rats fed a diet high in n-6 polyunsaturated fatty acids during pregnancy', *Journal of the National Cancer Institute*, 1996 Dec. 18;88(24):1821–7

70. N. Simonsen, et al., 'Adipose tissue omega-3 and omega-6 fatty acid content and breast cancer in the EURAMIC study. European Community Multicenter Study on Antioxidants, Myocardial Infarction, and Breast Cancer', *American Journal of Epidemiology*, 1998 Feb. 15;147(4):342–52

71. P. Terry, et al., 'Fatty fish consumption and risk of prostate cancer', *Lancet*, 2001 June 2;357(9270):1764–6

72. J. Kim, et al., 'Fatty fish and fish omega-3 fatty acid intakes decrease the breast cancer risk: A case-control study', *BMC Cancer*, 2009;9:216

73. Y.Y. Fan, et al., 'Proapoptotic effects of dietary (n-3) fatty acids are enhanced in colonocytes of manganese-dependent superoxide dismutase knockout mice', *Journal of Nutrition*, 2009 July;139(7):1328–32

74. C.A. Gogos, et al., 'Dietary omega-3 polyunsaturated fatty acids plus vitamin E restore immunodeficiency and prolong survival for severely ill patients with generalized malignancy: A randomized control trial', *Cancer*, 1998 Jan. 15;82(2):395–402

75. D.K. Banel and F.B. Hu, 'Effects of walnut consumption on blood lipids and other cardiovascular risk factors: A meta-analysis and systematic review', *American Journal of Clinical Nutrition*, 2009 July;90(1):56–63

76. C. La Vecchia, 'Association between Mediterranean dietary patterns and cancer risk', *Nutrition Reviews*, 2009 May;67 (Suppl 1):S126–S129

77. S. Frankel, et al., 'Childhood energy intake and adult mortality from cancer: the Boyd Orr Cohort Study', *British Medical Journal*, 1998 Feb. 14;316(7130):499–504

78. R.K. Peters, et al., 'Diet and colon cancer in Los Angeles County, California', *Cancer Causes and Control*, 1992 Sept.;3(5):457–73

79. Dr W.C. Willett, Symposium on Cancer Prevention, Annual meeting of the American Association for the Advancement of Science, March 2008

80. A. Tavani, et al., 'Consumption of sweet foods and breast cancer risk in Italy', *Annals of Oncology*, 2006 Feb.;17(2):341–5; and C.A. Krone and J.T. Ely, 'Controlling hyperglycemia as an adjunct to cancer therapy', *Integrative Cancer Therapies*, 2005 Mar.;4(1):25–31; and S.C. Larsson, et al., 'Glycemic load, glycemic index and breast cancer risk in a prospective cohort of Swedish women', *International Journal of Cancer*, 2009 July 1;125(1):153–7; and W. Wen, et al., 'Dietary carbohydrates, fiber, and breast cancer risk in Chinese

women', *American Journal of Clinical Nutrition*, 2009 Jan.;89(1):283–9; and S. Sieri, et al., 'Dietary glycemic index, glycemic load, and the risk of breast cancer in an Italian prospective cohort study', *American Journal of Clinical Nutrition*, 2007 Oct.;86(4):1160–6; and M. Lajous, et al., 'Carbohydrate intake, glycemic index, glycemic load, and risk of postmenopausal breast cancer in a prospective study of French women', *American Journal of Clinical Nutrition*, 2008 May;87(5):1384–91; and S.E. McCann, et al., 'Dietary patterns related to glycemic index and load and risk of premenopausal and postmenopausal breast cancer in the Western New York Exposure and Breast Cancer Study', *American Journal of Clinical Nutrition*, 2007 Aug.;86(2):465–71

81. M.L. Slattery, et al., 'Dietary sugar and colon cancer', *Cancer Epidemiology, Biomarkers and Prevention*, 1997 Sept.;6(9):677–85

82. D.S. Michaud, et al., 'Dietary sugar, glycemic load, and pancreatic cancer risk in a prospective study', *Journal of the National Cancer Institute*, 2002 Sept. 4;94(17):1293–300

83. S.A. Silvera, et al., 'Glycaemic index, glycaemic load and ovarian cancer risk: A prospective cohort study', *Public Health Nutrition*, 2007 Oct.;10(10):1076–81

84. G. Randi, et al., 'Glycemic index, glycemic load and thyroid cancer risk', *Annals of Oncology*, 2008 Feb.;19(2):380–3

85. S.A. Silvera, et al., 'Glycaemic index, glycaemic load and risk of endometrial cancer: A prospective cohort study', *Public Health Nutrition*, 2005 Oct.;8(7):912–9; and S.C. Larsson, et al., 'Carbohydrate intake, glycemic index and glycemic load in relation to risk of endometrial cancer: A prospective study of Swedish women', *International Journal of Cancer*, 2007 Mar. 1;120(5):1103–7

86. P. Bertuccio, et al., 'Dietary glycemic load and gastric cancer risk in Italy', *British Journal of Cancer*, 2009 Feb. 10;100(3):558–61

87. A.W. Barclay, et al., 'Glycemic index, glycemic load, and chronic disease risk: A meta-analysis of observational studies', *American Journal of Clinical Nutrition*, 2008 Mar.;87(3):627–37

88. A. Tavani, et al., 'Consumption of sweet foods and breast cancer risk in Italy', *Annals of Oncology*, 2006 Feb.;17(2):341–5; see also C.A. Krone and J.T. Ely, 'Controlling hyperglycemia as an adjunct to cancer therapy', *Integrative Cancer Therapies*, 2005 Mar.;4(1):25–31

89. G.C. Kabat, et al., 'Repeated measures of serum glucose and insulin in relation to postmenopausal breast cancer', *International Journal of Cancer*, 2009 June 2 [Epub ahead of print]; see also M.J. Gunter, et al., 'Insulin, insulin-like growth factor-I, and risk of breast cancer in postmenopausal women', *Journal of the National Cancer Institute*, 2009 Jan. 7;101(1):48–60

90. J. Ahn, et al., 'Adiposity, adult weight change, and postmenopausal breast cancer risk', *Archives of Internal Medicine*, 2007 Oct. 22;167(19):2091–102; see also A.H. Eliassen, et al., 'Adult weight change and risk of postmenopausal breast cancer', *Journal of the American Medical Association*, 2006 July 12;296(2):193–201

91. R. Huxley, et al., 'Type-II diabetes and pancreatic cancer: A meta-analysis of 36 studies', *British Journal of Cancer*, 2005 June 6;92(11):2076–83

92. S.C. Larsson, et al., 'Diabetes mellitus and risk of colorectal cancer: A meta-analysis', *Journal of the National Cancer Institute*, 2005 Nov. 16;97(22):1679–87; and S.C. Larsson, et al., 'Diabetes mellitus and risk of breast cancer: A meta-analysis', *International Journal of Cancer*, 2007 Aug. 15;121(4):856–62

93. World Cancer Research Fund/American Institute for Cancer Research, *Food, Nutrition, Physical Activity, and the Prevention of Cancer: A Global Perspective.* Washington, DC: AICR, 2007

94. R.K. Peters, et al., 'Diet and colon cancer in Los Angeles County, California', *Cancer Causes and Control*, 1992 Sept.;3(5):457–73

95. D. Royall, et al., 'Clinical significance of colonic fermentation', *American Journal of Gastroenterology*, 1990 Oct.;85(10):1307–12; G. Latella and R. Caprilli, 'Metabolism of large bowel mucosa in health and disease', *International Journal of Colorectal Disease*, 1991 May;6(2):127–32; R. Hoverstad, 'The normal microflora and short-chain fatty acids', *Proceedings of the Fifth Bengt E. Gustafsson Symposium, Stockholm* (1–4 June 1988)

96. J.M. Yuan, et al., 'Diet and breast cancer in Shanghai and Tianjin, China', *British Journal of Cancer*, 1995 June;71(6):1353–8

97. E. De Stefani, et al., 'Dietary fiber and risk of breast cancer: A case-control study in Uruguay', *Nutrition and Cancer*, 1997;28(1):14–19

98. E.F. Taylor, et al., 'Meat consumption and risk of breast cancer in the UK Women's Cohort Study', *British Journal of Cancer*, 2007 Apr. 10;96(7):1139–46

99. S.A. Smith-Warner, et al., 'Alcohol and breast cancer in women: A pooled analysis of cohort studies', *Journal of the American Medical Association*, 1998 Feb. 18;279(7):535–40

100. P. Boffetta and M. Hashibe, 'Alcohol and cancer', *Lancet Oncology*, 2006 Feb.;7(2):149–56

101. World Cancer Research Fund/American Institute for Cancer Research, *Food, Nutrition, Physical Activity, and the Prevention of Cancer: A Global Perspective.* Washington, DC: AICR, 2007

102. S.A. Glynn, et al., 'Alcohol consumption and risk of colorectal cancer in a cohort of Finnish men', *Cancer Causes and Control*, 1996 Mar.;7(2):214–23

103. A.J. Clifford, et al., 'Delayed tumor onset in transgenic mice fed an amino acid-based diet supplemented with red wine solids', *American Journal of Clinical Nutrition*, 1996 Nov.;64(5):748–56

104. 'Food, nutrition and the prevention of cancer', World Cancer Research Fund, American Institute for Cancer Research (1997)

105. K. Ishitani, et al., 'Caffeine consumption and the risk of breast cancer in a large prospective cohort of women', *Archives of Internal Medicine*, 2008 Oct. 13;168(18):2022–31

106. D. Panagiotakos, et al., 'The association between coffee consumption and plasma total homocysteine levels: The ATTICA Study', *Heart Vessels*, vol. 19(6), 2004, pp. 280–6

107. A 50 per cent higher level of one of the markers (known as Interleukin 6), a 30 per cent higher level of another (known as C-reactive protein) and a 28 per cent higher level of a third (known as TNF) compared to non-coffee consumers. A. Zampelas, et al., 'Associations between coffee consumption and inflammatory markers in healthy persons: The ATTICA Study', *American Journal of Clinical Nutrition*, vol. 80(4), 2004, pp. 862–7

108. G. Yang, et al., 'Prospective cohort study of green tea consumption and colorectal cancer risk in women', *Cancer Epidemiology, Biomarkers and Prevention*, 2007 June;16(6):1219–23

109. C.J. Dufresne and E.R. Farnworth, 'A review of latest research findings on the health promotion properties of tea', *Journal of Nutritional Biochemistry*, 2001 July;12(7):404–21

110. R. Ide, et al., 'A prospective study of green tea consumption and oral cancer incidence in Japan', *Annals of Epidemiology*, 2007 Oct.;17(10):821–6

Part 3

1. M.H. Repacholi, et al., 'Lymphomas in E mu-Pim1 transgenic mice exposed to pulsed 900 MHZ electromagnetic fields', *Radiation Research*, 1997 May;147(5):631–40

2. S. Roy, et al., 'The phorbol 12-myristate 13-acetate (PMA)-induced oxidative burst in rat peritoneal neutrophils is increased by a 0.1 mT (60 Hz) magnetic field', *FEBS Letters*, 1995 Dec. 4;376(3):164–6

3. J.A. Davidson, 'Brain tumours and mobile phones?', *Medical Journal of Australia*, 1998 Jan. 5;168(1):48

4. D. Carpenter and C. Sage (eds), 'BioInitiative Report: A rationale for a biologically-based public exposure standard for electromagnetic fields (ELF and RF)', 31 August 2007, see http://www.bioinitiative.org/report/docs/report.pdf.

5. L. Hardell, et al., Research carried out by scientists at University Hospital, Orebro, in Sweden and presented at a conference at the Royal Society of Radiation Research – reported in the *Independent* 24 September 2008

6. M.J. Gardner, et al., 'Follow-up study of children born to mothers resident in Seascale, West Cumbria (birth cohort)', *British Medical Journal (Clinical Research ed.)*, 1987 Oct. 3;295(6602):822–7; and M.J. Gardner, et al., 'Follow-up study of children born elsewhere but attending schools in Seascale, West Cumbria (schools cohort)', *British Medical Journal (Clinical Research ed.)*, 1987 Oct. 3;295(6602):819–22

7. S. Darby, et al., 'Risk of lung cancer associated with residential radon exposure in south-west England: a case-control study', *British Journal of Cancer*, 1998 Aug.;78(3):394–408

8. G.P. Studzinski and D.C. Moore, 'Sunlight – can it prevent as well as cause cancer?', *Cancer Research*, 1995 Sept. 15;55(18):4014–22

9. M.A. Pathak, 'Activation of the melanocyte system by ultraviolet radiation and cell transformation', *Annals of the New York Academy of Sciences*, 1985;453:328–39

10. P.J. McHugh and J. Knowland, 'Characterization of DNA damage inflicted by free radicals from a mutagenic sunscreen ingredient and its location using an in vitro genetic reversion assay', *Photochemistry and Photobiology*, 1997 Aug.;66(2):276–81

11. J. Thornton, 'Chlorine, human health and the environment: The breast cancer warning', Greenpeace, Washington DC (1993)

12. Collegium Ramazzini Statement, 'The Control of Pesticides in the European Union: A call for Action to Protect Human Health', Statement 13, 2008. Retrieved from: http://www.collegiumramazzini.org/download/13_ThirteenthCRStatement(2008).pdf. The Collegium Ramazzini (comprised of 180 physicians and scientists from 35 countries) is an international scientific society that examines critical issues in occupational and environmental medicine with a view towards action to prevent disease and to promote health.

13. Pesticide Action Network (PAN) UK, 'The List of Lists', 3rd edn, 2009

14. G. Lean, 'Massive crackdown on the use of scores of toxic pesticides', *Independent*, 21 December 2008

15. D. Charter, 'Crunch time for carrots as EU bans pesticides', *The Times*, 14 January 2009

16. W. Dunham, 'DDT-related chemical linked to testicular cancer', *Reuters,* 29 April 2008

17. New Zealand Total Diet Survey (1990/1991)

18. E. Gold, et al., 'Risk factors for brain tumors in children', *American Journal of Epidemiology*, 1979 Mar.;109(3):309–19

19. J.D. Buckley, et al., 'Occupational exposures of parents of children with acute nonlymphocytic leukemia: A report from the Children's Cancer Study Group', *Cancer Research*, 1989 July 15;49(14):4030–7

20. R.A. Lowengart, et al., 'Childhood leukemia and parents' occupational and home exposures', *Journal of the National Cancer Institute*, 1987 July;79(1):39–46

21. World Cancer Research Fund/American Institute for Cancer Research, *Food, Nutrition, Physical Activity, and the Prevention of Cancer: A Global Perspective.* Washington, DC: AICR, 2007

22. T. Hirayama, 'A large scale cohort study on cancer risks by diet – with special reference to the risk reducing effects of green-yellow vegetable consumption', *Princess Takamatsu Symposia*, 1985;16:41–53

23. R.B. Shekelle, et al., 'Dietary vitamin A and risk of cancer in the Western Electric study', *Lancet*, 1981 Nov. 28;2(8257):1185–90

24. World Cancer Research Fund/American Institute for Cancer Research, *Food, Nutrition, Physical Activity, and the Prevention of Cancer: A Global Perspective.* Washington, DC: AICR, 2007

25. H.A. Kahn, 'The Dorn study of smoking and mortality among U.S. veterans: Report on eight and one-half years of observation', *National Cancer Institute Monograph*, 1966 Jan.;19:1–125

26. S. Epstein, 'Winning the War Against Cancer? . . . Are they even fighting it?' *Ecologist*, 1998;28(2):69–80

27. G.H. Miller, et al., 'Women and lung cancer: A comparison of active and passive smokers with nonexposed nonsmokers', *Cancer Detection and Prevention*, 1994;18(6):421–30

28. A. Charloux, et al., 'Passive smoking and bronchial cancer: a difficult relation to establish', *Revue de Pneumologie Clinique*, 1996;52(4):227–34

29. A. Morabia, et al., 'Relation of breast cancer with passive and active exposure to tobacco smoke', *American Journal of Epidemiology*, 1996 May 1;143(9):918–28

30. D. Cadbury, *The Feminization of Nature*, Hamish Hamilton, pp. 180–3 (1997)

31. D. Spiegel, et al., 'Effect of psychosocial treatment on survival of patients with metastatic breast cancer', *Lancet*, 1989 Oct. 14;2(8668):888–91

32. J. Griffin and I. Tyrrell, *Dreaming Reality: How Dreaming Keeps Us Sane, or Can Drive Us Mad,* HG Publishing (2006)

33. D. Goleman, *Emotional Intelligence*, Bloomsbury paperbacks (1996)

34. D. Goleman, *Emotional Intelligence*, Bloomsbury paperbacks (1996)

35. A. Lutz, et al., 'Long-term meditators self-induce high-amplitude gamma synchrony during mental practice', *Proceedings of the National Academy of Sciences*, 2004 Nov. 16;101(46):16369–73

36. J.L. Glaser, et al., 'Elevated serum dehydroepiandrosterone sulfate levels in practitioners of the Transcendental Meditation (TM) and TM-Sidhi programs', *Journal of Behavioral Medicine*, 1992 Aug.;15(4):327–41; also see L.E. Carlson, et al., 'Mindfulness-based stress reduction in relation to quality of life, mood, symptoms of stress and levels of cortisol, dehydroepiandrosterone sulfate (DHEAS) and melatonin in breast and prostate cancer outpatients', *Psychoneuroendocrinology*, 2004 May;29(4):448–74; H. Wahbeh, et al., 'Binaural beat technology in humans: a pilot study to assess psychologic and physiologic effects', *Journal of Alternative and Complementary Medicine*, 2007 Jan.;13(1):25–32

Part 4

1. G.S. Omenn, et al., 'Effects of a combination of beta carotene and vitamin A on lung cancer and cardiovascular disease', *New England Journal of Medicine*, 1996 May 2;334(18):1150–5

2. World Cancer Research Fund/American Institute for Cancer Research, *Food, Nutrition, Physical Activity, and the Prevention of Cancer: A Global Perspective*, Washington, DC: AICR, 2007

3. World Cancer Research Fund, *Food Nutrition and the Prevention of Cancer,* 1997, p.138

4. B. Buijsse, et al., 'Plasma carotene and alpha-tocopherol in relation to 10-y all-cause and cause-specific mortality in European elderly: The Survey

in Europe on Nutrition and the Elderly, a Concerted Action (SENECA)', *American Journal of Clinical Nutrition*, 2005 Oct.;82(4):879–86

5. R.B. Shekelle, et al., 'Dietary vitamin A and risk of cancer in the Western Electric study', *Lancet*, 1981 Nov. 28;2(8257):1185–90

6. G.S. Omenn, et al., 'Effects of a combination of beta carotene and vitamin A on lung cancer and cardiovascular disease', *New England Journal of Medicine*, 1996 May 2;334(18):1150–5

7. D. Albanes, et al., 'Alpha-tocopherol and beta-carotene supplements and lung cancer incidence in the alpha-tocopherol, beta-carotene cancer prevention study: Effects of base-line characteristics and study compliance', *Journal of the National Cancer Institute*, 1996 Nov. 6;88(21):1560–70 ; and no authors listed, 'The effect of vitamin E and beta carotene on the incidence of lung cancer and other cancers in male smokers: The Alpha-Tocopherol, Beta Carotene Cancer Prevention Study Group', *New England Journal of Medicine*, 1994 Apr. 14;330(15):1029–35

8. M. Caraballoso, et al., 'Drugs for preventing lung cancer in healthy people', the Cochrane Database of Systematic Reviews 2005, issue 4, article no. CD002141

9. SuViMax study at www.news.bbc.co.uk/go/em/fr/-/1/hi/health/3122033.stm

10. J.A. Baron, et al., 'Neoplastic and antineoplastic effects of beta-carotene on colorectal adenoma recurrence: results of a randomized trial', *Journal of the National Cancer Institute*, 2003 May 21;95(10):717–22

11. S. Mannisto, et al., 'Dietary carotenoids and risk of lung cancer in a pooled analysis of seven cohort studies', *Cancer Epidemiology, Biomarkers and Prevention*, 2004 Jan.;13(1):40–8

12. I.D. Podmore, et al., 'Vitamin C exhibits pro-oxidant properties', *Nature*, 1998 Apr. 9;392(6676):559

13. G. Bjelakovic, et al., 'Antioxidant supplements for prevention of gastro-intestinal cancers: A systematic review and meta-analysis', *Lancet*, 2004 Oct. 2;364(9441):1219–28

14. J.A. Baron, et al., 'Neoplastic and antineoplastic effects of beta-carotene on colorectal adenoma recurrence: Results of a randomized trial', *Journal of the National Cancer Institute*, 2003 May 21;95(10):717–22

15. P. Correa, et al., 'Chemoprevention of gastric dysplasia: randomized trial of antioxidant supplements and anti-helicobacter pylori therapy', *Journal of the National Cancer Institute*, 2000 Dec. 6;92(23):1881–8

16. Letter from Dr P. Correa, September 2004

17. T.K. Basu, et al., 'Plasma vitamin A in patients with bronchial carcinoma', *British Journal of Cancer*, 1976 Jan.;33(1):119–21; G.W. Comstock, et al., 'The risk of developing lung cancer associated with antioxidants in the blood: Ascorbic acid, carotenoids, alpha-tocopherol, selenium, and total peroxyl radical absorbing capacity', *Cancer Epidemiology, Biomarkers and Prevention*, 1997 Nov.;6(11):907–16

18. R.B. Shekelle, et al., 'Dietary vitamin A and risk of cancer in the Western Electric study', *Lancet*, 1981 Nov. 28;2(8257):1185–90

19. G. Bond, et al., 'Dietary vitamin A and lung cancer: Results of a case-control study among chemical workers', *Nutrition and Cancer*, vol. 9(2/3), pp. 109–21 (1987); G.G. Bond, et al., 'Dietary vitamin A and lung cancer: Results of a case-control study among chemical workers', *Nutrition and Cancer*, 1987;9(2–3):109–21

20. T. Hirayama, 'Diet and Cancer', *Nutrition and Cancer*, 1979; 1(3):67–81

21. N.R. Cook, et al., 'Beta-carotene supplementation for patients with low baseline levels and decreased risks of total and prostate carcinoma', *Cancer*, 1999 Nov. 1;86(9):1783–92

22. C.L. Rock, et al., 'Responsiveness of carotenoids to a high vegetable diet intervention designed to prevent breast cancer recurrence', *Cancer Epidemiology, Biomarkers and Prevention*, 1997 Aug.;6(8):617–23

23. J.F. Dorgan, et al., 'Relationships of serum carotenoids, retinol, alpha-tocopherol, and selenium with breast cancer risk: results from a prospective study in Columbia, Missouri (United States)', *Cancer Causes and Control*, 1998 Jan.;9(1):89–97

24. H.F. Stich, et al., 'Response of oral leukoplakias to the administration of vitamin A', *Cancer Letters*, 1988 May;40(1):93–101

25. G.L. Sun, et al., 'Treatment of acute promyelocytic leukemia with all-trans retinoic acid. A five-year experience', *Chinese Medical Journal*, 1993 Oct.;106(10):743–8

26. F.R. Khuri, et al., 'Molecular epidemiology and retinoid chemoprevention of head and neck cancer', *Journal of the National Cancer Institute*, 1997 Feb. 5;89(3):199–211; S.M. Lippman and W.K. Hong, '13-cis-retinoic acid plus interferon-alpha in solid tumors: keeping the cart behind the horse', *Annals of Oncology*, 1994 May;5(5):391–3

27. S.T. Mayne, et al., 'Randomized trial of supplemental beta-carotene to prevent second head and neck cancer', *Cancer Research*, 2001 Feb. 15;61(4):1457–63

28. G. Block, 'Vitamin C and cancer prevention: The epidemiologic evidence', *American Journal of Clinical Nutrition*, 1991 Jan.;53(1 Suppl):270S–82S

29. G. Block, 'Epidemiologic evidence regarding vitamin C and cancer', *American Journal of Clinical Nutrition*, 1991 Dec.;54(6 Suppl):1310S–4S

30. E. Cameron and L. Pauling, 'Supplemental ascorbate in the supportive treatment of cancer: Prolongation of survival times in terminal human cancer', *Proceedings of the National Academy of Sciences of the United States of America*, 1976 Oct.;73(10):3685–9; E. Cameron and L. Pauling, 'Supplemental ascorbate in the supportive treatment of cancer: Reevaluation of prolongation of survival times in terminal human cancer', *Proceedings of the National Academy of Sciences of the United States of America*, 1978 Sept.;75(9):4538–42; M. Jaffey, 'Vitamin C and cancer: Examination of the Vale of Leven trial results using broad inductive reasoning', *Medical Hypotheses*, 1982 Jan.;8(1):49–84

31. A. Murata and F. Morishige, International Conference on Nutrition, Taijin, China 1981. Report in *Medical Tribune* (22/6/81) A. Murata, et al., 'Prolongation of survival times of terminal cancer patients by administration

of large doses of ascorbate', *International Journal for Vitamin and Nutrition Research,* (Suppl), 1982;23:103–13

32. E.T. Creagan, et al., 'Failure of high-dose vitamin C (ascorbic acid) therapy to benefit patients with advanced cancer: A controlled trial', *New England Journal of Medicine,* 1979 Sept. 27;301(13):687–90

33. K.A. Head, 'Ascorbic acid in the prevention and treatment of cancer', *Alternative Medicine Review,* 1998 June;3(3):174–86

34. M. Eichholzer, et al., 'Prediction of male cancer mortality by plasma levels of interacting vitamins: 17-year follow-up of the prospective Basel study', *International Journal of Cancer,* 1996 Apr. 10;66(2):145–50; C.M. Loria, et al., 'Vitamin C status and mortality in US adults', *American Journal of Clinical Nutrition,* 2000 July;72(1):139–45; K.T. Khaw, et al., 'Relation between plasma ascorbic acid and mortality in men and women in EPIC-Norfolk prospective study: a prospective population study. European Prospective Investigation into Cancer and Nutrition', *Lancet,* 2001 Mar. 3;357(9257):657–63

35. G. Block, 'Epidemiologic evidence regarding vitamin C and cancer', *American Journal of Clinical Nutrition,* 1991 Dec.;54(6 Suppl):1310S–4S

36. L.H. Kushi, et al., 'Intake of vitamins A, C, and E and postmenopausal breast cancer. The Iowa Women's Health Study', *American Journal of Epidemiology,* 1996 July 15;144(2):165–74

37. M.C. Ocke, et al., 'Repeated measurements of vegetables, fruits, beta-carotene, and vitamins C and E in relation to lung cancer: The Zutphen Study', *American Journal of Epidemiology,* 1997 Feb. 15;145(4):358–65; L.C. Yong, et al., 'Intake of vitamins E, C, and A and risk of lung cancer: The NHANES I epidemiologic follow-up study. First National Health and Nutrition Examination Survey', *American Journal of Epidemiology,* 1997 Aug. 1;146(3):231–43; E.V. Bandera, et al., 'Diet and alcohol consumption and lung cancer risk in the New York State Cohort (United States)', *Cancer Causes and Control,* 1997 Nov.;8(6):828–40; L.E. Voorrips, et al., 'A prospective cohort study on antioxidant and folate intake and male lung cancer risk', *Cancer Epidemiology, Biomarkers and Prevention,* 2000 Apr.;9(4):357–65

38. P. Knekt, et al., 'Serum vitamin E and risk of cancer among Finnish men during a 10-year follow-up', *American Journal of Epidemiology,* 1988 Jan.;127(1):28–41

39. R.E. Patterson, et al., 'Vitamin supplements and cancer risk: The epidemiologic evidence', *Cancer Causes and Control,* 1997 Sept.;8(5):786–802

40. N.J. Wald, et al., 'Plasma retinol, beta-carotene and vitamin E levels in relation to the future risk of breast cancer', *British Journal of Cancer,* 1984 Mar.;49(3):321–4

41. E. Negri, et al., 'Intake of selected micronutrients and the risk of breast cancer', *International Journal of Cancer,* 1996 Jan. 17;65(2):140–4

42. K. Nesaretnam, et al., 'Tocotrienols inhibit the growth of human breast cancer cells irrespective of estrogen receptor status', *Lipids,* 1998 May;33(5):461–9

43. O.P. Heinonen, et al., 'Prostate cancer and supplementation with alpha-tocopherol and beta-carotene: Incidence and mortality in a controlled trial', *Journal of the National Cancer Institute*, 1998 Mar. 18;90(6):440–6

44. W.J. Blot, et al., 'Nutrition intervention trials in Linxian, China: Supplementation with specific vitamin/mineral combinations, cancer incidence, and disease-specific mortality in the general population', *Journal of the National Cancer Institute*, 1993 Sept. 15;85(18):1483–92

45. M. Jaffey, 'Vitamin C and cancer: examination of the Vale of Leven trial results using broad inductive reasoning', *Medical Hypotheses*, 1982 Jan.;8(1):49–84

46. Q. Chen, et al., 'Pharmacologic doses of ascorbate act as a prooxidant and decrease growth of aggressive tumor xenografts in mice', *Proceedings of the National Academy of Sciences USA*, 2008 Aug. 12;105(32):11105–9; see also Q. Chen, et al., 'Pharmacologic ascorbic acid concentrations selectively kill cancer cells: Action as a pro-drug to deliver hydrogen peroxide to tissues', *Proceedings of the National Academy of Sciences USA*, 2005 Sept. 20;102(38):13604–9

47. S.J. Padayatty, et al., 'Intravenously administered vitamin C as cancer therapy: three cases', *Canadian Medical Association Journal*, 2006 Mar. 28;174(7):937–42

48. S. Hickey, et al., 'Pharmacokinetics of oral vitamin C', *Journal of Nutritional and Environmental Medicine*, 2008;17(3):169–177

49. J.M. Lappe, et al., 'Vitamin D and calcium supplementation reduces cancer risk: results of a randomized trial', *American Journal of Clinical Nutrition*, 2007 June;85(6):1586–91

50. C. Garland, et al., 'Dietary vitamin D and calcium and risk of colorectal cancer: A 19–year prospective study in men', *Lancet*, 1985 Feb. 9;1(8424):307–9

51. M. Elias, 'Vitamin D may help beat cancer', *USA Today*, 26 January 1989

52. Department of Health, 'Report of the Panel on Dietary Reference Values of the Committee on Medical Aspects of Food Policy', London: TSO (2003)

53. D.M. Freedman, et al., 'Prospective study of serum vitamin D and cancer mortality in the United States', *Journal of the National Cancer Institute*, 2007 Nov. 7;99(21):1594–602

54. E.D. Gorham, et al., 'Optimal vitamin D status for colorectal cancer prevention: A quantitative meta analysis', *American Journal of Preventive Medicine*, 2007 Mar.;32(3):210–6

55. N. Buyru, et al., 'Vitamin D receptor gene polymorphisms in breast cancer', *Experimental and Molecular Medicine*, 2003 Dec. 31;35(6):550–5

56. M.P. Saunders, et al., 'A novel cyclic adenosine monophosphate analog induces hypercalcemia via production of 1,25-dihydroxyvitamin D in patients with solid tumors', *Journal of Clinical Endocrinology and Metabolism*, 1997 Dec.;82(12):4044–8

57. C.F. Garland, et al., 'Vitamin D and prevention of breast cancer: pooled analysis', *Journal of Steroid Biochemistry and Molecular Biology*, 2007 Mar.;103(3–5):708–11

58. C.F. Garland, et al., 'The role of vitamin D in cancer prevention', *American Journal of Public Health*, 2006 Feb.;96(2):252–61; and E.D. Gorham, et al., 'Optimal vitamin D status for colorectal cancer prevention: a quantitative meta analysis', *American Journal of Preventive Medicine*, 2007 Mar.;32(3):210–6

59. C.F. Garland, et al., 'What is the dose-response relationship between vitamin D and cancer risk?', *Nutrition Reviews*, 2007 Aug.;65(8 Pt 2):S91–S95

60. H.G. Skinner, et al., 'Vitamin D intake and the risk for pancreatic cancer in two cohort studies', *Cancer Epidemiology, Biomarkers and Prevention*, 2006 Sept.;15(9):1688–95

61. B.A. Ingraham, et al., 'Molecular basis of the potential of vitamin D to prevent cancer', *Current Medical Research and Opinion*, 2008 Jan.;24(1):139–49

62. V. Fedirko, et al., 'Effects of vitamin D and calcium supplementation on markers of apoptosis in normal colon mucosa: A randomized, double-blind, placebo-controlled clinical trial', *Cancer Prevention Research (Phila Pa)*, 2009 Mar.;2(3):213–23

63. T.M. Beer and A. Myrthue, 'Calcitriol in the treatment of prostate cancer', *Anticancer Research*, 2006 July;26(4A):2647–51

64. M.F. Holick, 'Vitamin D: Importance in the prevention of cancers, type 1 diabetes, heart disease, and osteoporosis', *American Journal of Clinical Nutrition*, 2004 Mar.;79(3):362–71

65. G.E. Mullin and A. Dobs, 'Vitamin D and its role in cancer and immunity: A prescription for sunlight', *Nutrition in Clinical Practice*, 2007 June;22(3):305–22

66. R.P. Heaney, 'The case for improving vitamin D status', *Journal of Steroid Biochemistry and Molecular Biology*, 2007 Mar.;103(3–5):635–41

67. A. Zittermann, 'Vitamin D in preventive medicine: Are we ignoring the evidence?', *British Journal of Nutrition*, 2003 May;89(5):552–72

68. M.K. Thomas, et al., 'Hypovitaminosis D in medical inpatients', *New England Journal of Medicine*, 1998 Mar. 19;338(12):777–83

69. S. Gaugris, et al., 'Vitamin D inadequacy among post-menopausal women: A systematic review', *QJM.*, 2005 Sept.;98(9):667–76

70. R. Vieth, et al., 'The urgent need to recommend an intake of vitamin D that is effective', *American Journal of Clinical Nutrition*, 2007 Mar.;85(3):649–50

71. P. Tuohimaa, et al., 'Does solar exposure, as indicated by the non-melanoma skin cancers, protect from solid cancers: vitamin D as a possible explanation', *European Journal of Cancer*, 2007 July;43(11):1701–12

72. W. Zhou, et al., 'Vitamin D is associated with improved survival in early-stage non-small cell lung cancer patients', *Cancer Epidemiology, Biomarkers and Prevention*, 2005 Oct.;14(10):2303–9

73. O. Gillie (Editor), *'Sunlight, Vitamin D & Health: A report of a conference held at the House of Commons in November 2005'*, Health Research Forum Occasional Reports: No. 2 [Available as a free download at http://www.healthresearchforum.org.uk/reports/sunbook.pdf].

74. E. Hypponen and C. Power, 'Hypovitaminosis D in British adults at age 45 y: Nationwide cohort study of dietary and lifestyle predictors', *American Journal of Clinical Nutrition*, 2007 Mar.;85(3):860–8

75. E. Hypponen and C. Power, 'Hypovitaminosis D in British adults at age 45 y: Nationwide cohort study of dietary and lifestyle predictors', *American Journal of Clinical Nutrition*, 2007 Mar.;85(3):860–8

76. M.F. Holick, 'Vitamin D deficiency', *New England Journal of Medicine*, 2007 July 19;357(3):266–81

77. P.M. Kidd, 'Glutathione: Systemic protectant against oxidative and free radical damage', *Alternative Medicine Review*, 1997;2(3):155–75

78. B. Donnerstag, et al., 'Reduced glutathione and S-acetylglutathione as selective apoptosis-inducing agents in cancer therapy', *Cancer Letters*, 1996 Dec. 20;110(1–2):63–70

79. G. Ohlenschlager and G. Treusch, 'Reduced glutathione and anthocyans – redox recycling and redox reycling in biological systems', *Praxis-telegramm*

80. K. Folkers, 'Relevance of the biosynthesis of coenzyme Q10 and of the four bases of DNA as a rationale for the molecular causes of cancer and a therapy', *Biochemical and Biophysical Research Communications*, 1996 July 16;224(2):358–61; K. Folkers, et al., 'Activities of vitamin Q10 in animal models and a serious deficiency in patients with cancer', *Biochemical and Biophysical Research Communications*, 1997 May 19;234(2):296–9; see also P.R. Palan, et al., 'Plasma concentrations of coenzyme Q10 and tocopherols in cervical intraepithelial neoplasia and cervical cancer', *European Journal of Cancer Prevention*, 2003 Aug.;12(4):321–6

81. K. Lockwood, et al., 'Progress on therapy of breast cancer with vitamin Q10 and the regression of metastases', *Biochemical and Biophysical Research Communications*, 1995 July 6;212(1):172–7

82. K. Lockwood, et al., 'Apparent partial remission of breast cancer in "high risk" patients supplemented with nutritional antioxidants, essential fatty acids and coenzyme Q10', *Molecular Aspects of Medicine*, 1994;15 Suppl:s231–s240

83. L. Roffe, et al., 'Efficacy of coenzyme Q10 for improved tolerability of cancer treatments: A systematic review', *Journal of Clinical Oncology*, 2004 Nov. 1;22(21):4418–24

84. V.G. Premkumar, et al., 'Co-enzyme Q10, riboflavin and niacin supplementation on alteration of DNA repair enzyme and DNA methylation in breast cancer patients undergoing tamoxifen therapy', *British Journal of Nutrition*, 2008 Dec.;100(6):1179–82

85. S. Yuvaraj, et al., 'Effect of Coenzyme Q(10), Riboflavin and Niacin on Tamoxifen treated postmenopausal breast cancer women with special reference to blood chemistry profiles', *Breast Cancer Research and Treatment*, 2009 Mar.;114(2):377–84

86. J.T. Salonen, et al., 'Risk of cancer in relation to serum concentrations of selenium and vitamins A and E: Matched case-control analysis of prospective data', *British Medical Journal (Clinical Research Ed.)*, 1985 Feb. 9;290(6466):417–20

87. K.G. Losonczy, et al., 'Vitamin E and vitamin C supplement use and risk of all-cause and coronary heart disease mortality in older persons: The Established Populations for Epidemiologic Studies of the Elderly', *American Journal of Clinical Nutrition*, 1996 Aug.;64(2):190–6

88. E. White, et al., 'Relationship between vitamin and calcium supplement use and colon cancer', *Cancer Epidemiology, Biomarkers and Prevention*, 1997 Oct.;6(10):769–74

89. L.C. Yong, et al., 'Intake of vitamins E, C, and A and risk of lung cancer. The NHANES I epidemiologic follow-up study. First National Health and Nutrition Examination Survey', *American Journal of Epidemiology*, 1997 Aug. 1;146(3):231–43

90. G. Shklar, et al., 'The effectiveness of a mixture of beta-carotene, alpha-tocopherol, glutathione, and ascorbic acid for cancer prevention', *Nutrition and Cancer*, 1993;20(2):145–51

91. C. Ip and D.J. Lisk, 'Modulation of phase I and phase II xenobiotic-metabolizing enzymes by selenium-enriched garlic in rats', *Nutrition and Cancer*, 1997;28(2):184–8

92. W.C. Willett, et al., 'Prediagnostic serum selenium and risk of cancer', *Lancet*, 1983 July 16;2(8342):130–4

93. S.Y. Yu, et al., 'Regional variation of cancer mortality incidence and its relation to selenium levels in China', *Biological Trace Element Research*, 1985;7:21–9

94. C. Ip and D.J. Lisk, 'Efficacy of cancer prevention by high-selenium garlic is primarily dependent on the action of selenium', *Carcinogenesis*, 1995 Nov.;16(11):2649–52; C. Ip, et al., 'Selenium-enriched garlic inhibits the early stage but not the late stage of mammary carcinogenesis', *Carcinogenesis*, 1996 Sept.;17(9):1979–82

95. J.C. Fleet, 'Dietary selenium repletion may reduce cancer incidence in people at high risk who live in areas with low soil selenium', *Nutrition Reviews*, 1997 July;55(7):277–9

96. L.C. Clark, et al., 'Effects of selenium supplementation for cancer prevention in patients with carcinoma of the skin. A randomized controlled trial. Nutritional Prevention of Cancer Study Group', *Journal of the American Medical Association*, 1996 Dec. 25;276(24):1957–63

97. Interview with Dr Gerhard Schrauzer by Dr Richard Passwater in *Optimum Nutrition*, vol. 6(1) (1993)

98. S.M. Lippman et al., 'Effect of selenium and vitamin E on risk of prostate cancer and other cancers: the Selenium and Vitamin E Cancer Prevention Trial (SELECT)', *Journal of the American Medical Association*, 2009 Jan. 7;301(1):39–51

99. G. Bjelakovic, et al., 'Antioxidant supplements for prevention of gastrointestinal cancers: a systematic review and meta-analysis', *Lancet*, 2004 Oct. 2;364(9441):1219–28

100. M. Romanowska, et al., 'Effects of selenium supplementation on expression of glutathione peroxidase isoforms in cultured human lung adenocarcinoma cell lines', *Lung Cancer*, 2007 Jan.;55(1):35–42

101. S.A. Navarro Silvera and T.E. Rohan, 'Trace elements and cancer risk: a review of the epidemiologic evidence', *Cancer Causes and Control*, 2007 Feb.;18(1):7–27

102. M.P. Rayman, 'Dietary selenium: Time to act', *British Medical Journal*, 1997 Feb. 8;314(7078):387–8

103. E. Negri, et al., 'Intake of selected micronutrients and the risk of breast cancer', *International Journal of Cancer*, 1996 Jan. 17;65(2):140–4

104. K.K. Carroll, et al., 'Calcium and carcinogenesis of the mammary gland', *American Journal of Clinical Nutrition*, 1991 July;54(1 Suppl):206S–8S

105. E. Cho, et al., 'Dairy foods, calcium, and colorectal cancer: a pooled analysis of 10 cohort studies', *Journal of the National Cancer Institute*, 2004 July 7;96(13):1015–22

106. P. Whelan, et al., 'Zinc, vitamin A and prostatic cancer', *British Journal of Urology*, 1983 Oct.;55(5):525–8; F.K. Habib, et al., 'Metal-androgen inter-relationships in carcinoma and hyperplasia of the human prostate', *Journal of Endocrinology*, 1976 Oct.;71(1):133–41; I. Romics and L. Katchalova, 'Spectrographic determination of zinc in the tissues of adenoma and carcinoma of the prostate', *International Urology and Nephrology*, 1983;15(2):171–6; E. Ho, 'Zinc deficiency, DNA damage and cancer risk', *Journal of Nutritional Biochemistry*, 2004; 15:572–578

107. J.I. Anetor, et al., 'High cadmium/zinc ratio in cigarette smokers: Potential implications as a biomarker of risk of prostate cancer', *Nigerian Journal of Physiologcial Sciences*, 2008 June;23(1–2):41–9

108. M.F. Leitzmann, et al., 'Zinc supplement use and risk of prostate cancer', *Journal of the National Cancer Institute*, 2003 July 2;95(13):1004–7; see also E. Ho, 'Zinc deficiency, DNA damage and cancer risk', *Journal of Nutritional Biochemistry*, 2004 Oct.;15(10):572–8

109. A. Gonzalez, et al., 'Zinc intake from supplements and diet and prostate cancer', *Nutrition and Cancer*, 2009;61(2):206–15

110. A. Stuebe, et al., 'Lactation and incidence of premenopausal breast cancer: A longitudinal study', *Archives of Internal Medicine,* 2009 Aug. 10; 169(15):1364–71

111. M. S. Donaldson, 'Nutrition and cancer: A review of the evidence for an anti-cancer diet', *Nutrition Journal*, 2004;3(19):1–21

112. M. Hickson, et al., 'Use of probiotic *Lactobacillus* preparation to prevent diarrhoea associated with antibiotics: Randomised double blind placebo controlled trial', *British Medical Journal*, 2007 July 14;335(7610):80

113. R.K. Peters, et al., 'Diet and colon cancer in Los Angeles County, California', *Cancer Causes and Control*, 1992 Sept.;3(5):457–73

114. M.E. Sanders, 'Considerations for use of probiotic bacteria to modulate human health', *The Journal of Nutrition*, 2000 Feb.;130(2S Suppl):384S–90S

115. A.J. Burns and I.R. Rowland, 'Anti-carcinogenicity of probiotics and prebiotics', *Current Issues in Intestinal Microbiology*, 2000 Mar.;1(1):13–24

116. F.P. Martin, et al., 'Probiotic modulation of symbiotic gut microbial-host metabolic interactions in a humanized microbiome mouse model', *Molecular Systems Biology*, 2008;4:157

117. C. Fassler, et al., 'Fermentation of resistant starches: Influence of in vitro models on colon carcinogenesis', *Nutrition and Cancer*, 2007;58(1):85–92

118. J. Rafter, et al., 'Dietary synbiotics reduce cancer risk factors in polypectomized and colon cancer patients', *American Journal of Clinical Nutrition*, 2007 Feb.;85(2):488–96

119. L.J. Brady, et al., 'The role of probiotic cultures in the prevention of colon cancer', *The Journal of Nutrition*, 2000 Feb.;130(2S Suppl):410S–4S

120. I. Wollowski, et al., 'Protective role of probiotics and prebiotics in colon cancer', *American Journal of Clinical Nutrition*, 2001 Feb.;73(2 Suppl):451S–5S

121. G.T. Macfarlane, et al., 'Bacterial metabolism and health-related effects of galacto-oligosaccharides and other prebiotics', *Journal of Applied Microbiology*, 2008 Feb.;104(2):305–44

122. M. S. Donaldson, 'Nutrition and cancer: A review of the evidence for an anti-cancer diet', *Nutrition Journal*, 2004;3(19):1–21

123. M.C. Barc, et al., 'Effect of amoxicillin-clavulanic acid on human fecal flora in a gnotobiotic mouse model assessed with fluorescence hybridization using group-specific 16S rRNA probes in combination with flow cytometry', *Antimicrobial Agents and Chemotherapy*, 2004 Apr.;48(4):1365–8; and M.W. Pletz, et al., 'Ertapenem pharmacokinetics and impact on intestinal microflora, in comparison to those of ceftriaxone, after multiple dosing in male and female volunteers', *Antimicrobial Agents and Chemotherapy*, 2004 Oct.;48(10):3765–72

124. C.M. Velicer, et al., 'Antibiotic use in relation to the risk of breast cancer', *Journal of the American Medical Association*, 2004 Feb. 18;291(7):827–35

125. G.S. Kelly, 'Nutritional and botanical interventions to assist with the adaptation to stress', *Alternative Medicine Review*, 1999 Aug.;4(4):249–65

126. G.S. Kelly, 'Nutritional and botanical interventions to assist with the adaptation to stress', *Alternative Medicine Review*, 1999 Aug.;4(4):249–65

127. V. Coeuret, et al., 'Numbers and strains of lactobacilli in some probiotic products', *International Journal of Food Microbiology*, 2004 Dec. 15;97(2):147–56

128. P. Bourlioux, et al., 'The intestine and its microflora are partners for the protection of the host: Report on the Danone Symposium "The Intelligent Intestine", held in Paris, June 14, 2002', *American Journal of Clinical Nutrition*, 2003 Oct.;78(4):675–83; and C. Stanton, et al., 'Market potential for probiotics', *American Journal of Clinical Nutrition*, 2001 Feb.;73(2 Suppl):476S–83S

129. The University of Texas M. D. Anderson Cancer Center, 'Cat's claw Detailed Scientific Review', see: http://www.mdanderson.org/education-and-research/resources-for-professionals/clinical-tools-and-resources/cimer/therapies/herbal-plant-biologic-therapies/cats-claw-scientific.html [Accessed 20.11.09].

130. R. Cerri, et al., 'New Quinovic Acid Glycosides from Uncaria tomentosa', *Journal of Natural Products*, 1988;51(2):257–261

131. M. Erhard, et al., 'Effects of echinacea, aconium, lachesis and apis extracts and their combinations on phagocytosis of human granulocytes', *Phytotherapy Research*, vol. 8, pp. 14–17 (1994)

132. L. Zhang and I.R. Tizard, 'Activation of a mouse macrophage cell line by acemannan: The major carbohydrate fraction from Aloe vera gel', *Immunopharmacology*, 1996 Nov.;35(2):119–28

133. H. Nanba, 'MaitakeD-fraction: Healing and preventive potential for cancer', *Journal of Orthomolecular Medicine*, 1997;12(1):43–9

134. S.Y. Wang, et al., 'The anti-tumor effect of Ganoderma lucidum is mediated by cytokines released from activated macrophages and T lymphocytes', *International Journal of Cancer*, 1997 Mar. 17;70(6):699–705

135. J.M. Lin, et al., 'Radical scavenger and antihepatotoxic activity of Ganoderma formosanum, Ganoderma lucidum and Ganoderma neo-japonicum', *Journal of Ethnopharmacology*, 1995 June 23;47(1):33–41

136. K.S. Zhao, et al., 'Enhancement of the immune response in mice by Astragalus membranaceus extracts', *Immunopharmacology*, 1990 Nov.;20(3):225–33; D. Hoffman, *'Medical Herbalism: The science and practice of herbal medicine'*, Rochester, Vermont: Healing Arts Press (2003)

137. K. Krishnaswamy, et al., 'Retardation of experimental tumorigenesis and reduction in DNA adducts by turmeric and curcumin', *Nutrition and Cancer,* 1998;30(2):163–6

138. R. Kuttan, et al., 'Potential anticancer activity of turmeric (Curcuma longa)', *Cancer Letters*, 1985 Nov.;29(2):197–202; K.K. Soudamini and R. Kuttan, 'Inhibition of chemical carcinogenesis by curcumin', *Journal of Ethnopharmacology*, 1989 Nov.;27(1–2):227–33

139. B.B. Aggarwal, et al., 'Curcumin: The Indian solid gold', *Advances in Experimental Medicine and Biology*, 2007;595:1–75

140. H. Hatcher, et al., 'Curcumin: From ancient medicine to current clinical trials', *Cellular and Molecular Life Sciences: CMLS*, 2008 June;65(11):1631–52

141. B.B. Aggarwal, et al., 'Curcumin: The Indian solid gold', *Advances in Experimental Medicine and Biology*, 2007;595:1–75

142. S.M. Sagar, et al., 'Natural health products that inhibit angiogenesis: A potential source for investigational new agents to treat cancer-Part 2', *Current Oncology*, 2006 June;13(3):99–107

143. J.A. Bomser, et al., 'Inhibition of TPA-induced tumor promotion in CD-1 mouse epidermis by a polyphenolic fraction from grape seeds', *Cancer Letters*, 1999 Jan. 29;135(2):151–7; see also M. Kaur, et al., 'Grape seed extract induces cell cycle arrest and apoptosis in human colon carcinoma cells', *Nutrition and Cancer*, 2008; 60(Suppl 1): 2–11

144. H. Kamei, et al., 'Flavonoid-mediated tumor growth suppression demonstrated by in vivo study', *Cancer biotherapy & radiopharmaceuticals,* 1996 June;11(3):193–6

145. S.K. Katiyar, et al., 'Protective effects of silymarin against photocarcinogenesis in a mouse skin model', *Journal of the National Cancer Institute*, 1997 Apr. 16;89(8):556–66

146. X. Zi, et al., 'Anticarcinogenic effect of a flavonoid antioxidant, silymarin, in human breast cancer cells MDA-MB 468: induction of G1 arrest through an increase in Cip1/p21 concomitant with a decrease in kinase activity of cyclin-dependent kinases and associated cyclins', *Clinical Cancer Research*, 1998 Apr.;4(4):1055–64

147. G. Gerard, 'Therapeutique anti-cancreuse et bromelaines [Anticancer treatment and bromelains]', *Agressologie*, 1972;13(4):261–74

Part 6

1. L. Meacham, et al., 'Diabetes Mellitus in Long-term Survivors of Childhood Cancer', *Archives of Internal Medicine*, 2009; 169(15):1381–8

2. S. Epstein, D. Steinman, and S. LeVert, *The Breast Cancer Prevention Programme*, Macmillan, New York (1997)

3. No authors listed (Early Breast Cancer Trialists' Collaborative Group), 'Systemic treatment of early breast cancer by hormonal, cytotoxic, or immune therapy. 133 randomised trials involving 31,000 recurrences and 24,000 deaths among 75,000 women. Early Breast Cancer Trialists' Collaborative Group', *Lancet*, 1992 Jan. 4;339(8784):1–15

4. J. Raloff, 'Studies spark new tamoxifen controversy: Drug linked to endometrial cancer', *Science News* (26 February 1994)

5. C.B. Simone, 'Use of therapeutic levels of nutrients to augment oncology care', in P. Quillin, and M. Williams (eds), *Adjuvant Nutrition in Cancer Treatment*, Academic Press, Tulsa, OK, vol. 72 (1992); see also C.B. Simone, et al., 'Nutritional and lifestyle modification to augment oncology care: An overview', *Journal of Orthomolecular Medicine*, 1997;12(4):97–206

6. C.E. Myers, et al., 'Adriamycin: Amelioration of toxicity by alpha-tocopherol', *Cancer Treatment Reports*, 1976 July;60(7):961–2; and C.B. Simone, et al., 'Nutritional and lifestyle modification to augment oncology care: An overview', *Journal of Orthomolecular Medicine*, 1997;12(4):97–206.

7. K. Folkers and Y. Yamura, (eds), *Biomedical and Clinical Aspects of Coenzyme Q*, Amsterdam; Elsevier/Netherland Biomedical Press, vol. 2, pp. 333–47 (1980)

8. H.A. Nieper, 'Bromelain in der kontrolle malignen Waschstums', *Krebsgeschehen*, 1976;1:9–15

9. M. Muscaritoli, et al., 'Oral glutamine in the prevention of chemotherapy-induced gastrointestinal toxicity', *European Journal of Cancer*, 1997 Feb.;33(2):319–20

10. T.R. Ziegler, et al., 'Clinical and metabolic efficacy of glutamine-supplemented parenteral nutrition after bone marrow transplantation: A randomized, double-blind, controlled study', *Annals of Internal Medicine*, 1992 May 15;116(10):821–8

11. T.R. Austgen, et al., 'The effects of glutamine-enriched total parenteral nutrition on tumor growth and host tissues', *Annals of Surgery*, 1992

Feb.;215(2):107–13; W.W. Souba, 'Glutamine and cancer', *Annals of Surgery*, 1993 Dec.;218(6):715–28; K. Rouse, et al., 'Glutamine enhances selectivity of chemotherapy through changes in glutathione metabolism', *Annals of Surgery*, 1995 Apr.;221(4):420–6; V.S. Klimberg, et al., 'Glutamine facilitates chemotherapy while reducing toxicity', *Journal of Parenteral and Enteral Nutrition*, 1992 Nov.;16(6 Suppl):83S–7S

12. K.M. Skubitz and P.M. Anderson, 'Oral glutamine to prevent chemotherapy induced stomatitis: A pilot study', *Journal of Laboratory and Clinical Medicine*, 1996 Feb.;127(2):223–8; P.M. Anderson, et al., 'Oral glutamine reduces the duration and severity of stomatitis after cytotoxic cancer chemotherapy', *Cancer*, 1998 Oct. 1;83(7):1433–9

13. E. Barrett-Connor, et al., 'Effects of raloxifene on cardiovascular events and breast cancer in postmenopausal women', *New England Journal of Medicine*, 2006 July 13;355(2):125–37

14. M. Baum, et al., 'Anastrozole alone or in combination with tamoxifen versus tamoxifen alone for adjuvant treatment of postmenopausal women with early breast cancer: first results of the ATAC randomised trial', *Lancet*, 2002 June 22;359(9324):2131–9

15. L. Fallowfield, et al., 'Quality of life of postmenopausal women in the Arimidex, tamoxifen, alone or in combination (ATAC) adjuvant breast cancer trial', *Journal of Clinical Oncology*, 2004 Nov. 1;22(21):4261–71

16. M.J. Piccart-Gebhart, et al., 'Trastuzumab after adjuvant chemotherapy in HER2-positive breast cancer', *New England Journal of Medicine*, 2005 Oct. 20;353(16):1659–72

17. V. Guarneri, et al., 'Long-term cardiac tolerability of trastuzumab in metastatic breast cancer: The M.D. Anderson Cancer Center experience', *Journal of Clinical Oncology*, 2006 Sept. 1;24(25):4107–15

18. P. Lichtenstein, et al., 'Environmental and heritable factors in the causation of cancer-analyses of cohorts of twins from Sweden, Denmark, and Finland', *New England Journal of Medicine*, 2000 July 13;343(2):78–85

19. Professor J. Plant, *Your Life in Your Hands*, Virgin Books Ltd., (2007); data from WHO International Agency for Research on Cancer (IARC)

20. World Cancer Research Fund/American Institute for Cancer Research, 'Food, Nutrition, Physical Activity, and the Prevention of Cancer: A Global Perspective', Washington, DC: AICR, 2007

21. D.W. Voskuil, et al., 'Insulin-like growth factor (IGF)-system mRNA quantities in normal and tumor breast tissue of women with sporadic and familial breast cancer risk', *Breast Cancer Research and Treatment*, 2004 Apr.;84(3):225–33

22. M. Jain, et al., 'Premorbid diet and the prognosis of women with breast cancer', *Journal of the National Cancer Institute*, 1994 Sept. 21;86(18):1390–7

23. R.T. Chlebowski, et al., 'Dietary fat reduction and breast cancer outcome: Interim efficacy results from the Women's Intervention Nutrition Study', *Journal of the National Cancer Institute*, 2006 Dec. 20;98(24):1767–76; J.P. Pierce, et al., 'Greater survival after breast cancer in physically active women

with high vegetable-fruit intake regardless of obesity', *Journal of Clinical Oncology*, 2007 June 10;25(17):2345–51

24. E. Ho, et al., 'Dietary influences on endocrine-inflammatory interactions in prostate cancer development', *Archives of Biochemistry and Biophysics*, 2004 Aug. 1;428(1):109–17

25. A.J. Pantuck, et al., 'Phase II study of pomegranate juice for men with rising prostate-specific antigen following surgery or radiation for prostate cancer', *Clinical Cancer Research*, 2006 July 1;12(13):4018–26

26. S. Rohrmann, et al., 'Fruit and vegetable consumption, intake of micro-nutrients, and benign prostatic hyperplasia in US men', *American Journal of Clinical Nutrition*, 2007 Feb.;85(2):523–9

27. J. Stanford, et al., 'Prostate cancer trends 1973–1995', Bethesda, MD:SEER Program, *National Cancer Institute*, 1998

28. J.M. Chan, et al., 'Insulin-like growth factor-I (IGF-I) and IGF binding pro-tein-3 as predictors of advanced-stage prostate cancer', *Journal of the National Cancer Institute*, 2002 July 17;94(14):1099–106

29. P. Terry, et al., 'Fatty fish consumption and risk of prostate cancer', *Lancet*, 2001;357(9270):1764–1766

30. Y. Li, et al., 'Regulation of FOXO3a/beta-catenin/GSK-3beta signaling by 3,3'-diindolylmethane contributes to inhibition of cell proliferation and induction of apoptosis in prostate cancer cells', *Journal of Biological Chemistry*, 2007 July 20;282(29):21542–50; and D. Kong, et al., 'Inhibition of angiogenesis and invasion by 3,3'-diindolylmethane is mediated by the nuclear factor-kappaB downstream target genes MMP-9 and uPA that regu-lated bioavailability of vascular endothelial growth factor in prostate cancer', *Cancer Research*, 2007 Apr. 1;67(7):3310–9

31. D. Ornish, et al., 'Intensive lifestyle changes may affect the progression of prostate cancer', *Journal of Urology*, 2005 Sept.;174(3):1065–9

32. W.H. Goldmann, et al., 'Saw palmetto berry extract inhibits cell growth and Cox-2 expression in prostatic cancer cells', *Cell Biology International*, 2001;25(11):1117–24

33. T.L. Wadsworth, et al., 'Saw palmetto extract suppresses insulin-like growth factor-I signaling and induces stress-activated protein kinase/c-Jun N-terminal kinase phosphorylation in human prostate epithelial cells', *Endocrinology*, 2004 July;145(7):3205–14

34. F. Yablonsky, et al., 'Antiproliferative effect of Pygeum africanum extract on rat prostatic fibroblasts', *Journal of Urology*, 1997 June;157(6):2381–7

Resources

∾

Nutrition, exercise and well-being

The Institute for Optimum Nutrition (ION) offers a three-year foundation degree course in nutritional therapy, which includes training in the optimum-nutrition approach to mental health. There is a clinic, a list of nutrition practitioners across the UK, an information service and a quarterly journal, *Optimum Nutrition*. Visit www.ion.ac.uk; address: Avalon House, 72 Lower Mortlake Road, Richmond, TW9 2JY, UK; tel.: +44 (0)20 8614 7800.

Nutritional therapy and consultations To find a nutritional therapist near you whom I recommend, visit www.patrickholford.com. This service gives details on who to see in the UK as well as internationally. If there is no one available nearby, you can always complete an online assessment – see below.

Online 100% Health Programme Are you 100 per cent healthy? Find out with my FREE health check and comprehensive 100% Health Programme, giving you a personalised action plan, including diet and supplements. Visit www.patrickholford.com.

Zest4Life is a health and nutrition club, based on low-GL principles, which provides advice, coaching and support for losing weight and gaining health through a series of weekly meetings. For more information, visit www.zest4life.eu.

Psychocalisthenics is an excellent exercise system that takes less than 20 minutes a day, and develops strength, suppleness and stamina as well as generating vital energy which brings peace of mind, mental vitality and well-being. The best way to learn it is to do the Psychocalisthenics Training. See www.patrickholford.com/psychocalisthenics for details. Also available is the book *Master Level Exercise: Psychocalisthenics* and the *Psychocalisthenics* CD and DVD available from www.patrickholford.com (shop). For further information about Psychocalisthenics, please see www.pcals.com.

Yoga As well as stretching the body, which helps it become more supple and the joints more flexible, yoga is a good way to relax and relieve stress. The British Wheel of Yoga can put you in touch with a yoga school or teacher in your area. Visit www.bwy.org.uk; tel.: 01529 306851; email: office@bwy.org.uk.

T'ai chi and qigong (chi gung) Both these forms of exercise are known as 'chi-generating martial arts'. They exercise the body as well as bringing peace of mind, mental vitality and well-being. Because of this, they are excellent destressors. The Tai Chi Union for Great Britain provides details of teachers near you, events and news. Visit www.taichiunion.com. Also contact The London School of T'ai Chi Chuan and Traditional Health Resources, visit http://taichi.gn.apc.org; tel.: 020 8566 1677.

Five Rhythms is a system that uses music and movement to tap deeply into unexpressed emotions and then to release them. For more information about Gabrielle Roth and the Five Rhythms globally, visit www.gabrielleroth.com. To find a Five Rhythms teacher or class in London, visit www.acalltodance.com.

Psychotherapy To find a psychotherapist or counsellor in your area, contact the United Kingdom Council for Psychotherapy. Visit www. psychotherapy.org.uk; tel.: 020 7014 9955; email: info@ukcp.org.uk.

I have been particularly impressed by psychotherapists and counsellors trained at the Psychosynthesis and Education Trust, 92–94 Tooley Street, London Bridge, London SE1 2TH. They also have an excellent workshop called The Essentials, which enables you to look at your life, how you would like it to be and what needs to change. Essentials is run either as a five-day intensive programme or over two long weekends. Visit www.psychosynthesis.edu; tel.: 020 7403 2100; email: enquiries@petrust.org.uk.

Hoffman Institute UK The Hoffman Process is an eight-day intensive residential course in which you're shown how to let go of the past, release pent-up stress, self-limiting behaviours and resentments, and start creating the future you desire. Visit www.hoffmaninstitute. co.uk, Box 72, Quay House, River Road, Arundel, West Sussex, BN18 9DF; tel.: 080 0068 7114 or +44 (0) 1903 88 99 90; email: info@ hoffmaninstitute.co.uk. Courses are also offered in South Africa, Australia, Singapore and other parts of the world. For details of these and other international centres visit www.hoffmaninstitute.com.

Finding exercise groups locally You will probably find a list of exercise, yoga, Pilates or movement classes in your local newspaper, or ask at your doctor's surgery, local school or gym. Many schools and gyms hold classes for all levels of fitness.

Support organisations

Cancer Options is a private cancer consultancy where you can obtain consultancy, research and coaching for all the different cancer treatments and therapies. You will find the best of orthodox and complementary approaches evaluated by Britain's leading experts in the integrative field. They are the only professional service with the knowledge and experience of all approaches to cancer to guide you to safe and effective treatment choices. The Cancer Options team are committed to helping their clients make confident, informed decisions about their cancer care.

The founder of Cancer Options, Patricia Peat, was an oncology nurse for many years and saw the need for people to have access to good-quality information about all approaches to treatment so that they could take charge of their cancer decisions. She is a medical adviser to the Yes To Life Charity (see below) and the Integrated Healthcare Trust, patron of the Cancer Active Charity and has a regular column in *ICON* magazine (*Integrative Cancer and Oncology News* – see below). She is also co-author of *The Frontier Guide to Medicine* with Professor Karol Sikora. Visit: www.canceroptions.co.uk; email: enquiries@canceroptions.co.uk; tel.: 0845 009 2041; international: +44 1623 438733, or write to: Cancer Options, PO Box 6778, Kirkby in Ashfield, Nottingham, NG17 7QU, UK.

Yes to Life is a UK charity dedicated to empowering people with cancer by directly supporting them in obtaining an integrated approach to treatment, one that allies the best of complementary and alternative medicine (CAM) with orthodox approaches. In addition to the help centre services, Yes to Life offers an online directory of CAM treatments, as well as loaning out equipment and running free Wellbeing Workshops. Yes to Life is working to influence the focus of NHS cancer care towards a more integrated approach. Visit: www. yestolife.org.uk; email: helpcentre@yestolife.org.uk; helpline tel.: 0870 163 2990; or write to: Yes to Life, Unit 7, Block C, Imperial Works, Perren Street, London NW5 3ED.

CANCERactive is the UK's number-one charity for scientifically researched complementary cancer therapies and new and alternative treatments, not just orthodox ones. It has a comprehensive website (www.canceractive.com), which also extensively covers factors that may cause and maintain a cancer. The founders pride themselves on being independent – having no vested interests and being the patients' champion. Every three months they produce *ICON*, an easy-to-read magazine that reflects this patient-friendly stance.

CancerWise (formerly Wessex Cancer Help Centre) offers hope and support to all cancer patients and carers living in West Sussex and South East Hampshire, providing a wide range of complementary therapies, counselling and emotional support, an information library and regular talks on cancer-related subjects. Contact: Diane Townson, (Centre Manager), CancerWise, Tavern House, 4 City Business Centre, Basin Road, Chichester, PO19 8DU 01243 778516; email: enquiries@cancerwise.org.uk; or visit: www.cancerwise.org.uk.

Penny Brohn Cancer Care (formerly Bristol Cancer Help Centre) The centre offers advice on a wide range of therapies that form the Bristol Approach, a holistic approach to living well with cancer. A variety of courses offer support to those with cancer and their carers. They offer one-day courses or three- and five-day residential courses where they provide theory and information as well as practical experience. Therapies available at the centre – as part of the courses or as single appointments – include sessions with an integrative doctor, as well as nutritional therapy, counselling, art therapy, healing and body work, such as massage and shiatsu. Tel.: 0845 123 23 10; email: info@pennybrohn.org; or write to: Penny Brohn Cancer Care, Chapel Pill Lane, Pill, Bristol, BS20 0HH; or visit: www.pennybrohncancercare.org.

Genetic Health is a UK company based in a state-of-the-art diagnostic clinic in Harley Street, London. Tests for men at the clinic are for the risks of various cancers, including the prostate and bowel; for women, the risks of ovarian and breast cancer. Specific single-gene panels are used for the detection of BRAC1 and BRAC2 for breast cancer. Testing of a group of cytochrome P450 genes can predict further risks. Genetic Health is a company run by doctors who work with a group of UK genetic counsellors that also provides client support. Visit: www.genetic-health.co.uk; tel.: +44(0)870 043 5551.

Photodynamic therapy (PDT) (see page 310) For further information, contact the charity KILLING Cancer, Charles Bell House, 67–73 Riding House Street, London, W1W 7EJ. They have a detailed website at www.killingcancer.co.uk, or email: killing.cancer@virgin.net. PDT has been used for a number of years at the National Medical Laser Centre based at University College Hospital, London and many other UK hospitals. PDT is also widely available across other world territories.

Laboratory tests

Food Allergy (IgG ELISA) tests, and testing for homocysteine, plus GLCheck (measures your level of glycosylated haemoglobin, also called HbA1C) and Livercheck tests are available through York Test Laboratories. You will be sent a home-test kit where you can take your own pinprick blood sample and return it to the lab for analysis. Visit www.yorktest.com, or call freephone (UK) 0800 074 6185. These test kits are also available from www.totallynourish.com.

Intestinal permeability (leaky gut) test This test is available from the following labs through qualified nutrition consultants and doctors: Biolab Medical Unit (doctor's referral only): visit www.biolab.co.uk or tel.: +44 (0)20 7636 5959/5905. Genova Diagnostics: visit www.gdx.uk.net or tel.: +44 (0)20 8336 7750.

Adrenal stress index uses saliva samples to measure a person's levels of cortisol, and another key stress hormone called DHEA (the anti-ageing adrenal hormone and a precursor for stress hormones). Both are good indicators of adrenal stress and are best measured in saliva. This standard stress test involves providing four saliva samples at different intervals over a 24-hour period, which are then sent for analysis. Such tests, available through nutritional therapists (see Nutritional Therapy and Consultations above), can determine whether a person needs to pursue a nutritional or hormonal strategy, or perhaps other therapies such as meditation, to restore the body so that it can respond to stress in a healthy way.

Health products

Nutritional supplement drinks

Get Up & Go A delicious low-GL breakfast shake powder. It contains a range of vitamins and minerals, one-third of your daily protein requirements, and relevant levels of essential fatty acids. It is made from the best-quality wholefoods, ground into a powder.

Sugar alternative Xylitol is a low-GL natural sugar alternative, available from high street health-food stores. Also available by mail order from Totally Nourish (see below), sold as XyloBrit.

CherryActive is sold in a highly concentrated juice format. Mix a 30ml serving with 250ml water to make a deliciously healthy, low-GL cherry juice. Each 946ml bottle contains the juice from over 3,000 cherries – that's half a tree's worth – and contains a month's supply. CherryActive is also available as a dried cherry snack and in capsules. For more information and to order, visit www.totallynourish.com (see below).

Transdermal skin cream This form of 'natural progesterone' HRT, called Projuven, is only available on prescription in the UK, so you should consult a doctor who is trained in its use (see NPIS below). Although it is available over the counter in other countries, I do not recommend that you use it without supervision.

The Natural Progesterone Information Service (NPIS) provides women and their doctors with information on natural progesterone and details of how to obtain information packs as well as books and other resources relating to natural hormone health. Visit www.npis. info for more information; tel: 07000 784849, address: NPIS, PO Box 24, Buxton, SK17 9FB.

Water filters There are many water filters on the market. One of the best is offered by the Fresh Water Filter Company, who produce mains-attached water-filtering units using gravity rather than reverse osmosis (which can filter out some useful minerals as well). You can buy a whole-house filter or an under-sink version. Visit www.totallynourish. com or www.freshwaterfilter.com.

Supplements

Nutritional supplements are available from a wide variety of companies. Two companies that provide an extensive range, between them covering the speciality supplements referred to in this book, are Solgar and BioCare (see below).

Finding your own perfect supplement programme can be confusing, but my website, www.patrickholford.com, offers useful guidance. The backbone of a good supplement programme is:

● A high-strength multivitamin

● Additional vitamin C

● An essential-fat supplement containing omega-3 and omega-6 oils

In this section are examples of supplements that provide the herbs and nutrients at the levels discussed in this book. The addresses of the companies whose products we've referred to are given under Supplement Suppliers.

Antioxidants

A good all-round antioxidant complex should provide vitamin A (beta-carotene and/or retinol), vitamins C and E, zinc, selenium, glutathione or cysteine, anthocyanidins of berry extracts, lipoic acid and coenzyme Q_{10}. Two products that fulfil this criteria are BioCare's AGE Antioxidant or Solgar's Advanced Antioxidant Nutrients. AGE Antioxidant contains resveratrol as well as glutathione and other essential antioxidants. Complexes of bioflavonoids, often found together with vitamin C, are available from both companies.

Digestive enzymes and support

A good digestive enzyme combination should contain protease, amylase and lipase, which digest protein, carbohydrate and fat respectively. Some also contain amyloglucosidase (which helps to digest glucosides found in certain beans and vegetables) and lactase (which helps to digest milk sugars). If you get bloated after lentils or beans, such as soya products, choose an enzyme that contains alpha-galactosidase. Try Solgar's Vegan Digestive Enzymes. You can also buy digestive enzymes with probiotics – BioCare's DigestPro contains all these enzymes and probiotics, together with some glutamine.

Essential fats and fish-oil supplements

The most important omega-3 fats are DHA, DPA and EPA, found both in oily fish and in cod liver oil. The most important omega-6 fat is GLA, the richest source being borage (also known as star-flower) oil. Try BioCare's Essential Omegas, which provides a highly concentrated mix of EPA, DHA, DPA and GLA. They also produce Mega-EPA, a high potency omega-3 fish oil supplement. Seven Seas produce Extra High Strength Cod Liver Oil.

Homocysteine-lowering nutrients

A good methyl nutrient complex should contain at least B_6, B_{12} and folic acid. Some formulas also contain vitamin B_2, trimethylglycine (TMG), zinc, and N-acetyl-cysteine. Three products that fulfil this criteria are BioCare's Connect, which contains them all, or Solgar's Gold Specifics Homocysteine Modulators, which contains TMG, vitamin B_6, vitamin B_{12} and folic acid; or Higher Nature's 'H Factors', which contains TMG, vitamins B_2, B_6, B_{12}, folic acid and zinc (see www.highernature.co.uk).

Multivitamin and mineral supplements

Supplementing the right multivitamin is the most important supplement decision you make. Most multis are based on RDA levels of nutrients, which are not the same as optimum nutrition levels. A good multivitamin based on optimum nutrition levels is BioCare's Advanced Optimum Nutrition Formula. Another is Solgar's VM2000. Both of these recommend taking two tablets a day. Advanced Optimum Nutrition Formula has higher mineral levels, especially of calcium and magnesium. Ideally, take a multivitamin and mineral with an extra 1g of vitamin C.

Probiotics

Probiotics are supplements of beneficial bacteria, the two main strains being *Lactobacillus acidophilus* and *Bifidobacterium bifidus*. There are various types of strains within these two; some more important in children, others in adults. There is quite some variability in amounts of bacteria (some labels say things like 'a billion viable organisms per capsule') and quality. A good product is BioCare's Bio-Acidophilus and also Digestpro, which also contains digestive enzymes.

Salvestrols

Maintenance dosage levels of salvestrols are available from BioCare (see below). For higher, therapeutic dosage levels, contact: Nature's Defence (UK) Ltd, Charnwood Science Centre, 103 High Street, Syston, Leicester, LE7 1GQ; email: info@naturesdefence.com; tel.: 01162 602963, to find a practitioner near you who is knowledgeable in the use of salvestrols.

Sugar balance

Look for a product that contains 200mcg of chromium, either as chromium polynicotinate or chromium picolinate, ideally with a cinnamon high in MCHP, such as BioCare's Cinnachrome. (Cinnulin PF is the name of a concentrated extract of cinnamon that is especially high in MCHP.)

Vitamin C

Liposomal vitamin C If you wish to use a liposomal form of vitamin C, see www.livonlabs.com (Lipo-Spheric Vitamin C). For orders within Europe, South Africa, Greenland and United Arab Emirates: tel.: +44 1580-201-687; email: vms@simply-nature.co.uk, or write to: Simply Nature Ltd, Unit 11, Old Factory Buildings, Battenhurst Road, Stonegate, East Sussex, TN5 7DU.

Skincare, personal care and household care products

Environ products were developed by the cosmetic surgeon Dr Des Fernandes to address the damaging effects of the environment on our skin to prevent skin cancer. Environ help to maintain a normal healthy skin or effectively treat and prevent the signs of ageing, pigmentation, problem skin and scarring. It is formulated with scientifically proven active ingredients, including vitamin A and antioxidant vitamins C, E and beta-carotene, which are used in progressively higher concentrations. Environ products are available from www.totallynourish.com or direct from an Environ skincare therapist. Call +44(0)20 8450 2020 to find an Environ skincare therapist near you in the UK. For international enquiries email tollfree@environ.co.za or visit www.environ.co.za.

RAD is a revolutionary sunscreen containing sun filters and sun reflectants giving an SPF 16 to provide protection from both UVA and UVB irradiation. RAD also contains antioxidant vitamins to combat the effects of the sun and pollution on the skin. It is suitable for all skin types and ages, including babies.

Neways International operates in 29 countries and has a range of cosmetic, personal health care and household care products free from undesirable chemicals. (Endorsed by Dr Samuel Epstein in *Unreasonable Risk – How to Avoid Cancer from Cosmetics and Personal Care Products: The Neways Story*, 2001.) Visit: www.neways.com.

Supplement suppliers

The following companies produce good-quality supplements that are widely available in the UK.

BioCare offers an extensive range of nutritional and herbal sup-plements, including daily 'packs', which are good for travelling or when you are away from home. Their products are stocked by most good health-food stores. Visit www.biocare.co.uk; tel.: +44 (0)121 433 3727. They are also available by mail order from Totally Nourish (www.totallynourish.com).

Totally Nourish is an 'e'-health shop that stocks many high-quality health products, including home test kits and supplements. Visit www.totallynourish.com; tel.: 0800 085 7749 (freephone within the UK).

Solgar Available in most independent health-food stores or visit www.solgar-vitamins.co.uk; tel.: +44 (0) 1442 890355.

Herbal products

Herbal products

MediHerb offers an extensive range of high-quality herbal products, including liquid extracts and tablets. Their distributors in the UK and Eire are Balance Healthcare Ltd., 7–10 Langston Priory Mews, Station Road, Kingham, Oxfordshire, OX7 6UP. Freephone Order Line: 0800 072 0202; email: sales@balancehealthcare.com; visit: www.mediherb.co.uk. They also have distributors in South Africa, Australia, New Zealand, USA and Canada (see below).

And in other regions:

South Africa

Bioharmony produce a wide range of products in South Africa and other African countries. For details of your nearest supplier visit www.bioharmony.co.za; tel.: 0860 888 339.

MediHerb (see above) distributors in South Africa are Natura Laboratory. Visit: www.mediherb.co.za; tel.: 012 813 9434.

Australia

Solgar supplements are available in Australia. Visit www.solgar.com.au; tel.: 1800 029 871 (free call) for your nearest supplier. Another good brand is Blackmores.

MediHerb (see above) – purchase direct from Mediherb Australia Head Office. Visit: www.mediherb.com.au, tel.: +61 7 4661 0700; toll free: 1800 639 122.

New Zealand

BioCare products (see above) are available in New Zealand through Aurora Natural Therapies. Visit www.aurora.org.nz; address: 12a Battys Road, Springlands, Blenheim 7201, New Zealand.

MediHerb (see above) distributors in New Zealand are Proherb. Visit: www.proherb.co.nz; tel.: +64 3 381 2255 or enquiries@proherb.co.nz.

Singapore

BioCare (see above) and **Solgar** products are available in Singapore through Essential Living. Visit www.essliv.com; tel.: 6276 1380.

UAE

BioCare supplements (see above) are available in Dubai from Nutripharm FZCO; address: Post Box: 71246, Dubai, United Arab Emirates; tel.: +971-4-3410008; fax.: +971-4-3410009.

Canada

MediHerb (see above) distributors in Canada are Promedics Neutraceutical Ltd. Visit: www.mediherb.ca; tel. (toll free): 877 268 5057.

USA

MediHerb (see above) distributors in the USA are Standard Process. Visit: www.mediherb.com; tel.: 800 848 5061 or email info@standardprocess.com.

Recommended Reading

Bland, Jeffrey, *Genetic Nutritioneering*, Keats Publishing (1999)

Cadbury, Deborah, *The Feminization of Nature*, Hamish Hamilton (1997)

Colborn, Theo, John Peterson Myers and Diane Dumanoski, *Our Stolen Future*, Little, Brown (1996)

Daniel, Rosy, *The Cancer Directory*, Harper Thorsons (2005)

Hickey, Steve and Hilary Roberts, *Ascorbate: The Science of Vitamin C*, Lulu.com (2004)

Holford, Patrick, *Beat Stress and Fatigue*, Piatkus (1999)

Holford, Patrick, *New Optimum Nutrition Bible*, Piatkus (2004)

Holford, Patrick, *Ten Secrets of 100% Healthy People* (2009)

Lee, John, *What Your Doctor May Not Tell You About Breast Cancer*, Warner (2002)

Passwater, Richard, *Cancer and its Nutritional Therapies*, Keats Publishing (1983)

Pauling, Linus, *How to Live Longer and Feel Better*, Oregon State University Press (2006)

Pert, Candice, *Molecules of Emotion*, Pocket Books (1999)

Plant, Jane, *Your Life in Your Hands: Understand, Prevent and Overcome Breast Cancer and Ovarian Cancer*, Virgin Books (2007)

Plant, Jane, *Prostate Cancer: Understand, Prevent and Overcome Prostate Cancer*, Virgin Books (2007)

Siegel, Bernie, *Love, Medicine and Miracles*, Rider & Co. (1999)

Simonton, O. Carl, Stephanie Matthews Simonton and James L. Creighton, *Getting Well Again*, Bantam Books (1986)

Index

Page numbers in italic indicate illustrations.